Review Questions & Answers For Veterinary Boards

Basic Sciences

Edited by

Paul W. Pratt, VMD

Production Manager:
Elisabeth S. Stein

American Veterinary Publications, Inc.
5782 Thornwood Drive
Goleta, CA 93117

© 1993

Library of Congress Card Number: 93-70147

ISBN 0-939674-39-4

Printed in the United States of America

Authors

Introduction

Dean C. Frey, DVM
Animal Clinic, 1823 16th Avenue SW, Cedar Rapids, IA 52404

Biochemistry

Hara P. Misra, BVSc, MS, PhD
Professor, Department of Biomedical Sciences, Director, University
Center of Toxicology, Virginia-Maryland Regional College of Veterinary
Medicine, Virginia, Polytechnic Institute, Blacksburg, VA 24061

Embryology

Alexander de Lahunta, DVM, PhD, Dipl ACVIM
James Law Professor, Department of Anatomy, College of Veterinary
Medicine, Cornell University, Ithaca, NY 14853

Gross Anatomy

Donald R. Adams, PhD
Professor, Department of Veterinary Anatomy, College of Veterinary
Medicine, Iowa State University, Ames, IA 50011

Fredric L. Frye, DVM, MS
Fellow, Royal Society of Medicine, Former Clinical Professor of Medicine,
Department of Medicine, School of Veterinary Medicine,
University of California, Davis, CA 95616

Nani G. Ghoshal, DVM
Professor, Department of Veterinary Anatomy, College of Veterinary
Medicine, Iowa State University, Ames, IA 50011

Microbiology

Gordon R. Carter, DVM, MS, DVSc, Dipl ACVM
Professor Emeritus, Department of Pathobiology, Virginia-Maryland
Regional College of Veterinary Medicine, Virginia Polytechnic Institute,
Blacksburg, VA 24061

Muhammed Ikram, DVM, MS, PhD
Animal Health Technology Program, Fairview College, Box 3000,
Fairview, Alberta, Canada T0H 1L0

Microscopic Anatomy

Sheryl J. Morgan, DVM, PhD, Dipl ACVP
Veterinary Pathologist, Division of Drug Safety Evaluation, Abbott
Laboratories, D-469, AP-13A, One Abbott Park Road,
Abbott Park, IL 60064

Neuroanatomy

Alexander de Lahunta, DVM, PhD, Dipl ACVIM
James Law Professor, Department of Anatomy, College of Veterinary
Medicine, Cornell University, Ithaca, NY 14853

Parasitology

Dwight D. Bowman, PhD, MS
Assistant Professor, Department of Microbiology, Immunology &
Parasitology, College of Veterinary Medicine, Cornell University,
Ithaca, NY 14853

Pathology

Ronald D. Hunt, DVM
Professor, New England Regional Primate Research Center, Harvard
Medical School, POB 9102, Southborough, MA 01772

Continued

Physiology

James E. Breazile, DVM, PhD
Professor, Director of Laboratory Animal Resources, College of Veterinary
Medicine, Oklahoma State University, Stillwater, OK 74078

Thomas P. Colville, DVM, MS
Director, Veterinary Technology Program, Department of Veterinary and
Microbiological Sciences, North Dakota State University, Fargo, ND 58105

Terminology

Paul W. Pratt, VMD
Editor and Publisher, American Veterinary Publications,
5782 Thornwood Drive, Goleta, CA 93117

Preface

This series of review books was developed to help candidates prepare for scholastic, licensure and certification examinations. While the books are not definitive texts, they can help candidates organize their preparations, and detect areas in which more study is required.

Time and again while editing the thousands of questions, I found myself saying, "I wish I had these books when I was in veterinary school, and studying for Boards."

I am indebted to our group of 112 contributors, who have taken the time from their busy professional and personal lives to carefully craft questions on their respective subject areas. Their enthusiasm and ingenuity in developing challenging questions are evident throughout the 5 volumes. While I had considered myself fairly well read in our field, I was humbled by the depth and breadth of knowledge illustrated in their questions.

This series contains over 9,400 questions, with accompanying answers. We have gone to great effort to root out all errors and ambiguous statements. Despite these precautions, however, a number of flaws undoubtedly have escaped notice.

We would be grateful if readers would notify us of any errors, ambiguities or questionable statements in these books. We also encourage readers to send their comments/criticism on any aspect of the books. In this way we can improve the quality of future editions. For your convenience, a postage-paid Comments form is included at the back of each book.

Paul W. Pratt, VMD
Editor and Publisher

Contents

Introduction

D.C. Frey

State and national board examinations have long been surrounded with an air of mystery, misunderstanding and anxiety. *Review Questions & Answers For Veterinary Boards*, a series of 5 volumes, was written to alleviate much of this confusion.

These volumes are not textbooks, nor are they meant to supplant textbooks. Rather, they are guides designed to help readers review, in convenient form, current information on the various subject areas within the scope of a veterinarian's duties.

Who Should Use These Books?

Veterinary Students: Veterinary students can use *Review Questions & Answers For Veterinary Boards* as a review in preparing for final examinations, as each course is concluded.

New Graduates: Graduates can use these books at the conclusion of their veterinary education in preparing for the National Board Examination, and in preparing for licensure examinations required by many states and provinces (see the following section on Licensing of Veterinarians).

Practicing Veterinarians: Veterinarians now working in practice will find these books useful in continuing education. Graduates re-entering the profession will find them helpful in updating their knowledge on various topics. Licensed veterinarians moving to a new locale can use the books to prepare for the licensing examination in their new state or province. The books are also useful in preparing for the American Board of Veterinary Practitioners examination.

Foreign Graduates: Graduates of non-accredited foreign veterinary colleges can use these books in preparing for Education Commission for Foreign Veterinary Graduates (ECFVG) certification.

What Is Covered In These Books?

Review Questions & Answers For Veterinary Boards is a series of 5 volumes covering nearly every aspect of veterinary medicine. The series includes volumes on *Basic Sciences, Clinical Sciences, Small Animal Medicine and Surgery, Large Animal Medicine and Surgery,* and *Ancillary Topics.*

These 5 books contain more than 9,400 questions, divided into the following subject areas:

Anesthesiology: This section covers equipment, techniques and agents used to anesthetize animals. Included are questions on sedation, tranquilization, and general, local and spinal anesthesia.

Behavior: Questions on normal and abnormal behavior of domestic species are included in this section.

Biochemistry: This section contains questions relating to biochemical reactions involved in metabolic processes in animals.

Cage/Aviary Bird Medicine: These questions relate to diseases and husbandry of cage/aviary birds.

Cardiology: These questions concern diagnosis and management of heart disorders.

Clinical Pathology: This section covers all aspects of laboratory diagnosis.

Cytology: This section includes questions on cytologic evaluation of various types of specimens.

Dentistry: This section includes questions on dental anatomy, terminology, periodontal disease, prophylaxis, floating, extraction, endodontics, orthodontics and other dental procedures.

Dermatology: These questions concern skin disease.

Diagnostic Imaging and Recordings: Questions in this section relate to equipment and techniques used in radiography, ultrasonography, endoscopy, electrocardiography, electroencephalography and electromyography.

Diseases of Aquarium Fish: These questions relate to care of freshwater and saltwater aquarium fish.

Embryology: These questions relate to embryonic development of mammals and birds.

Epidemiology: These questions relate to the dynamics of disease in animal populations.

Ethics, Jurisprudence and Animal Welfare: Ethical, legal and animal welfare issues in veterinary medicine are explored in this section.

Gross Anatomy: These questions relate to gross anatomy of all body tissues. Species covered include small animals (dogs, cats), monogastric ungulates (horses, pigs), ruminants (cattle, sheep, goats), and avian/exotics (birds, reptiles).

Hematology: This section includes questions on hematopoiesis, blood and bone marrow cell morphology and coagulation.

Immunology: This section includes questions on immune system structure, function and disorders.

Laboratory Animal Medicine: These questions relate to diseases and husbandry of common laboratory species.

Medical Diseases: These sections contain questions on diagnosis and nonsurgical management of infectious and noninfectious diseases in small and large animals. Disciplines include cardiology, dermatology, neurology, oncology, ophthalmology and urology. Questions cover history taking, physical examination, diagnostic techniques, medical care, followup care and emergency care.

Microbiology: These questions relate to morphology, physiology, culture and identification of bacteria, fungi and viruses of veterinary importance.

Microscopic Anatomy: These questions relate to microscopic anatomy of all body tissues, including blood cells, bone marrow cells and spermatozoa.

Necropsy: Included are questions on techniques used in necropsy of domestic animals.

Neuroanatomy: This section contains questions on gross and microscopic anatomy of the central and peripheral nervous systems.

Neurology: These questions relate to disorders of the central and peripheral nervous systems.

Nutrition: Nutritional requirements and feeding domestic animals are the focus of this section.

Oncology: These questions relate to types and treatment of neoplasia.

Ophthalmology: These questions concern diseases of the eye.

Parasitology: These questions relate to the life cycle, pathologic effects and identification of arthropods, protozoans and helminths of veterinary importance.

Pathology: These questions relate to pathologic processes in various body systems.

Pharmacology: These questions concern the actions of various classes of drugs, calculation of dosages and dilutions, and procedures used in the pharmacy.

Physiology: This section covers the physical and metabolic functions of the various body systems.

Poultry Medicine: These questions relate to diseases and husbandry of domestic fowl and wild waterfowl.

Practice Management: These questions relate to clinic management, practice administration and client relations.

Preventive Medicine: This section focuses on procedures used to prevent disease in domestic species, including use of biologics, anthelmintics, disinfectants and quarantine procedures.

Principles of Surgery: These questions concern wound healing and infection, antimicrobial use, hemostasis, asepsis, sterilization, instruments, suture materials, drains and dressings.

Public Health and Regulatory Medicine: This section covers zoonoses, meat and milk hygiene, and drug residues in animal tissues.

Surgical Diseases: These sections contain questions relating to surgical management of conditions involving the various body systems of small and large animals. Questions cover preoperative preparation, operative technique and postoperative care.

Terminology: This section reviews surgical, medical, anatomic and directional terms, terms used in microbiology and pharmacology, and universally accepted abbreviations.

Theriogenology: This section includes questions on reproductive physiology, function and disease in male and female animals.

Toxicology: These questions relate to toxicants of veterinary importance.

Urology/Nephrology: This section covers diseases of the urinary system.

Zoo, Exotic and Marine Animal Medicine: These questions relate to diseases and care of zoo species, companion exotic species, and marine mammals.

What Types of Questions Are Included In These Books?

The questions in these books were prepared by highly qualified authors, including veterinary educators, content-area specialists and experienced clinicians. The questions have been carefully constructed to test factual knowledge, reasoning skills and clinical judgment. They will also help pinpoint deficiencies in a candidate's studies. The questions are original, and none have been knowingly "recycled" from previous national or state licensure examinations; however, certain overlap is unavoidable and not necessarily a disadvantage.

All of the questions are multiple choice. This format was chosen because it is most commonly used in licensure examinations. Also, it is similar to the format used in the National Board Examination. Questions in these books present 5 answer choices. Each question has only 1 correct answer. There are no "trick" questions.

Multiple-choice questions offer several advantages. Many questions covering a broad range of subjects can be presented in a limited testing period. Also, multiple-choice examinations can be quickly and accurately graded (often by automated optical scanner). Finally, a candidate's answers to multiple-choice questions are not subject to differences of interpretation by the grading examiner, as in essays.

Questions are presented in several styles:

Completion: Together with the question stem, the appended answer forms a complete sentence. For example,

1. *The last nucleated stage of maturing mammalian erythrocytes is the:*

    a. rubricyte
    b. metarubricyte
    c. reticulocyte

    d. mature erythrocyte
    e. prorubricyte

    (The correct answer is b.)

Selection: The question is presented as a complete sentence, and the reader selects the best answer. For example,

2. *Which stage of maturing mammalian erythrocytes is the last nucleated stage?*

    a. rubricyte
    b. metarubricyte
    c. reticulocyte
    d. mature erythrocyte
    e. prorubricyte

    (The correct answer is b.)

Association: Several answer choices are listed, followed by a series of questions relating to these choices. For example,

    a. prorubricyte
    b. metarubricyte
    c. reticulocyte
    d. erythrocyte
    e. rubricyte

3. *The final stage of erythrocyte maturation.*

4. *The last nucleated stage of maturing erythrocytes.*

5. *The first non-nucleated stage of maturing erythrocytes.*

6. *The earliest functional stage of maturing erythrocytes.*

*7. The stage of maturing erythrocytes **least** commonly seen in peripheral blood.*

(Correct answers: 3. d, 4. b, 5. c, 6. e, 7. a)

Case History: A clinical case is described, and questions pertain to case management. For example,

Questions 8 through 11

A 3-month-old mixed-breed puppy is presented because of diarrhea and coughing. The puppy was recently obtained from an animal shelter, and has been vaccinated (DHLP) but never dewormed. The puppy has a dull haircoat and slight fever, but is well hydrated, alert and playful.

8. The most appropriate initial procedure is to:

  a.   make thoracic and abdominal radiographs

  b.   perform a physical examination

  c.   obtain blood samples for serum chemistry assays

  d.   perform an electrocardiographic examination

  e.   euthanize the puppy because of probable distemper

9. You examine a fecal sample and find roundworm eggs. The most appropriate drug for deworming this puppy is:

  a.   niclosamide

  b.   piperazine

  c.   sulfadimethoxine

  d.   praziquantel

  e.   fenbendazole

10. Considering this dog's history and origin, the most likely cause of the coughing is:

  a.   infectious tracheobronchitis

  b.   lungworm infection

  c.   heartworm disease

  d.   congenital heart defect

  e.   tracheal collapse

11. The most reasonable course of action is to:

  a.   hospitalize the puppy for elimination of adult heartworms

  b.   hospitalize the puppy for angiocardiographic studies

  c.   deworm the puppy and dispense antibacterials

  d.   hospitalize the puppy for intravenous antibacterial and fluid therapy

  e.   administer dexamethasone and dispense prednisolone

Answers

8. **b** This first step can help guide subsequent diagnostic procedures and treatments.

9. **b** None of the other drugs listed is appropriate for treating roundworm infection.

10. **a** "Kennel cough" is a common problem in commingled dogs obtained from pounds and shelters.

11. **c** This treatment should resolve these relatively minor problems.

How To Use These Books

Review Questions & Answers For Veterinary Boards was meant to be used in reviewing for final examinations or licensure examinations. Before you begin a section, review your texts and course notes pertaining to that subject area. Then, approach each section as you would an actual examination:

- *Carefully read each question.* Look for such key words as "most," "best," "least," "always," "never" and "except." Consider only the facts presented in the question, and don't make assumptions and inferences that may not be true.

- *Carefully evaluate each answer choice.* Each question has only 1 correct answer, with 4 incorrect answers or "distractors." If more than 1 answer choice appears to be correct, closely examine them for clues that would eliminate any as incorrect.

  Most of the questions ask you to find a single correct answer among 4 incorrect answers. However, some questions ask you to find an *exception*. For these questions, the answer you are seeking is the single *incorrect* answer among 4 *correct* answers.

- *Select an answer* by circling the letter preceding your answer choice. If you do not wish to mark the book, use the blank answer sheets in the back of the book for practice tests.

- *Compare your answers with the correct answers.* The correct answers are listed separately at the end of each section. Many answers are accompanied by an explanation as to why a specific answer is correct or incorrect.

- *Identify your "weak" areas.* If you cannot correctly answer most of the questions in a particular subject area, it may be wise to spend extra time reviewing that subject before your actual examination. If you do not understand the rationale of why certain answers are correct or incorrect, consult the references in the Recommended Reading list at the beginning of each section.

Preparing for final examinations, licensure examinations and specialty board examinations can be an intimidating task. Faced with stacks of textbooks and lecture notes, you may find it difficult to know where to begin and how to study in an organized, productive fashion. Also, anxiety about examinations can interfere with your preparations.

We hope *Review Questions & Answers For Veterinary Boards* will assist you in preparing for examinations and in updating your knowledge on the many subject areas of veterinary medicine. Good luck in your preparations.

According to Earl Nightingale, "Luck is what happens when preparedness meets opportunity." You have always had the opportunity to succeed. With these books, you can better prepare for success.

Dean C. Frey, DVM
Cedar Rapids, Iowa

This page intentionally left blank.

Licensing of Veterinarians

D.C. Frey

History of Veterinary Licensing

During the early years of the United States, there was no organized system of veterinary education or licensing. Almost anybody could claim to be an "animal doctor" or "healer of animals."

The American Veterinary Medical Association (AVMA) directory lists 42 veterinary teaching institutions in existence during the period of 1852 to 1947. All of these were closed by 1947. The first veterinary school established at a land-grant college was at Iowa State College in 1878. In those early years, there was a great diversity in education and training in what was to become the veterinary profession.

New York was the first state to pass a law, in 1886, requiring prospective veterinary practitioners to pass an examination. In 1888, the U.S. Supreme Court ruled that a state could protect its citizens by imposing licensing conditions upon members of the medical professions.

The National Board Examination

Before 1954, all states and provinces developed their own licensing examinations. In 1954, 3 states first administered the National Board Examination in Veterinary Medicine (NBE) to 210 veterinary candidates.

The AVMA's Consultant Advisory Board and the NBE Committee work with the Professional Examination Service in developing the NBE and Clinical Competency Test. Construction of each examination is a very thorough and exacting process.

Questions are developed at item development workshops held throughout the country each year. Validation workshops and psychometric reviews are conducted until the final printing of the examination by the Professional Examination Service. The NBE is prepared by the Professional Examination Service under contract to the AVMA. It is available for purchase by state and provincial licensing boards.

A companion test, the Clinical Competency Test (CCT), was first administered in 1979. As opposed to the multiple-choice questions of the NBE, the CCT consists of 14 case management problems. Each problem presents an opening clinical scenario, and questions pertain to a sequence of steps in diagnosis and treatment of the animal's problem.

The NBE is a 400-item multiple-choice examination. The content of the NBE is based on a job analysis for entry-level veterinarians. It is administered in 2 parts of 200 questions each. Only 360 questions are used in the final scoring; the 40 questions on which candidates score lowest are deleted in final scoring.

Until December, 1992, the NBE was scored on a "norm-referenced" basis. In this system, candidates scoring 1 or 1.5 standard deviations below the mean of the "criterion population" were failed. The criterion population consisted of candidates taking the examination for the first time in the year in which they were graduating from accredited veterinary colleges.

The philosophy of norm-referenced scoring was that the public interest and the integrity of the profession were protected by failing (not licensing) the lowest-scoring candidates. With this relative-standard system, a given percentage of candidates automatically failed the NBE.

"Criterion-referenced" scoring has since replaced norm-referenced scoring of the NBE. With criterion-referenced scoring, a passing score is based on an absolute standard delineating the qualifications for licensure. All candidates have an opportunity to pass because their scores are compared to a standard, not to the scores of other candidates taking the NBE.

Currently the NBE is required for licensure in nearly every state in the United States, and in 4 Canadian provinces. The CCT is currently required for licensure in 52 states and provinces. Candidates should contact the licensing board of the state or province in which they desire licensure to obtain information on licensing requirements.

In Canada, the Canadian Veterinary Medical Association is responsible for developing examinations. The individual Canadian provinces are responsible for registering qualified veterinarians within the provincial association.

Candidates moving from one state to another can have their NBE and CCT scores reported to their new state by contacting the Interstate Reporting Service, Professional Examination Service, 475 Riverside Drive, New York, NY 10015; telephone (212) 870-3169.

United States

For the convenience of candidates seeking information on licensure, the addresses of state licensing boards follow:

Alabama

Executive Officer
Board of Veterinary Medicine
PO Box 1767
Decatur AL 35602

Alaska

Division of Occupational Licensing
Department of Commerce & Economic
  Development
PO Box D-LIC
Juneau AK 99881

Arizona

Executive Director
Veterinary Medical Examining Board
Room 410
1645 W. Jefferson
Phoenix AZ 85007

Arkansas

Executive Secretary
Arkansas Veterinary Medical Examining
  Board
1 Natural Resources Drive
Little Rock AR 72215

California

Executive Officer
Board of Examiners in Veterinary Medicine
Suite 6
1420 Howe Ave.
Sacramento CA 95825

Colorado

Colorado Veterinary Medical Examining
  Board
Suite 1310
1560 Broadway
Denver CO 80202

Connecticut

Connecticut Board of Veterinary Medicine
150 Washington St.
Hartford CT 06106

Delaware

Board of Veterinary Medicine
PO Box 1401
Dover DE 19903

District of Columbia

District of Columbia Board of Veterinary
  Examiners
Room 923
614 H St. NW
Washington DC 20001

Florida

Executive Director
Florida Board of Veterinary Medicine
1910 N. Monroe St.
Tallahassee FL 32399

Georgia

Executive Director
State Examining Boards
166 Pryor St. SW
Atlanta GA 30303

Hawaii

Executive Secretary
Board of Veterinary Examiners
Box 3469
1010 Richards St.
Honolulu HI 96801

Idaho

Board of Veterinary Medicine
PO Box 7249
Boise ID 83707

Illinois

Veterinary Licensing and Disciplinary Board
Department of Professional Regulation
320 W. Washington
Springfield IL 62786

Indiana

Board Director
Health Professions Bureau
Room 041
402 W. Washington St.
Indianapolis IN 46204

Iowa

Secretary
Iowa Board of Veterinary Medicine
2nd Floor
Wallace Building
Des Moines IA 50319

Kansas

Executive Director
Kansas Board of Veterinary Examiners
North Star Route
Lakin KS 67860

Kentucky

Kentucky Board of Veterinary Examiners
PO Box 456
Frankfort KY 40602

Louisiana

Executive Secretary
Board of Veterinary Medical Examiners
PO Box 15191
Baton Rouge LA 70895

Maine

Division of Licensing and Enforcement
Department of Professional and Financial
    Regulation
State House Station 35
Augusta ME 04333

Maryland

President
State Board of Veterinary Medical
    Examiners
50 Truman Hwy.
Annapolis MD 21401

Massachusetts

Secretary
Board of Registration in Veterinary
    Medicine
Room 1516
100 Cambridge St.
Boston MA 02202

Michigan

Licensing Administrator
Michigan State Board of Veterinary
    Medicine
Department of Commerce
PO Box 30018
Lansing MI 48909

Minnesota

Executive Director
Board of Veterinary Medicine
Room 102
2700 University Ave. West
St. Paul MN 55114

Mississippi

Executive Secretary
Mississippi Board of Veterinary Medicine
209 S. Lafayette St.
Starkville MS 39759

Missouri

Executive Director
Missouri Veterinary Medical Board
PO Box 633
Jefferson City MO 65102

Montana

Board of Veterinary Medicine
Department of Commerce
Lower Level, Arcade Building
111 N. Last Chance Gulch
Helena MT 59620

Nebraska

Director
Bureau of Examining Boards
Department of Health
PO Box 95007
Lincoln NE 68509

Nevada

Nevada State Board of Veterinary Medical
    Examiners
Suite 246
1005 Terminal Way
Reno NV 89502

New Hampshire
Secretary-Treasurer
New Hampshire Board of Veterinary
  Medicine
Caller Box 2042
Concord NH 03302

New Jersey
New Jersey State Board of Veterinary
  Medical Examiners
PO Box 45020
Newark NJ 07101

New Mexico
Executive Director
New Mexico Board of Veterinary Examiners
Suite 400-C
1650 University Blvd. NE
Albuquerque NM 87102

New York
Executive Secretary
New York State Board of Veterinary
  Medical Examiners
Room 3043
Cultural Education Center
Albany NY 12230

North Carolina
Executive Director
North Carolina Veterinary Medical Board
PO Box 12587
Raleigh NC 27605

North Dakota
North Dakota Veterinary Medical
  Examining Board
c/o Board of Animal Health
1st Floor, J Wing
600 East Blvd.
Bismarck ND 58505

Ohio
Executive Secretary
Ohio Veterinary Medical Board
16th Floor
77 S. High St.
Columbus OH 43266

Oklahoma
Executive Secretary
Board of Veterinary Medical Examiners
PO Box 18256
Oklahoma City OK 73154

Oregon
Executive Secretary
Veterinary Medical Examining Board
PO Box 231
Portland OR 97207

Pennsylvania
Chairman
Pennsylvania State Board of Veterinary
  Medicine
PO Box 2649
Harrisburg PA 17104

Rhode Island
Administrator
Division of Professional Regulation
Department of Health
Room 104
3 Capitol Hill
Providence RI 02908

South Carolina
Secretary-Treasurer
State Board of Veterinary Medical
  Examiners
PO Box 11293
Columbia SC 29211

South Dakota
Executive Secretary
State Board of Veterinary Medical
  Examiners
411 S. Fort St.
Pierre SD 57501

Tennessee
Registration Boards Administrator
Board of Veterinary Medical Examiners
283 Plus Park Blvd.
Nashville TN 37217

Texas
Executive Director
Texas State Board of Veterinary Medical
  Examiners
Suite 306
1946 South Interstate Hwy 35
Austin TX 78704

Utah
Division of Occupational and Professional
  Licensing
PO Box 45802
Salt Lake City UT 84145

Vermont
State Veterinary Board
Office of Professional Regulations
109 State St.
Montpelier VT 05609

Virginia
Virginia Board of Veterinary Medicine
1601 Rolling Hills Dr.
Richmond VA 23229

Washington
Program Manager
Veterinary Board of Governors
1300 E. Quince
Olympia WA 98504

West Virgina
Executive Secretary
Board of Veterinary Medicine
712 McCorkle Ave.
South Charleston WV 25303

Wisconsin
Bureau Director
Veterinary Examining Board
PO Box 8935
Madison WI 53708

Wyoming
Secretary-Treasurer
Wyoming Board of Veterinary Medicine
Herschler Bldg.
Cheyenne WY 82002

Canada

Candidates interested in practicing in Canadian provinces should contact those licensing boards at the following addresses:

Alberta
Secretary-Treasurer
Board of Veterinary Medical Examiners
#100
8615 149th St.
Edmonton, Alberta T5R 1B3

British Columbia
Board of Veterinary Medical Examiners
Suite 155
1200 W. 73rd Ave.
Vancouver, British Columbia V6P 6G5

Manitoba
Registrar
Veterinary Medical Board
Agricultural Services Complex
545 University Crescent
Winnipeg, Manitoba R3T 5S6

New Brunswick
Secretary-Treasurer
Board of Veterinary Medical Examiners
PO Box 1065
Moncton, New Brunswick E1C 8P2

Nova Scotia
Board of Veterinary Medical Examiners
Agricultural Centre
Kentville, Nova Scotia B4N 1J5

Ontario
Registrar
College of Veterinarians
Suite 24-25
340 Woodlawn Rd. West
Guelph, Ontario N1H 2X1

Quebec
General Director and Secretary
Board of Veterinary Medical Examiners
Suite 200
795 Avenue du Palais
St. Hyacinthe, Quebec J2S 5C6

Saskatchewan
Secretary-Treasurer
Board of Veterinary Medical Examiners
Suite 11
1025 Boychuk Dr.
Saskatoon, Saskatchewan S7H 5B2

This page intentionally left blank.

Biochemistry

H.P. Misra

Recommended Reading

Clarenburg R: *Physiological Chemistry of Domestic Animals.* Mosby Year Book, St. Louis, 1992.
Devlin TM: *Textbook of Biochemistry.* 3rd ed. John Wiley & Sons, New York, 1992.
Montgomery *et al: Biochemistry: A Case-Oriented Approach.* 5th ed. Mosby, St. Louis, 1990.

> *Practice answer sheets are on pages 251-252.*

Questions

1. *All of the following subcellular organelles can be isolated essentially intact **except***:

    a. mitochondria
    b. nuclei
    c. peroxisomes
    d. lysosomes
    e. endoplasmic reticulum

2. *Lysosomes may:*

    a. secrete their enzymes from the cell for digestion of complex carbohydrates
    b. combine with mitochondria to provide additional oxidative phosphorylation potential for synthesis of ATP
    c. combine with phagocytic vacuoles to become digestive vacuoles
    d. combine with peroxisomes to become digestive vacuoles
    e. secrete digestive enzymes to degrade microtubules for exocytosis of enzymes and hormones.

3. *Which reagent is used for quantitative determination of amino acids in general?*

    a. Pauly's reagent
    b. Sakaguchi reagent
    c. ninhydrin
    d. periodic acid
    e. methylene blue

Correct answers are on pages 23-26.

4. When protein subunits combine to form a quaternary structure, all of the following interactions may occur **except**:

   a. hydrogen bonding
   b. hydrophobic interaction
   c. van der Waal's force
   d. disulfide bond formation
   e. electrostatic interaction

5. Proteins may be separated according to size by:

   a. ion-exchange chromatography
   b. isolectric focusing
   c. polyacrylamide gel density gradient
   d. molecular exclusion chromatography
   e. ammonium sulfate precipitation

6. Blacktongue in dogs is caused by a deficiency of:

   a. thiamin
   b. riboflavin
   c. pantothenic acid
   d. niacin
   e. alpha-tocopherol

7. Trypsin digests:

   a. sucrose
   b. unsaturated fatty acids
   c. proteins
   d. complex carbohydrates
   e. lipopolysaccharides

8. Vitamin K is necessary for:

   a. platelet aggregation
   b. activation of thromboplastin
   c. modification of prothrombin
   d. synthesis of hemoglobin
   e. activation of fibrinogen

9. As compared with nonruminants, ruminants derive more volatile fatty acids from:

   a. vegetable proteins
   b. carbohydrates
   c. vitamins
   d. lipoproteins
   e. nucleic acids

10. When it binds to oxygen, hemoglobin exhibits:

    a. negative cooperativity
    b. a sigmoid saturation curve
    c. a beta-barrel structure
    d. an alpha-helix structure
    e. an allosteric conformational state

11. When the plasma activity of an intracellular enzyme is abnormally high, all of the following are possible **except**:

    a. tissue damage may have occurred
    b. the enzyme may have been activated
    c. the enzyme's rate of removal from the plasma may be depressed
    d. quantitation may yield valuable diagnostic information
    e. a competitive inhibitor is usually given to reduce it to normal levels

12. Metal ions may:

    a. participate in oxidation-reduction processes
    b. compete with substrate for the active sites of enzymes
    c. serve as rate-limiting steps in enzyme activity
    d. participate in the committed step in enzyme synthesis
    e. activate enzyme degradation

13. Types of physiologic regulation of enzyme activity include all of the following **except**:

    a. covalent modification
    b. competitive inhibition
    c. change in rate of synthesis of the enzyme
    d. allosteric activation
    e. covalent catalysis

14. *Cell membranes typically contain all of the following* **except***:*

   a. cholesterol
   b. phospholipids
   c. transmembrane and surface proteins
   d. free glucose or glucose attached to gangliosides
   e. carbohydrates in the form of glycoproteins and glycoplipids

15. *Membrane channels:*

   a. may form clusters that create gap junctions between 2 cells
   b. are closed when the transmembrane potential is changed
   c. commonly contain an amphipathic beta-barrel structure
   d. have a nonselective permeable gate for cations
   e. have protein structure largely impermeable to cations

16. *The transport system that maintains the Na$^+$ and K$^+$ gradients across the cell membrane:*

   a. is a symport system
   b. involves ATPase
   c. is an electrically neutral system
   d. allows Na$^+$ into the cell
   e. requires cAMP for activation

17. *If mitochondria are exposed to rotenone,:*

   a. succinate oxidation remains normal
   b. the rate of NADH oxidation is diminished to two-thirds of normal value
   c. electron flow is inhibited at coenzyme Q level
   d. oxidative phosphorylation is uncoupled
   e. electron flow ceases but ATP synthesis from NADH continues at two-thirds of normal value

18. *If tightly coupled mitochondria that actively oxidize succinate are exposed to cyanide,:*

   a. electron flow ceases but ATP synthesis continues
   b. electron flow ceases but ATP synthesis can be restored by subsequent addition of rotenone
   c. subsequent addition of oligomycin causes greater oxygen uptake
   d. subsequent addition of 2,4-dinitrophenol causes ATP hydrolysis
   e. subsequent addition of azide restores ATP synthesis

19. *Which tricarboxylic acid cycle intermediate may be added or removed by another metabolic pathway?*

   a. isocitrate
   b. oxalosuccinate
   c. alpha-ketoglutarate
   d. cis-aconitate
   e. fumarate

20. *Which common nutrient in animal feed does* **not** *provide energy?*

   a. protein
   b. fat
   c. sucrose
   d. complex carbohydrates
   e. vitamins

21. *When the supply of glucose is more than the immediate need, the bulk excess is stored as:*

   a. cholesterol
   b. phospholipids
   c. glycogen
   d. structural proteins
   e. neutral fat

22. *All of the following enzyme or vitamin antioxidants remove reactive species of oxygen* **except***:*

   a. superoxide dismutase
   b. xanthine oxidase
   c. catalase
   d. glutathione peroxidase
   e. ascorbate

Correct answers are on pages 23-26.

23. *Optimal activity of the pyruvate dehydrogenase complex requires all of the following essential cofactors **except**:*

    a. vitamin B₁ (thiamin)
    b. vitamin B₂ (riboflavin)
    c. niacin
    d. lipoic acid
    e. ATP

24. *All of the following antibiotics inhibit prokaryotic protein synthesis **except**:*

    a. streptomycin
    b. cycloheximide
    c. tetracycline
    d. chloramphenicol
    e. erythromycin

25. *Ultraviolet radiation can covalently modify DNA by producing:*

    a. thiamin dimers
    b. lethal mutations
    c. deamination of cytosine residues
    d. free radicals that disrupt covalent bonds
    e. inactive polymerase I

26. *The major action of aspirin is by:*

    a. inhibiting phospholipase C
    b. inhibiting diacylglycerol lipase
    c. augmenting the action of phospholipase A₂
    d. inhibiting cyclooxygenase
    e. blocking lipoxygenase

27. *The Lesch-Nyham syndrome is characterized by hyperuricemia and neurologic problems, and is caused by a failure or defect in:*

    a. pyrimidine degradation
    b. pyrimidine recycling
    c. purine degradation
    d. purine recycling
    e. choline esterase inhibition

28. *Oubain and digoxin are cardiac glycosides that have been used in treatment of chronic cardiac failure. These glycosides act by:*

    a. making a tight link between neurotransmitter and receptor
    b. reducing $Na^+ - K^+$ ATPase activity
    c. inhibiting the breakdown of cAMP
    d. opening the ion-gated channels
    e. inhibiting choline esterase

29. *Enzymes:*

    a. are less specific than inorganic catalysts
    b. increase reaction rate by decreasing the activation barrier
    c. that have competitive inhibitors are physiologically important
    d. are always synthesized as proenzymes
    e. have one or more subunits that undergo denaturation before becoming active

30. *In glycolysis, ATP synthesis is catalyzed by:*

    a. hexokinase
    b. phosphoglycerate kinase
    c. phosphofructokinase
    d. pyruvate dehydrogenase
    e. triose phosphate isomerase

31. *In an enzyme-catalyzed reaction, NAD^+ can be regenerated in the cytoplasm if NADH reacts with any of the following **except**:*

    a. pyruvate
    b. oxaloacetate
    c. dihydroacetone phosphate
    d. malate
    e. 1,3-bisphosphoglycerate

32. *Gluconeogenic enzymes include all of the following **except**:*

    a. phosphoglucomutase
    b. pyruvate carboxylase
    c. fructose 1,6-bisphosphatase
    d. phosphoenolpyruvate carboxy kinase
    e. glucose 6-phosphatase

---

33. A major non-nitrogenous source for net glucose synthesis in liver and adipose tissue is:

   a. methionine
   b. glycerol
   c. acetic acid
   d. palmitic acid
   e. unsaturated fatty acids

34. A major function of the pentose phosphate shunt in endocrine cells is to provide:

   a. NADPH for fat synthesis
   b. pentoses for nucleic acid production and protein synthesis
   c. pentoses for quick release of energy
   d. NADPH for production of 3 ATPs
   e. glucolactone for conversion of prohormones to active forms of hormones

35. The hormone that enhances glycogenolysis in muscle is:

   a. glucagon
   b. epinephrine
   c. growth hormone
   d. adrenocorticotropic hormone
   e. secretion

36. The enzyme responsible for modification of structures of certain key enzymes that simultaneously stimulate glycogenolysis while inhibiting glycogenesis is:

   a. phosphoprotein phosphatase
   b. phosphorylase
   c. glycogen synthetase
   d. UDP-glucokinase
   e. cAMP-dependent protein kinase

37. In the liver, the effects of glucagon are more immediate than those of glucocorticoids because:

   a. glucagon acts via nuclear events that lead to protein synthesis

   b. glucagon converts an inactive form of an already-synthesized enzyme into the active form
   c. glucagon is quickly synthesized, while glucocorticoids require more time to be released from vesicles
   d. glucocorticoids must be synthesized before they can be effective
   e. glucocorticoids are stored in vesicles in an inactive form and require several minutes to be activated and released

38. The high glucagon/insulin ratio seen in starvation promotes all of the following **except**:

   a. beta-oxidation by inhibiting production of malonyl CoA
   b. increased concentrations of ketone bodies in the blood
   c. production of volatile fatty acids for quick production of energy
   d. mobilization of fatty acids from adipose stores
   e. increased utilization of ketone bodies by the brain

39. In dogs, fatty acids:

   a. are not required in the diet
   b. containing double bonds cannot be synthesized
   c. must be supplied entirely by the diet
   d. other than palmitate must be supplied in the diet
   e. can be synthesized from excess dietary carbohydrate or protein

40. Triacylglycerols:

   a. yield about the same amount of ATP on complete oxidation as an equivalent weight of glycogen
   b. represent sufficient energy to sustain life for several weeks in an average individual
   c. are good emulsifying agents
   d. are stored as hydrated molecules
   e. are generally negatively charged molecules at physiologic pH

Correct answers are on pages 23-26.

41. *Of the following amino acids, which has the greatest hydrophobicity?*

   a. phenylalanine
   b. arginine
   c. glycine
   d. glutamic acid
   e. proline

42. *Polymerization of amino acids into polypeptide chains does **not** involve:*

   a. catalysis by enzymes
   b. RNA
   c. ribosomes
   d. a dehydration reaction
   e. ATP

43. *The amino acid sequence of a polypeptide chain in a protein is known as the:*

   a. primary structure
   b. secondary structure
   c. tertiary structure
   d. quaternary structure
   e. helical structure

44. *Amino acids whose R groups contain nitrogen atoms are known as:*

   a. acidic amino acids
   b. basic amino acids
   c. resonance isomers
   d. aromatic amino acids
   e. monocarboxylic amino acids

45. *The ionic form of an amino acid in which the positive charge from positively charged ionized groups is exactly equal to the negative charge from negatively charged ionized groups is called the:*

   a. resonance isomer
   b. amino acid residue
   c. zwitterion form
   d. trans conformation
   e. cis conformation

46. *The pH at which an amino acid is electrically neutral is the:*

   a. isohydric pH
   b. isozyme pH
   c. isoelectric pH
   d. electrostatic pH
   e. ionic pH

47. *Proteins may be separated based on pI values by:*

   a. molecular exclusion chromatography
   b. polyacrylamide gel electrophoresis in the presence of sodium dodecyl sulfate
   c. ion-exchange chromatography
   d. affinity chromatography
   e. ammonium sulfate precipitation

48. *Generalized amino aciduria associated with hypophosphatemia and excretion of glucose are signs of:*

   a. cystinuria
   b. phenylketonuria
   c. Hartnup disease
   d. Fanconi's syndrome
   e. diabetes mellitus

49. *All of the following reagents cleave polypeptides at specific points for sequencing purposes **except**:*

   a. silver nitrate
   b. cyanogen bromide
   c. trypsin
   d. chymotrypsin
   e. o-iodobenzoic acid

50. *Substitution of an amino acid by another acid of similar polarity is termed:*

   a. invariant residual substitution
   b. conservative substitution
   c. nonconservative substitution
   d. primary substitution
   e. homology

51. *The secondary structure of a protein refers to the:*

    a. local conformation of the polypeptide chain
    b. amino acid sequence
    c. total 3-dimensional structure of the polypeptide units
    d. structure and interactions of the noncovalent association of discrete polypeptide sub-units into a multi sub-unit protein
    e. covalent structure

52. *In sickle-cell anemia, the variant form of hemoglobin (HbS) is:*

    a. an analogous mutation
    b. an invariant residue
    c. a conservative mutation
    d. a native conformation
    e. a nonconservative mutation

53. *The bond between the nitrogen and alpha carbon in a polypeptide chain is the:*

    a. ionic bond
    b. phi bond
    c. hydrogen bond
    d. noncovalent bond
    e. psi bond

54. *The distance between repeating turns of a protein helix or a line drawn parallel to the axis is the:*

    a. fingerprint
    b. regular secondary structure
    c. beta structure
    d. distance matrix
    e. helix pitch

55. *All of the following are characteristics of an alpha-helical conformation of a protein* ***except***:

    a. 3.6 amino acid residues per 360-degree turn
    b. the planes of the peptide bonds are approximately parallel to the axis of the helix
    c. each peptide forms a hydrogen bond to the peptide bond of the fourth amino acid above and below in the primary structure
    d. the hydrogen bonds between the peptide groups, donor atom, acceptor atom and hydrogen atom are approximately colinear
    e. the helical structure has symmetric properties correlating with no optical activity

56. *The tertiary structure of a protein refers to the:*

    a. total 3-dimensional structure of the protein
    b. amino acid sequence
    c. arrangement of polypeptide chain units in a multi-chain protein
    d. local comformation of the polypeptide chain
    e. specific ordering of structural motifs

57. *All of the following are characteristic of collagen* ***except***:

    a. constitutes over one-third of all animal proteins
    b. synthesized as preprocollagen, which is extensively modified posttranslationally
    c. every third amino acid in an alpha chain of the helical portion of collagen is glycine; hence, glycine can limit growth in young animals
    d. considered a low-quality protein because it lacks or contains low concentrations of certain essential amino acids
    e. about 5% of the amino acids in collagen are proline or hydroxyproline

58. *In a protein quaternary structure, all of the following associations may occur* ***except***:

    a. hydrogen bonding
    b. noncovalent interaction
    c. hydrophobic interaction
    d. van der Waal's forces
    e. disulfide bonding

Correct answers are on pages 23-26.

59. Fibrous proteins are characterized by all of the following **except**:

   a. large amounts of regular secondary structure
   b. a long, cylindric shape
   c. low solubility in water
   d. a dynamic role in the cell
   e. a structural role in function

60. Which of the following has quaternary structure?

   a. trypsin
   b. hemoglobin
   c. myoglobin
   d. elastase
   e. insulin

61. The amino acid hydroxyproline is unique to:

   a. collagen
   b. alpha-keratin
   c. tropomyosin
   d. elastin
   e. actin

62. Tropomyosin is a component of:

   a. muscle tissue
   b. lung tissue
   c. cartilage
   d. skin, hair and claw/hooves
   e. vascular tissue

63. Alpha-keratin is a component of:

   a. the aorta
   b. skin, hair and claws/hooves
   c. muscle
   d. the liver
   e. cartilage

64. Purified protein components of a lipoprotein are called:

   a. telopeptides
   b. desmosines
   c. chylomicrons
   d. apolipoproteins
   e. isodesmosines

65. Which of the following contains the highest percentage of total protein?

   a. high-density lipids
   b. low-density lipids
   c. intermediate-density lipids
   d. very-low-density lipids
   e. chylomicrons

66. Absence of chylomicrons, very-low-density lipids and low-density lipids and accumulation of lipid droplets in small intestine cells, malabsorption of fat, and acanthocytosis are all characteristic of:

   a. hypercholesterolemia
   b. hyperlipidemia
   c. beta-lipoproteinemia
   d. Tangier disease
   e. lecithin deficiency

67. Which of the following is **not** a glycoprotein?

   a. interferon
   b. immunoglobulin
   c. follicle-stimulating hormone
   d. thyroid-stimulating hormone
   e. albumin

68. HbA$_{IC}$ is:

   a. the hemoglobin that causes sickle-cell anemia
   b. a glycosylated hemoglobin
   c. normal adult hemoglobin
   d. normal fetal hemoglobin
   e. oxygenated hemoglobin

69. *Of the following bond types, which has the highest bond strength?*

   a. covalent bonds
   b. hydrogen bonds
   c. ionic bonds
   d. van der Waal's interactions
   e. hydrophobic interactions

70. *The most important noncovalent forces that cause a randomized polypeptide conformation to fold into its native structure is:*

   a. van der Waal's interactions
   b. ionic bonding
   c. hydrophobic interactions
   d. hydrogen bonding
   e. electrostatic interactions

71. *A protein can be denatured by any of the following* **except**:

   a. urea
   b. detergents
   c. strong acids or bases
   d. heating to temperatures above 60 C
   e. a conservative mutation

72. *Circular dichroism is caused by:*

   a. differences in refractive index
   b. differences in light absorption
   c. quenchers
   d. excitation energy transfers
   e. fluorescence emission

73. *Posttranslational processing of a newly synthesized protein includes all of the following* **except**:

   a. hydroxylation of lysine and proline
   b. methylation of histidine in muscle proteins
   c. conversion of zymogens into active enzymes
   d. cross-linking of peptide chains as in collagen
   e. incorporation of methionine at the N-terminal of peptides

74. *Materials that evoke antibody production are called:*

   a. serine proteases
   b. haptens
   c. immunoglobulins
   d. antigens
   e. heavy chains

75. *Complementary determining regions are:*

   a. C_L regions
   b. hypervariable sequences
   c. constant regions
   d. C_H2 regions
   e. C_H3 regions

76. *All of the following are protein families* **except**:

   a. immunoglobulins
   b. serine proteases
   c. hemoglobins
   d. DNA binding proteins
   e. fibrous proteins

77. *An inactive precursor form of an enzyme is termed:*

   a. a fragment
   b. an isotype
   c. a zymogen
   d. a hapten
   e. a serpin

78. *Natural serine protease inhibitors are called:*

   a. haptens
   b. serpins
   c. zymogens
   d. proenzymes
   e. exons

Correct answers are on pages 23-26.

79. *A leucine zipper is characterized by all of the following **except**:*

    a. alpha-helices containing at least 4 leucines
    b. leucines separated by 6 amino acids
    c. interdigitation of the leucine helix with a second leucine helix
    d. alignment of the leucines on one edge of the helix
    e. direct interaction with DNA

80. *How many O_2 binding sites does myoglobin contain?*

    a. 1
    b. 2
    c. 3
    d. 4
    e. 5

81. *A complete protein with its prosthetic group is:*

    a. an apoprotein
    b. a holoprotein
    c. a ligand
    d. a hemoglobin
    e. a serpin

82. *The binding of 4 O_2 molecules in hemoglobin is:*

    a. additive
    b. simultaneous
    c. positively cooperative
    d. complementary
    e. noncooperative

83. *The deoxy conformation of hemoglobin is referred to as the:*

    a. T conformational state
    b. alpha-helical conformation
    c. R conformational state
    d. beta-strand conformation
    e. psi conformation

84. *Serine proteases:*

    a. hydrolyze peptide bonds involving the amino groups of serine residues
    b. are inactivated by reacting with one molecule of diisopropylfluorophosphate per molecule of protein
    c. are endopeptidases
    d. are synthesized in an active form in prodaryotes
    e. have several active sites, each containing a serine residue

85. *All of the following relate to the structure and/or function of proteins **except**:*

    a. receptors in membranes
    b. certain hormones, such as estrogen and testosterone
    c. structural elements, such as collagen and cytoskeleton
    d. blood clotting factors
    e. lubricants, such as mucus

86. *The active sites of serine proteases contain which amino acids?*

    a. lysine and arginine
    b. r-carboxyglutamate and proline
    c. serine and hydroxyproline
    d. cysteine and valine
    e. aspartate and histidine

87. *Concerning immunoglobulins, which statement is **least** accurate?*

    a. The chains are linked by disulfide bonds.
    b. There are 2 copies of each chain.
    c. There are 4 polypeptide chains.
    d. Carbohydrates are covalently linked to the proteins.
    e. One molecule of heme is bound per globin chain.

88. *All of the following are classes of immunoglobulin **except**:*

    a. IgM
    b. IgG

c. IgH
d. IgE
e. IgD

89. Which class of immunoglobulin plays a role in allergic responses, hay fever, asthma and anaphylactic shock?

a. IgM
b. IgG
c. IgH
d. IgE
e. IgD

90. Which immunoglobulin is the first to be produced in a normal immune response?

a. IgM
b. IgG
c. IgH
d. IgE
e. IgD

91. Restriction endonucleases are enzymes that make specific cuts in:

a. protein tertiary structure
b. mRNA
c. DNA
d. tRNA
e. rRNA

92. Palindromes can be recognized by:

a. DNA polymerase
b. reverse transcriptase
c. DNA-dependent RNA polymerase
d. restriction endonucleases
e. methylases

93. During DNA replication, the daughter strands that are synthesized continuously and discontinuously are called, respectively, the:

a. leading strand and lagging strand
b. lagging strand and leading strand
c. Okazaki fragment and lagging strand
d. primary strand and secondary strand

e. replication strand and replication fork

94. The enzyme responsible for DNA synthesis in both replication and repair is called:

a. RNA polymerase
b. DNA-dependent DNA polymerase
c. reverse transcriptase
d. DNA ligase
e. endonuclease

95. The enzyme that seals nicks in the DNA helix during DNA synthesis and repair is:

a. DNA primase
b. DNA polymerase
c. DNA ligase
d. replicase
e. RNA polymerase

96. Concerning Okazaki fragments, which statement is *least* accurate?

a. They consist of 100-200 deoxyribonucleotides in eukaryotes.
b. They consist of 1000-2000 deoxyribonucleotides in *E coli*.
c. They are also called nascent DNA.
d. They are also called precursor fragments.
e. They result in congenital defects.

97. The process of copying a segment of DNA into RNA is known as:

a. translation
b. transcription
c. transformation
d. transition
e. elongation

98. RNA synthesis begins at a region in the DNA molecule known as the:

a. initiator
b. promoter
c. enhancer
d. repressor
e. stimulator

Correct answers are on pages 23-26.

99. The enzyme that couples each amino acid to its appropriate tRNA molecule is:

a. tRNA synthetase
b. acyl-tRNA synthetase
c. aminoacyl-tRNA synthetase
d. peptidyl transferase
e. RNA polymerase

100. The genetic code is said to be degenerate because:

a. most of the amino acids are represented by more than one codon
b. one codon represents many amino acids
c. genes degenerate at the time of protein synthesis
d. many genes are not coded
e. the genetic code is ambiguous

101. Peptide bond formation is catalyzed by peptidyl transferase, a catalytic activity that is thought to be mediated by:

a. tRNA
b. a major rRNA molecule in the large ribosomal unit
c. a minor rRNA molecule in the small ribosomal unit
d. a minor tRNA molecule in the intermediate ribosomal unit
e. mRNA

102. Concerning RNA polymerase, which statement is most accurate?

a. Bacterial cells use many types of RNA polymerase to transcribe all classes of RNA, whereas eukaryotic cells use only one type of RNA polymerase.
b. Bacterial cells use one type of RNA polymerase to transcribe all classes of RNA, whereas eukaryotic cells use 3 different types of RNA polymerase.
c. Bacterial cells use RNA polymerase to transcribe all classes of DNA.
d. RNA polymerase is not present in bacteria.
e. RNA polymerase is not required to transcribe RNA in bacteria but is required in eukaryotes.

103. The termination of protein synthesis is coded by the amino acid sequence:

a. UAG, GGA or AAG
b. UAA, AGU or GGU
c. UGA, GAA or UUG
d. UAG, UAA or UGA
e. GAU, AGU or UUG

104. Many antibiotics used in modern medicine selectively inhibit bacterial protein synthesis by exploiting the structural and functional difference between prokaryotic and eukaryotic:

a. nuclei
b. mitochondria
c. ribosomes
d. mRNA
e. hnRNA

105. The energy required for protein synthesis is supplied in the form of:

a. ATP
b. GTP
c. amino acyl-tRNA
d. GDP
e. NADP

106. The direction of mRNA transcription and translation is:

a. 3' to 5'
b. 5' to 3'
c. first 3' to 5' and then 5' to 3'
d. first 4' to 6' and then 6' to 4'
e. 4' to 6'

107. An enzyme that recognizes the difference between $tRNA_i^{met}$ and $tRNA_m^{met}$ is:

a. tRNA synthetase
b. rRNA
c. transformylase
d. formylase
e. methyltransferase

108. *Patients with thalassemia syndromes have:*

 a. an abnormally low level of hemoglobin
 b. an excessive amount of hemoglobin
 c. sickle-shaped red blood cells
 d. an abnormally low level of myoglobin
 e. excessively fragile myoglobin

109. *After the intron sequence has been cut out, the coding RNA sequences on either side of the intron are joined to each other in a reaction known as:*

 a. RNA ligation
 b. RNA splicing
 c. recombination
 d. transcription
 e. transference

110. *Error-prone DNA repair is a process that allows:*

 a. DNA replication to take place in a stop-gap manner until the damage is permanently repaired by another mechanism
 b. DNA damage to be repaired instantaneously by DNA ligase
 c. incorporation of many unwanted nucleotides to the daughter strand
 d. DNA replication with a substitute daughter strand that is later substituted
 e. DNA damage to be repaired instantaneously by RNA ligation

111. *Which of the following is a frame-shift mutagen?*

 a. acridine orange
 b. lithium bromide
 c. benz(a) anthracene
 d. epoxide
 e. methyl cryptyline acetate

112. *Southern blotting is used to detect disease characterized by:*

 a. frame-shift mutation
 b. point mutations

 c. deletion or insertion mutations
 d. transposition mutations
 e. tertiary strand mutations

113. *Skin cells from patients with xeroderma pigmentosum are unable to repair DNA damage produced by:*

 a. epoxide
 b. sunlight
 c. ultraviolet light
 d. x-rays
 e. gamma-rays

114. *Clinically, the most important missense mutation known is the change from A to U in the GAA or GAG codon for glutamate, resulting in a GUA or GUG codon to valine in the sixth position of the beta chain in:*

 a. IgG
 b. hemoglobin
 c. insulin
 d. beta-glucuronidase
 e. growth hormone

115. *General recombination is catalyzed by a protein known as:*

 a. rec A
 b. lex A
 c. recombinase
 d. protease
 e. integrase

116. *The catabolism of odd-chain fatty acids ultimately results in formation of propionyl CoA molecules, which are further oxidized following carboxylation, rearrangement and conversion to:*

 a. acetyl CoA
 b. succinyl CoA
 c. butyryl CoA
 d. HMG CoA
 e. acyl CoA

Correct answers are on pages 23-26.

117. *Phosphatidic acid is a biochemical intermediate in which biosynthetic pathway?*

 a. cholesterol
 b. leukotrienes
 c. sphingolipids
 d. phospholipids
 e. prostaglandins

118. *Dietary ergosterol is converted in the skin by ultraviolet radiation to:*

 a. vitamin A
 b. vitamin B
 c. vitamin C
 d. vitamin D
 e. vitamin E

119. *Energy in the form of NADPH is required in all of the following metabolic pathways **except**:*

 a. fatty acid metabolism
 b. phospholipid metabolism
 c. cholesterol metabolism
 d. sphingolipid metabolism
 e. triacylglycerol metabolism

120. *Long-chain fatty acids (≥16 carbons) are metabolized by a scheme involving:*

 a. alpha oxidation
 b. beta oxidation
 c. delta oxidation
 d. sigma oxidation
 e. theta oxidation

121. *The most important dietary precursor of prostaglandins is the essential fatty acid:*

 a. linolenic acid
 b. linoleic acid
 c. palmitic acid
 d. arachidic acid
 e. arachidonic acid

122. *One of the pathways for cholesterol disposal by the liver involves incorporation into the plasma lipoproteins of:*

 a. very-low-density and low-density lipids
 b. low-density and intermediate-density lipids
 c. intermediate-density and high-density lipids
 d. very-low-density and intermediate-density lipids
 e. low-density and high-density lipids

123. *The most common and primary bile acids in the body are:*

 a. glycocholic and taurocholic acids
 b. deoxycholic and lithocholic acids
 c. cholic and deoxycholic acids
 d. deoxycholic and chenodeoxycholic acids
 e. cholic and chenodeoxycholic acids

124. *The lipid that is produced by type-II pneumocytes and is required for normal pulmonary function to prevent atelectasis is:*

 a. cardiolipin
 b. lecithin
 c. surfactant
 d. phosphatidic acid
 e. sterol

125. *Formation of cholesterol-rich and/or bile pigment gallstones usually results from impaired production and/or secretion of:*

 a. triacylglycerols
 b. phospholipids
 c. sphingolipids
 d. fatty acids
 e. leukotrienes

126. *The enzymes responsible for hydrolysis of triacylglycerols are termed:*

 a. thioesterases
 b. lipases
 c. oxidases
 d. reductases
 e. fatty acylases

127. The biomolecules produced in the intestines that function in absorption and transport of dietary fat are:

    a. plasma lipoproteins
    b. ketone bodies
    c. chylomicrons
    d. serum albumins
    e. serum lipoproteins

128. Decarboxylation of phosphatidylserine in liver mitochondria results in production of:

    a. phosphatidylcholine
    b. phosphatidylleucine
    c. phosphatidylglycerol
    d. phosphatidylinositol
    e. phosphatidylethanolamine

129. In the presence of thromboxane A synthetase, thromboxane A2 is biosynthesized from the endoperoxide:

    a. prostaglandin E2
    b. prostaglandin F2
    c. prostaglandin G2
    d. prostaglandin H2
    e. prostaglandin I2

130. Which ketone body accumulates in the blood of ketoacidotic diabetics and can be detected in the breath?

    a. acetone
    b. acetoacetate
    c. beta-hydroxybutyrate
    d. valerate
    e. propionate

131. Beta-hydroxy-beta-methyl-glutaryl coenzyme A (HMG CoA) is a biochemical intermediate in which biosynthetic pathway?

    a. phospholipids
    b. sphingolipids
    c. cholesterol
    d. prostaglandins
    e. triacylglycerols

132. Fatty acids at the 1 and/or 3 positions of triacylglycerols and diacyglycerols are hydrolyzed by:

    a. acyltransferase
    b. hydrolase
    c. lipoprotein lipase
    d. hormone-sensitive lipase
    e. phosphatase

133. Biosynthesis of oleic acid (18:1) requires the equivalent energy of:

    a. 49 ATP molecules
    b. 54 ATP molecules
    c. 56 ATP molecules
    d. 61 ATP molecules
    e. 63 ATP molecules

134. Which phospholipid plays a role in activation of the enzyme beta-hydroxybutyrate dehydrogenase, which reversibly converts acetoacetate to beta-hydroxybutyrate?

    a. phosphatidylserine
    b. phosphatidylglycerol
    c. phosphatidylinositol
    d. phosphatidylcholine
    e. phosphatidylethanolamine

135. Prostaglandins are manufactured by nearly all mammalian cells **except**:

    a. monocytes
    b. lymphocytes
    c. macrophages
    d. platelets
    e. red blood cells

136. Tay-Sachs disease results from a metabolic deficiency of hexosaminidase A, which causes cerebral accumulation of:

    a. globoside
    b. sulfatide
    c. cerebroside
    d. ganglioside G_{M1}
    e. ganglioside G_{M2}

Correct answers are on pages 23-26.

137. Glucocerebroside accumulation in the viscera causes:

   a. Fabry's disease
   b. Krabbe's disease
   c. Gaucher's disease
   d. Niemann-Pick disease
   e. metachromatic leukodystrophy

138. Generalized gangliosidosis is a metabolic disease that results in visceral and cerebral accumulation of ganglioside G_{M1} due to a lack of:

   a. sphingomyelinase
   b. beta-galactosidase
   c. galactocerebrosidase
   d. arylsulfatase A
   e. hexosaminidase A

139. All of the following are nonessential fatty acids **except**:

   a. oleic acid
   b. linolenic acid
   c. arachidonic acid
   d. palmitoleic acid
   e. palmitic acid

140. Phosphatidylcholine can be formed in the liver by repeated methylation of:

   a. phosphatidylserine
   b. phosphatidylglycerol
   c. phosphatidylethanolamine
   d. phosphatidylinositol
   e. dipalmitoyllecithin

141. In synthesis of fatty acids, branched-chain fatty acids are manufactured when malonyl CoA is substituted by:

   a. propionyl CoA
   b. methylmalonyl CoA
   c. acetylmalonyl CoA
   d. butyrylmalonyl CoA
   e. succinyl CoA

142. The major site for control of cholesterol synthesis is the enzyme beta-hydroxy-beta-methyl-glutaryl coenzyme A (HMG CoA) reductase, which catalyzes the rate-limiting reaction that produces:

   a. mevalonic acid
   b. farnesyl pyrophosphate
   c. squalene
   d. lanosterol
   e. cholesterol

143. Ketone body production occurs in the:

   a. intestines and lungs
   b. liver and intestines
   c. kidney and intestines
   d. lungs and liver
   e. liver and kidney

144. Which compound is **not** a corticosteroid that blocks phospholipase A_2?

   a. hydrocortisone
   b. prednisone
   c. betamethasone
   d. indomethacin
   e. dexamethasone

145. The backbone of sphingolipids found in highest concentration in the white matter of the central nervous system is provided by the long-chain amino alcohol:

   a. dihydrosphingosine
   b. phosphocholine
   c. CDP-phosphocholine
   d. sphinganine
   e. sphingosine

146. Primary bile acids are metabolized in the gut to the deconjugated and dehydroxylated secondary bile acids:

   a. glycocholic and taurocholic acids
   b. deoxycholic and lithocholic acids
   c. cholic and deoxycholic acids
   d. deoxycholic and chenodeoxycholic acids
   e. cholic and chenodeoxycholic acids

147. Biosynthesis of palmitic acid (16:0) requires the equivalent energy of:

  a. 49 ATP molecules
  b. 54 ATP molecules
  c. 56 ATP molecules
  d. 61 ATP molecules
  e. 63 ATP molecules

148. A severe biotin deficiency is most likely to affect:

  a. amino acid biosynthesis
  b. amino acid catabolism
  c. fatty acid biosynthesis
  d. fatty acid oxidation
  e. carbohydrate catabolism

149. A severe pantothenic acid deficiency is most likely to affect:

  a. amino acid biosynthesis
  b. fatty acid catabolism
  c. fatty acid biosynthesis
  d. fatty acid oxidation
  e. amino acid catabolism

150. Which of the following is a 20-carbon straight-chain fatty acid with 4 double bonds?

  a. palmitic acid
  b. palmitoleic acid
  c. oleic acid
  d. arachidic acid
  e. arachidonic acid

151. Nonsteroidal antiinflammatory drugs, such as aspirin, indomethacin and phenylbutazone, irreversibly inhibit:

  a. peroxidase
  b. lipoxygenase
  c. phospholipase
  d. cyclooxygenase
  e. prostaglandin synthetase

152. All of the following fatty acids are commonly found in sphingomyelin **except**:

  a. palmitic acid
  b. stearic acid
  c. lignoceric acid
  d. nervonic acid
  e. sphingonic acid

153. Fatty alcohols are the building blocks of ether-linked chains of fatty acids commonly found in:

  a. ketone bodies
  b. phospholipids
  c. sphingolipids
  d. triglycerides
  e. triacylglycerols

154. Fatty acids subject to auto-oxidation include all of the following **except**:

  a. saturated fatty acids
  b. mono-unsaturated fatty acids
  c. di-unsaturated fatty acids
  d. tri-unsaturated fatty acids
  e. polysaturated fatty acids

155. Activated fatty acyl CoA molecules are carried across the inner mitochondrial membrane by an efficient shuttle system involving:

  a. anserine
  b. carnosine
  c. carnitine
  d. ornithine
  e. lecithin cholesterol acyltransferase

156. Covalent stabilizing elements that increase the rigidity of polypeptide chains include:

  a. hydrogen bonds
  b. ionic interactions
  c. disulfide cross-links
  d. hydrophobic interactions
  e. electostatic bridges

Correct answers are on pages 23-26.

157. *All of the following amino acids are considered essential* **except**:

   a. tyrosine
   b. histidine
   c. threonine
   d. arginine
   e. tryptophan

158. *All of the following nonessential amino acids can be biosynthesized in the body* **except**:

   a. asparagine
   b. glutamine
   c. hydroxyproline
   d. phenylalanine
   e. alanine

159. *Several clinical chemistry determinations are based on use of blood serum versus plasma. For tests requiring serum, blood should be collected in a vacuum tube without anticoagulant, so serum becomes separated from blood cells. These "clot" tubes have a top colored:*

   a. red
   b. green
   c. purple
   d. blue
   e. gray

160. *Collagen contains which amino acid at every third residue?*

   a. proline
   b. hydroxyproline
   c. glycine
   d. hydroxylysine
   e. lysine

161. *Tyrosine condenses under the influence of tyrosine hydroxylase to form L-dopa, which has been used with great success in people to treat the symptoms of:*

   a. Parkinson's disease
   b. Alzheimer' disease
   c. Lou Gehrig's disease

   d. alkaptonuria
   e. phenylketonuria

162. *Biosynthesis of protein begins at the amino end of a growing peptide and progresses by addition of amino acids to the:*

   a. amino end
   b. carboxyl end
   c. A-terminus
   d. N-terminus
   e. phosphoryl end

163. *While the first 2 letters of a codon are very specific, the wobble hypothesis speculates that often the same amino acid is coded, regardless of the base pairing in the third nucleotide position at the:*

   a. 1' end of the mRNA codon
   b. 2' and of the mRNA codon
   c. 3' end of the mRNA codon
   d. 4' end of the mRNA codon
   e. 5' end of the mRNA codon

164. *The antibiotic that specifically inhibits protein biosynthesis in mammalian cells, but* **not** *in microbial cells, is:*

   a. chloramphenicol
   b. streptomycin
   c. cycloheximide
   d. tetracycline
   e. puromycin

165. *The transmethylation of norepinephrine produces:*

   a. epinephrine
   b. L-dopa
   c. dopamine
   d. serotonin
   e. 5-hydroxytryptamine

166. *All of the following plasma proteins are biosynthesized in the liver* **except**:

   a. albumin

b. fibrinogen

c. alpha-globulins

d. beta-globulins

e. gamma globulins

167. *Effective routes of administration for the peptide antibiotic bacitracin include all of the following* **except**:

a. topically

b. orally

c. intramuscularly

d. subcutaneously

e. intravenously

168. *Lathyrism (sweet pea poisoning) is characterized by inhibited formation of aldehyde groups necessary for stable cross-links in mature collagen fibrils. This results when the enzyme peptidyl lysyl oxidase is inhibited by:*

a. alpha-aminitin

b. beta-aminitin

c. alpha-aminobutyrlnitrile

d. beta-aminopropionitrile

e. alpha, beta-aminitinitrile

169. *Proflavin blocks mRNA chain elongation by binding to deoxyribonucleotides other than:*

a. deoxyadenosine residues

b. deoxyguanosine residues

c. deoxycytidine residues

d. deoxythymidine residues

e. deoxyuridine residues

170. *Ingestion of the toxin alpha-amanitin present in the poisonous mushroom* Amanita phalloides *blocks the elongation phase of transcription by inhibiting:*

a. DNA polymerase I

b. DNA polymerase II

c. DNA polymerase III

d. RNA polymerase I

e. RNA polymerase II

171. *The complete regulatory unit of a set of clustered genes is called the:*

a. operator

b. inducer

c. repressor

d. operon

e. promoter

172. *Polyamines are low-molecular-weight organic cations present in nongrowing tissues (pancreas, prostate gland, lactating mammary gland) that are active in protein biosynthesis. All of the following are considered polyamines* **except**:

a. spermine

b. putrescine

c. cadaverine

d. spermidine

e. odorine

173. *Production of histamine in mast cells during anaphylaxis and allergic reactions results from decarboxylation of:*

a. glutamine

b. asparagine

c. histidine

d. hydroxylysine

e. 5-hydroxytryptamine

174. *Excess dietary phenylalanine can be converted into tyrosine under the influence of phenylalanine hydroxylase. Tyrosine serves as a precursor to all of the following* **except**:

a. glutathione

b. dopamine

c. thyroxine

d. epinephrine

e. norepinephrine

Correct answers are on pages 23-26.

175. All of the following clinicopathogic measurements reflect abnormal changes in protein and/or nitrogen metabolism **except**:

a. serum protein level
b. serum creatine level
c. serum creatinine level
d. plasma ammonia level
e. serum urea nitrogen level

176. An operon includes:

a. mRNA, structural genes and control elements
b. a regulatory gene, mRNA and structural genes
c. structural genes, regulatory genes and control elements
d. tRNA, mRNA and control elements
e. mRNA, a regulatory gene and control elements

177. Concerning the design of a recombinant DNA molecule to synthesize an active eukaryotic polypeptide in bacteria, which statement is **least** accurate?

a. The eukaryotic gene may contain its usual complement of introns.
b. The foreign polypeptide should be resistant to degradation by bacterial proteases.
c. Glycosylation of the polypeptide should be unnecessary.
d. The foreign polypeptide should be nontoxic to the bacteria.
e. Bacterial controlling elements are necessary.

178. Catabolic activator protein:

a. is a structural protein that, when combined with NADP, inhibits transcription of the lac operon
b. is monosteric in nature
c. is a regulatory protein that, when combined with cAMP, can control transcription of the lac operon
d. competitively inhibits the cis operon but synergistically enhances synthesis of peptides

e. promotes degradation of damaged DNA strands and, when combined with NADP, can be used as a structural protein

179. Oxytocin and vasopressin are synthesized in the:

a. neuronal cell bodies of the hypothalamus
b. argentaffin cells of the posterior pituitary
c. cortical cells of the adrenal glands
d. interstitial cells of Leydig in the testes
e. chromophobe vacuoles of thyroid gland cells

180. Follicle-stimulating hormone operates through the protein kinase A pathway, which acts in the:

a. seminiferous tubules and ovarian follicle
b. endometrium and posterior pituitary
c. hypothalamus and epididymis
d. posterior pituitary and oviducts
e. testicular interstitium and corpus luteum

181. The direct effect of cAMP in the protein kinase A pathway is to:

a. activate adenylate cyclase
b. phosphorylate certain cellular proteins
c. phosphorylate protein kinase A
d. dissociate regulatory subunits from protein kinase
e. release hormones from a target issue

182. When a hormone interacts with its receptor,

a. only one polypeptide chain is necessary
b. only one second messenger is generated
c. an array of transmembrane helices may form the binding site for the hormone
d. receptors have a greater affinity for hormones than for synthetic agonists or antagonists
e. receptors have a greater affinity for synthetic agonists than for natural antagonists

183. The precursor of steroid hormones is:

a. cholesterol

b. benzene
c. a triglyceride
d. cortisol
e. oxybenzene

184. *Concerning aldosterone, which statement is* **least** *accurate?*

 a. It enhances uptake of sodium ions via conductance channels.
 b. It induces diuresis.
 c. It increases blood pressure.
 d. It increased blood volume.
 e. Secretion of aldosterone is increased during periods of stress.

185. *In the presence of estradiol, progesterone maintains:*

 a. the uterine endometrium for implantation
 b. the differentiation factor for the ovaries
 c. cellular phenotypic expressions
 d. glycogen levels in the homeostatic range
 e. genotypic expressions in embryonic cells

186. *Monoamine oxidase catalyzes:*

 a. oxidative deamination of peptides to aldehydes
 b. conversion of choline to acetylcholine
 c. oxidative deamination of amines, whether or not they have been subjected to alteration by the methyltransferase reaction
 d. conversion of NADPH to NADP
 e. reduction of peroxides after the action of methyltransferase of the eye

187. *The lens of the eye contains the enzyme:*

 a. galactose reductase
 b. aldose dehydrogenase
 c. sorbitol transferase
 d. transketo carboxylase
 e. ornithine oxidase

188. *Troponin complex consists of 3 dissimilar subunits. One of the subunits (Tn-C) binds calcium, which:*

 a. alters the conformation of tropomyosin, resulting in exposure of actin-myosin binding sites
 b. combines with Tn-T and induces muscle contraction
 c. inhibits free myosin
 d. combines with Tn-A and promotes muscle relaxation
 e. binds with actin-myosin sites and promotes muscle relaxation

189. *Platelet aggregation:*

 a. is initiated at the site of an injury by conversion of prothrombin to thrombin
 b. is inhibited in uninjured blood vessels by secretion of prostacyclin by intact vascular endothelium
 c. induces release of serotonin
 d. is facilitated by release of ADP and thromboxane A_2
 e. is inhibited in bone marrow by fibrinase production in megakaryocytes

190. *Functions of cytochrome P450 include all of the following* **except**:

 a. synthesis of steroid hormones
 b. conversion of some chemicals to mutagens
 c. hydroxylation of amino acids
 d. inactivation of some hydrophobic drugs
 e. metabolism of fatty acid derivatives

191. *Induction of cytochrome P450:*

 a. occurs only by endogenous compounds
 b. occurs only at the transcriptional level
 c. may occur by posttranscriptional processes
 d. necessitates formation of an inducer-receptor protein complex
 e. initiates an irreversible cascade of cellular energy depletion

Correct answers are on pages 23-26.

192. Concerning metabolism of aminolevulinic acid, which statement is most accurate?

a. In acute intermittent porphyria, activity of aminolevulinic acid synthetase decreases.
b. In variegate porphyria, activity of aminolevulinic acid synthetase decreases.
c. In lead poisoning, activity of aminolevulinic acid synthetase decreases.
d. Decarboxylation of aminolevulinic acid results in porphoblingenuria.
e. Aminolevulinic acid is unrelated to porphyria.

193. The increase in acidity of hemoglobin as it binds to O_2 is known as:

a. the Bohr effect
b. allosteric equilibrium
c. the acidemic shift
d. the heterotrophic effect
e. the Hill coefficient

194. The primary result of consumption of excessive protein, beyond the body's immediate needs, is:

a. excretion of the excess protein in the urine
b. increased storage pool of protein
c. increased synthesis of muscle protein
d. increased levels of plasma proteins
e. increased adipose tissue

195. Which dietary regimen most effectively reduces serum cholesterol levels?

a. restrict dietary proteins
b. increase the ratio of dietary polyunsaturated to saturated fatty acids
c. decrease dietary fiber content
d. restrict dietary energy
e. increase the ratio of dietary fat to fiber

196. The major function of the pancreas in digestion and nutrient absorption in the bowels is elaboration of:

a. bicarbonate and enzymes for intraluminal digestion
b. bile acids
c. hormones that facilitate absorption of electrolytes
d. insulin
e. hydrochloric acid to catabolize ingesta

197. Pancreatic secretions are especially rich in the proenzyme for:

a. phospholipase C
b. phospholipase A_2
c. phosphatidyl choline
d. phospholipase D
e. phosphatidyl alanine

198. Basal metabolic rate is defined as the:

a. rate of energy utilization during exercise
b. rate of energy utilization in the resting state
c. rate at which protein is metabolized
d. rate at which energy is produced in maintenance of homeostasis during exercise
e. rate at which calories are released from carbohydrates

199. Kwashiorkor is:

a. a disease caused by inadequate intake of protein in the presence of adequate energy intake
b. the most common form of protein-calorie malnutrition in tropical areas
c. a deficiency of essential amino acids despite intake of sufficient amounts of protein
d. the most common form of biotin deficiency
e. a common manifestation of intestinal malabsorption

200. Deposition of excessive iron in tissues characterizes a condition called:

a. hemochromatosis
b. hypertransferrinosis
c. Menke's syndrome
d. Wilson's disease
e. ferratosis pigmentum

Answers

1. **e** Gentle disruption of cells does not destroy mitochondria, nuclei, peroxisomes or lysosomes. However, when the endoplasmic reticulum is disrupted, it forms small vesicles called microsomes.

2. **c**

3. **c**

4. **d** The quaternary structure is stabilized exclusively by noncovalent interaction. Disulfide bonds are covalent.

5. **d** Ion-exchange chromatography and isoelectric focusing separate proteins on the basis of charge. Polyacrylamide gel is used for electrophoresis to separate proteins according to size in the presence of sodium dodecyl sulfate, not for density gradient.

6. **d**

7. **c**

8. **c** The modification of prothrombin and factors VII, IX and X to form the glutamic acid residues occurs during synthesis by a carboxylase enzyme located on the luminal side of the rough endoplasmic reticulum. Vitamin K is an essential cofactor for this carboxylase enzyme.

9. **b**

10. **b**

11. **e** Competitive inhibitors are often toxic to animals.

12. **a**

13. **e** Covalent catalysis involves a covalent bond between an enzyme and a portion of the substrate.

14. **d**

15. **a** Membrane channels are quite specific. Voltage-gated channels are controlled by a change in the transmembrane potential, but nicotinic acetylcholine channels are chemically regulated.

16. **b** Na^+-K^+ ATPase regulates Na^+-K^+ transport. It is an antiport, vectorial (Na^+-out), electrogenic system and does not require cAMP.

17. **a** Rotenone inhibits at site I, preventing all electron flow and all ATP synthesis from NADH. Succinate feeds electrons at site II, and thus is not affected.

18. **d** Cyanide inhibits electron transport at site III, blocking electron flow and ATP synthesis. Subsequent addition of an uncoupler activates ATPase to hydrolyze ATP unless it is inhibited by a phosphorylase inhibitor, such as oligomycin.

19. **c** Alpha-ketoglutarate can be formed from glutamate.

20. **e**

21. **c**

22. **b** Xanthine oxidase makes both hydrogen peroxide and superoxide radicals. Superoxide dismutase removes superoxide radicals, and catalase and glutathione peroxidase removes hydrogen peroxide. Ascorbate (vitamin C) removes superoxide radicals.

23. **e**

24. **b**

25. **a**

26. **d**

27. **d** This disorder is associated with a very severe or complete deficiency of HGPRTase activity (adenine + PRPP → AMP + PP). The gene for HGPRTase is on the X chromosome; hence, the deficiency is virtually limited to males.

28. **b** These glycosides are some of the most active Na^+-K^+ ATPase inhibitors.

29. **b**

30. **b** Hexokinase and phosphofructokinase use ATP. Both reactions are irreversible, whereas phosphoglycerate kinase synthesizes ATP and the reaction is reversible.

31. **d** Malate dyhydrogenase uses NAD^+ and malate to generate NADH and oxaloacetate.

32. **a**

33. **b**

34. **b**

35. **b** Epinephrine affects glycogenolysis in both muscle and liver. Glucagon can selectively mobilize glucose from hepatic glycogen stores without depleting muscle glycogen.

36. **e** cAMP protein kinase phosphorylates proteins. Phosphorylation converts glycogen phosphorylase, phosphorylase kinase and phosphatase inhibitor-1 from their inactive phosphorylase form to their active phosphoprotein phosphatase form. Simultaneously, it converts glucogen synthetase from its active form to its inactive phosphorylase form. The phosphoprotein phosphatase form has opposite effects.

37. **b** Glucocorticoids act via nuclear events that lead to increased enzyme protein synthesis. Glucagon converts an inactive form of an already-synthesized enzyme into the active form. Glucagon is synthesized and stored in vesicles and, therefore, can be immediately released. Glucocorticoids are synthesized upon demand.

38. **c** A high glucagon/insulin ratio results in cAMP-mediated phosphorylation that activates hormone-sensitive lipase and inhibits acetyl CoA carboxylase. This leads to increased ketone body production in mitochondria by greatly increased acetyl CoA production, thereby ensuring efficient uptake and utilization by the brain.

39. **e**

40. **b** Triacylglycerols are neutral, hydrophobic molecules with no hydrophilic portion. They are not good emulsifying agents and are stored anhydrously. They are more energy rich than carbohydrates.

41. **a**

42. **e**

43. **a**

44. **b**

45. **c**

46. **c**

47. **c**

48. **d**

49. **a**

50. **b**

51. **a**

52. **e**

53. **b**

54. **e**

55. **e**

56. **a**

57. **e** Collagen contains about 25% of amino acids as proline or hydroxyproline.

58. **e** Disulfide bonds are covalent.

59. **d**

60. **b**

61. **a**

62. **a**

63. **b**

64. **d**

65. **a**

66. **c**

67. **e**

68. **b**

69. **a**

70. **c**

71. **e**

72. **b**

73. **e**

74. **d**

75. **b**

76. **e**

77. **c**

78. **b**

79. **e**

80. **a**

81. **b**

82. **c**

83. **a**

84. **b**

85. **b**

86. **e**

87. **e**

88. **c**

89. **d**

90. **a**

91. **c**

92. **d**

93. **a**
94. **b**
95. **c**
96. **e**
97. **b**
98. **b**
99. **c**
100. **a**
101. **b**
102. **b** Bacterial cells use one type of RNA polymerase to transcribe all classes of RNA, whereas eukaryotic cells use 3 different types of RNA polymerase for mRNA, tRNA and rRNA synthesis.
103. **d**
104. **c**
105. **b**
106. **b**
107. **c**
108. **a**
109. **b**
110. **a**
111. **a**
112. **c**
113. **c**
114. **b**
115. **a**
116. **b**
117. **d**
118. **d**
119. **b**
120. **b**
121. **b**
122. **a**
123. **e**
124. **c**
125. **b**
126. **b**
127. **c**
128. **e**
129. **d**
130. **a**
131. **c**
132. **c**
133. **c**
134. **d**
135. **e**
136. **e**
137. **c**
138. **b**
139. **b**
140. **c**
141. **b**
142. **a**
143. **e**
144. **d**
145. **e**
146. **b**
147. **a**
148. **c**
149. **d**
150. **e**
151. **d**
152. **e**
153. **d**
154. **c**
155. **c**
156. **c**
157. **a**
158. **d**
159. **a**
160. **c**
161. **a**
162. **b**
163. **c**
164. **c**
165. **a**
166. **e**
167. **b**
168. **d**
169. **b**
170. **e**
171. **d**
172. **e**
173. **c**

174. **a**	188. **a**
175. **b**	189. **d**
176. **c**	190. **c**
177. **a**	191. **c**
178. **c**	192. **c**
179. **a**	193. **a**
180. **a**	194. **e**
181. **d**	195. **b**
182. **c**	196. **a**
183. **a**	197. **b**
184. **b**	198. **b**
185. **a**	199. **a**
186. **c**	200. **a**
187. **b**	

Notes

Embryology

A. de Lahunta

Recommended Reading

Noden DM and de Lahunta A: *The Embryology of Domestic Animals: Developmental Mechanisms and Malformations*. Williams & Wilkins, Baltimore, 1985.

> ***Practice answer sheet is on page 253.***

Questions

1. *A recent paper described a left cranial vena cava in a 25-year-old Arabian mare that was being dissected by veterinary students in a gross anatomy laboratory. Where would you expect this vessel to enter the heart?*

   a. through the left atrium
   b. at the normal site of the right cranial vena cava
   c. ventral to the opening of the caudal vena cava
   d. with the right azygos vein
   e. through the tip of the right auricle

2. *Surgical examination of a bilaterally cryptorchid Miniature Schnauzer with an otherwise normal male phenotype and a karyogram of 100% 78XY lymphocytes (normal: 76 autosomes) reveals a completely developed uterus, with uterine tubes adjacent to the epididymis and ductus deferens. What would explain this duct system?*

   a. insufficient testosterone
   b. interstitial-cell hypertrophy
   c. inadequate paramesonephric duct-inhibiting substance
   d. unrecognized gonadal 78XX cells
   e. lack of 5-alpha reductase receptors

3. *The nucleus pulposus of intervertebral disks is a remnant of the embryonic:*

   a. sclerotomes
   b. notochord
   c. primitive node
   d. primitive streak
   e. perichordal mesenchyme

Correct answers are on pages 30-32.

4. *If the inherited abnormality that results from breedings to produce the "new look" Eastern type of Burmese cat is due to a disturbance in the prosencephalon and/or its associated neural crest, which change would **not** be expected?*

    a. meningoencephalocele
    b. brachygnathia
    c. microphthalmos
    d. atlantooccipital malformation
    e. duplicated maxillary processes

5. *A 3-year-old female Morgan horse with increased respiratory effort during stress or exercise was small at birth and grew poorly. The horse is in poor physical condition, and has increased heart and respiratory rates. Auscultation reveals a prominent systolic murmur over the left cranioventral thorax, with a palpable thrill at that site. Mild exercise provokes respiratory distress and cyanosis of the oral mucosa. Which primary lesion would be the most likely cause of these signs?*

    a. valvular pulmonic stenosis
    b. tetralogy of Fallot
    c. left atrioventricular valve dysplasia
    d. left to right shunting patent ductus arteriosus
    e. subvalvular aortic stenosis

6. *Which of the following would **not** be expected to be related to the inherited abnormalities that result from the breeding that produces Manx cats?*

    a. acaudatus
    b. failure of urorectal septal development
    c. meningomyelocele
    d. spina bifida
    e. omphalocele

7. *Which embryonic structure is **not** involved in the condition of anodontia?*

    a. pharyngeal arch 1
    b. labiogingival lamina
    c. neural crest
    d. enamel organ
    e. pharyngeal pouch 1

8. *Which structures are found in the fetal median ligament of the bladder?*

    a. urachus and umbilical veins
    b. yolk sac and vitelline vessels
    c. yolk sac and umbilical veins
    d. urachus and umbilical arteries
    e. urachus and vitelline vessels

9. *What is the fate of the visceral layer of the vaginal process that surrounds the extra-abdominal gubernaculum proper in males before descent of the testis?*

    a. it becomes the visceral layer of peritoneum on the testis
    b. it is incorporated in the ligament of the tail of the epididymis
    c. it becomes the mesoductus deferens
    d. it is incorporated in the proper ligament of the testis
    e. it becomes the mesorchium

10. *Mesodiverticula, umbilical fistulas and ileal diverticula represent:*

    a. abnormal development of the allantoic and vitelline vessels
    b. abnormal development of the allantoic and umbilical arteries
    c. abnormal development of the yolk sac and umbilical veins
    d. abnormal development of the yolk sac and vitelline vessels
    e. abnormal rotation of the embryonic intestinal loop

11. *In female embryos, the urogenital sinus contributes to all of the following **except** the:*

    a. cervix
    b. vagina
    c. urethra
    d. bladder
    e. vestibule

12. *A cranial cervical swelling could be caused by any of the following **except**:*

    a. craniopharyngioma

b. salivary mucocele

c. abscess

d. pharyngeal (branchial) cyst

e. thyroid cyst

13. *Improper development of the nasolacrimal duct relates to faulty development of the:*

a. medial and lateral palatine processes

b. nasolateral and nasomedial processes

c. choanae

d. maxillary process and nasolateral process

e. lens placode and optic cup

14. *The left recurrent laryngeal nerve is found caudal to the ligamentum arteriosum on the left, but the right recurrent laryngeal nerve is found caudal to the right subclavian artery because of:*

a. loss of connection of the right 6th aortic arch to the dorsal aortic root

b. loss of the dorsal aortic root between the right 3rd and 4th aortic arches

c. the origin of the aorta from the left 4th aortic arch

d. loss of the right distal (caudal) dorsal aortic root at its attachment to the single descending dorsal aorta

e. migration of the left 7th dorsal cervical intersegmental artery cranially on the left dorsal aortic root

15. *Based on developmental relationships, which of the following is most likely to be found in the spermatic cord near the testis in the scrotum of a stallion?*

a. prostate gland

b. adrenal cortex

c. bulbourethral gland

d. pancreatic exocrine tissue

e. gallbladder mucosal epithelium

16. *The muscles of the tongue are derived from the:*

a. neural crest

b. most rostral somitomeres

c. occipital myotomes

d. 1st pharyngeal arch mesoderm

e. mesoderm of the first 3 pharyngeal arches

17. *At birth of a foal, 2 membranes are associated with the umbilical cord. The one attached to the cord near the foal and that formerly covered the fetus in the uterus is composed of:*

a. amnion internally (next to the fetus) and yolk sac externally

b. amnion internally and chorion externally

c. allantois internally and chorion externally

d. allantois internally and amnion externally

e. amnion internally and allantois externally

18. *Phocomelia is:*

a. synonymous with micromelia

b. an abnormality of the spinal cord

c. a depression in the sternum

d. absence of part of a limb

e. a multiple fusion of digits

19. *The embryonic ventral hepatic diverticulum gives rise to the:*

a. left lobe of the pancreas

b. cystic duct

c. liver sinusoids

d. minor duodenal papilla

e. spleen

20. *Throughout fetal development, oxygen saturation is higher in the left ventricle than in the right ventricle because the:*

a. ductus arteriosus carries oxygenated blood to the aorta

b. pulmonary veins return oxygenated blood to the left atrium

c. right ventricular blood mixes with left ventricular blood via the interventricular foramen

d. caudal vena caval blood enters the left atrium via the foramen ovale

e. cranial vena caval blood enters the left atrium

Correct answers are on pages 30-32.

21. *At 9 months of age, a dog begins to have episodes of collapse in the pelvic limbs, with occasional cyanosis and syncope following severe exercise. There is no obvious cardiac murmur. The most likely cause of these signs is:*

   a. tetralogy of Fallot
   b. pulmonic stenosis
   c. patent ductus arteriosus, with reverse flow
   d. persistent right 4th aortic arch
   e. persistent foramen secundum

22. *Peritoneopericardial communication has its genesis in:*

   a. failed closure of the embryonic peritoneopericardial orifice
   b. failed development of pleuroperitoneal membranes
   c. failed development of pleuropericardial membranes
   d. improper development of the liver and septum transversum
   e. retarded growth of the lungs into the lateral body wall

23. *Concerning salivary mucoceles and pharyngeal (branchial) cysts, which statement is **least** accurate?*

   a. Both can be located in the cranial neck region.
   b. Salivary mucoceles lack an epithelial lining.
   c. Pharyngeal cysts contain fluid with the consistency of saliva.
   d. Both refill if the fluid is drained off.
   e. Sialography shows radiopaque dye in a pharyngeal cyst.

24. *Hepatic encephalopathy has been reported in dogs with various malformations of the portal vein, caudal vena cava and azygos vein. Which of the following would **not** be implicated in these malformations?*

   a. vitelline vein
   b. subcardinal vein
   c. cranial cardinal vein
   d. supracardinal vein
   e. umbilical vein

25. *In development of the interatrial septum, the septum secundum forms:*

   a. the foramen ovale, directed at the cranial vena cava
   b. a valve-like structure to the left of the septum primum
   c. craniocaudally on the right side of the septum primum
   d. simultaneously with the atrioventricular endocardial cushions and closure of the atrioventricular canal
   e. a foramen secundum in its dorsal wall

Answers

1. **c** One would expect it to enter ventral to the opening of the caudal vena cava, in common with the cardiac venous drainage, which is the remnant of the left common and cranial cardinal veins.

2. **c** Inadequate paramesonephric duct-inhibiting substance accounts for persistence of a uterus with uterine tubes. The testis-determining factor on the Y chromosome accounts for the male gonads, with testosterone being produced by the interstitial cells to form the male duct system and male external genitalia via their 5-alpha reductase receptors. Cryptorchidism follows insufficient testicular secretions.

3. **b** Notochord. Perichordal mesenchyme forms the anulus fibrosus and vertebral body.

4. **d** Atlantooccipital malformation. These bones are derived from the occipital and cranial cervical somites.

---

5. **b** Tetralogy of Fallot. The pulmonic stenosis accounts for the systolic murmur in the left cranial thorax. This prevents normal oxygenation. The persistent interventricular septal defect and dextroaorta permit shunting of unoxygenated blood into the systemic circulation, causing cyanosis.

6. **e** Omphalocele, which is a defect in closure of the body wall at the site of the amnion in which abdominal organs protrude and are covered by amnion. The characteristics of Manx cats relate to inheritance of absent tail vertebrae and the derivatives of the caudal aspect of the primitive streak (neural tube, hind gut).

7 **e** Pharyngeal pouch 1 is an endoderm-lined evagination of the pharynx that forms the auditory tube and middle ear. Anodontia is a lack of teeth, which normally develop from pharyngeal and oral ectoderm (labiogingival lamina, enamel organs) and related neural crest mesenchyme.

8. **d** The urachus and umbilical arteries course through the fetal ventral mesentery, which becomes the median ligament of the bladder. The umbilical vein courses cranially in the falciform ligament. In the fetus, the yolk sac and vitelline vessels attach to the small intestine.

9. **b** It is incorporated in the ligament of the tail of the epididymis. The testis descends with its covering of visceral peritoneum that formed at its site of development. The gubernaculum regresses into 2 ligaments. The cranial, intraabdominal part forms the proper ligament of the testis. The extraabdominal part forms the ligament of the tail of the epididymis.

10. **d** The yolk sac and its vitelline vasculature connect with the endodermal gut tube and its dorsal mesentery at the site of the beginning of the ileum.

11. **a** The cervix is formed from the paramesonephric (Mullerian) duct. The vagina is considered to be derived from both this duct and the urogenital sinus.

12. **a** Craniopharyngiomas are derived from abnormal differentiation of the hypophyseal (Rathke's) pouch and are found intracranially at the site of the pituitary gland.

13. **d** Where the maxillary process and the nasolateral process are adjacent, a cord of ectodermal cells becomes buried in the mesenchyme and then hollows out to form the nasolacrimal duct.

14. **a** Loss of connection of the right 6th aortic arch to the dorsal aortic root allows the right recurrent laryngeal nerve to move cranially to the right 4th aortic arch as no 5th arch develops. The right 4th aortic arch becomes the origin of the right subclavian artery.

15. **b** Adrenocortical tissue is derived from intermediate mesoderm cranial to the mesonephros and the site of gonad development.

16. **c** Occipital myotomes are the origin of the tongue muscles that migrate rostrally into the swellings on the floor of the pharynx.

17. **e** Amnion internally and allantois externally form the membrane closest to the fetus that contains amniotic fluid.

18. **d** Usually this refers to absence of the proximal components of a limb, leaving the short distal components attached to the body and forming a flipper-like appendage (*phoco*=seal, *melia*=limb).

19. **b** Cystic duct is derived from the ventral hepatic diverticulum, which arises from the duodenum at the major papilla. The bile duct, hepatic ducts, hepatocytes, gallbladder and right lobe of the pancreas are also derived from it.

20. **d** Caudal vena caval blood enters the left atrium via the foramen ovale and carries oxygenated blood that entered it via the ductus venosus and umbilical vein.

21. **c** Patent ductus arteriosus with reverse flow allows unoxygenated pulmonary arterial blood to enter the systemic circulation caudal to the aortic vessels that supply the forelimbs, head and neck (brachiocephalic trunk and subclavian arteries). This results in unoxygenated blood circulating initially to the more caudal trunk and pelvic limbs. The usual patent ductus arteriosus carries blood from the higher-pressure systemic circulation (aorta) to the lower-pressure pulmonic circulation. This is reversed under conditions of pulmonary hypertension.

22. **d** Improper development of the liver and septum transversum causes a secondary defect that results in communication between the pericardial and peritoneal cavities. There is never a normal communication here, as between the pleural and peritoneal cavities.

23. **e** Lack of an epithelial lining in the mucocele distinguishes it from a pharyngeal cyst, in which the epithelial lining is the source of the saliva-like secretion. Sialography shows a leak in the salivary duct system involved in producing a mucocele but not a pharyngeal cyst.

24. **c** The cranial cardinal vein gives rise to the venous drainage of the head, neck, thoracic limbs and heart. All of the others listed are involved in forming the portal vein, caudal vena cava and/or azygos vein.

25. **c** The septum secundum's caudal margin demarcates the foramen ovale and is directed at the caudal vena cava like a baffle that directs about 60% of the caudal vena caval blood (most oxygenated) into the tube-like channel between the 2 septa and into the left atrium via the foramen secundum.

Notes

Gross Anatomy

Recommended Reading

Adams DR: *Canine Anatomy*. Iowa State University Press, Ames, 1986.

Baumel JJ *et al: Nomina Anatomica Avium*. Academic Press, New York, 1979.

Constantinescu GM: *Clinical Dissection Guide for Large Animals*. Mosby Year Book, St. Louis, 1991.

Cooper JE and Jackson OF: *Diseases of the Reptilia*. Academic Press, New York, 1981.

de Lahunta A and Habel RE: *Applied Veterinary Anatomy*. Saunders, Philadelphia, 1986.

Dyce KM *et al: Textbook of Veterinary Anatomy*. Saunders, Philadelphia, 1987.

Dyce KM and Wensing CJG: *Essentials of Bovine Anatomy*. Lea & Febiger, Philadelphia, 1971.

Evans HE and Christensen GC: *Miller's Anatomy of the Dog*. 2nd ed. Saunders, Philadelphia, 1979.

Frye FL: *Biomedical and Surgical Aspects of Captive Reptile Husbandry*. 2nd ed. Krieger Publishing, Melbourne, FL, 1991.

Getty R: *Sisson and Grossman's Anatomy of the Domestic Animals*. Saunders, Philadelphia, 1975.

Harrison GJ and Harrison LR: *Clinical Avian Medicine and Surgery*. Saunders, Philadelphia, 1986.

Jennings PB: *The Practice of Large Animal Surgery*. Saunders, Philadelphia, 1984.

King AS and McLelland J: *Form and Function in Birds*. Academic Press, New York, 1979.

King AS and McLelland J: *Outlines of Avian Anatomy*. Bailliere Tindall, London, 1975.

Marcus LC: *Veterinary Biology and Medicine of Captive Amphibians and Reptiles*. Lea & Febiger, Philadelphia, 1981.

Nickel R *et al: Anatomy of Domestic Birds*. Verlag Paul Parey, Berlin, 1977.

Nickel R *et al: The Viscera of the Domestic Mammals*. 2nd ed. Verlag Paul Parey, Berlin, 1979.

Nickel R *et al: The Anatomy of the Domestic Animals*. Vol 1. Verlag Paul Parey, Berlin, 1986.

Petrak ML: *Diseases of Cage and Aviary Birds*. 2nd ed. Lea & Febiger, Philadelphia, 1982.

Sack WO: *Essentials of Pig Anatomy*. Veterinary Textbooks, Ithaca, NY, 1982.

Sack WO: *Rooney's Guide to the Dissection of the Horse*. 6th ed. Veterinary Textbooks, Ithaca, NY, 1991.

Smallwood JE: *A Guided Tour of Veterinary Anatomy*. Saunders, Philadelphia, 1992.

Stashak TS: *Adams' Lameness in Horses*. 4th ed. Lea & Febiger, Philadelphia, 1987.

Practice answer sheets are on pages 255-257.

Correct answers are on pages 89-99.

Dogs and Cats

D.R. Adams

Questions

1. A complete fracture of a tuber calcaneus (with separation of the tuber frum the remainder of the calcaneus) would most greatly impair an animal's ability to:

   a. flex the digits
   b. flex the hock
   c. extend the digits
   d. extend the hock
   e. extend the stifle

2. Upon observing in a standing dog that the vertebral border of the right scapula projects dorsally above the tips of the spinous processes of the thoracic vertebrae, you might most correctly suspect a:

   a. rupture of the subscapular muscle
   b. fracture of the neck of the scapula
   c. paralysis of the trapezius muscle
   d. rupture of the serratus ventralis muscle
   e. paralysis of the supraspinatus muscle

3. The primary combined action of the internal obturator, external obturator and gemellus muscles is to:

   a. flex the hip
   b. extend the hip
   c. abduct the pelvic limb
   d. adduct the pelvic limb
   e. rotate the pelvic limb

4. The primary action of the triceps brachii is to:

   a. flex the shoulder
   b. extend the shoulder
   c. flex the elbow
   d. extend the elbow
   e. abduct the thoracic limb

5. The paired muscle that opens the jaw is the:

   a. buccinator
   b. masseter
   c. digastricus
   d. temporalis
   e. medial pterygoid

6. A pin placed in the calcaneus to stabilize the tuber calcanei would most likely pass through tendons of the:

   a. gastrocnemius and superficial digital flexor
   b. gastrocnemius and deep digital flexor
   c. superficial and deep digital flexors
   d. anconeus and popliteus
   e. cranial tibial and fibularis longus

7. Transecting the patellar ligament, parapatellar retinacula, and fascia lata of the right pelvic limb would most likely result in:

   a. overextension of the right stifle joint
   b. hyperflexion of the hip joint
   c. cranial drawer movement of the stifle joint
   d. caudal drawer movement of the stifle joint
   e. increased tension on the long digital extensor tendon

8. To inject a drug into the stifle joint of a dog, such that the injected solution would enter the synovial space between patella and femur, femur and tibia, and tibia and proximal fibula (without having to diffuse through synovial membranes), what is the minimum number of injections that could be given?

   a. 1
   b. 2
   c. 3

d. 4

e. 5

9. *The muscle that most completely covers the distolateral surface of the femur is the:*

   a. gastrocnemius
   b. vastus lateralis
   c. biceps femoris
   d. tensor fasciae latae
   e. adductor

10. *The cranial preputial muscle is a partially isolated portion of the:*

   a. external abdominal oblique
   b. internal abdominal oblique
   c. transversus abdominis
   d. rectus abdominis
   e. cutaneus trunci

11. *Most growth in height of a young dog occurs in the distal portion of the humerus and femur. This growth occurs in the:*

   a. physes
   b. metaphyses
   c. diaphyses
   d. articular cartilages
   e. primary ossification centers

12. *Accommodation for near and far vision is accomplished by contraction or relaxation of muscles in the:*

   a. ciliary body
   b. conjunctiva
   c. iris
   d. limbus
   e. retina

13. *The muscle most closely in contact with the ventral surface of cervical vertebrae and intervertebral disks is the:*

   a. sternohyoideus
   b. sternothyroideus
   c. sternocephalicus

d. longus colli

e. longus capitis

14. *The cervical vertebra with large ventrolaterally projecting transverse processes, each subdivided into 2 projections, is the:*

   a. first cervical vertebra
   b. second cervical vertebra
   c. third cervical vertebra
   d. sixth cervical vertebra
   e. seventh cervical vertebra

15. *Concerning the stifle joint, which statement is **least** accurate?*

   a. The medial meniscus and medial collateral ligament are in contact with each other.
   b. The tibial attachment of the cranial cruciate ligament is cranial to that of the caudal cruciate ligament.
   c. The patella is attached to right and left fabellae by connective tissue.
   d. The popliteal tendon of origin crosses the deep surface of the lateral collateral ligament.
   e. The tendon of origin of the deep digital flexor is attached to the distal end of the femur.

16. *The portion of the mandible that articulates with the temporal bone is the:*

   a. retroarticular process
   b. coronoid process
   c. angle
   d. condylar process
   e. zygomatic process

17. *From a lateral approach, separation of which 2 muscles from each other would expose the lateral surface of the femoral bone?*

   a. triceps surae and semitendinosus
   b. semitendinosus and biceps femoris
   c. biceps femoris and vastus lateralis
   d. vastus lateralis and sartorius
   e. semimembranosus and adductor

Correct answers are on pages 89-99.

Dogs and Cats, continued

18. *When removing the entire distal phalanx of each digit during declawing of cats, you sever the tendons of insertion of the:*

    a. gastrocnemius and deep digital flexor muscles

    b. superficial and deep digital flexor muscles

    c. cranial tibial and long digital extensor muscles

    d. deep digital flexor and long digital extensor muscles

    e. superficial digital flexor and long digital extensor muscles

19. *Which condition would most likely result in "sinking" of the right carpal pad toward the floor surface when the limb supports weight?*

    a. detached lateral epicondyle of the humerus

    b. torn common digital extensor tendons

    c. stretched biceps brachii tendon

    d. separated transverse humeral ligament

    e. fractured accessory carpal bone

20. *Which muscle of dogs does **not** normally have a sesamoid bone associated with its tendon?*

    a. popliteus

    b. long abductor of the first digit

    c. superficial digital flexor

    d. cranial tibial

    e. gastrocnemius

21. *A needle passed into the shoulder joint from a lateral approach would most likely pass through the:*

    a. subscapularis muscle

    b. lateral head of the triceps brachii muscle

    c. deltoideus muscle

    d. omotransversarius muscle

    e. brachialis muscle

22. *Concerning the anatomic structure and function of the limbs, which statement is **least** accurate?*

    a. The deep digital flexor in the pelvic limb is also an extensor of the tarsus.

    b. The superficial digital flexor in the thoracic limb is also a flexor of the carpus.

    c. The long digital extensor also provides some stability to the stifle joint.

    d. The triceps brachii also flexes the shoulder joint.

    e. The gastrocnemius also flexes the digits.

23. *The tendon of the infraspinatus muscle may be best revealed by detaching and retracting the tendon of insertion of which muscle?*

    a. supraspinatus

    b. subscapularis

    c. teres minor

    d. triceps brachii

    e. deltoideus

24. *To most completely reveal the dorsal aspect of the hip joint, which muscle must be detached and its tendon of insertion retracted?*

    a. tensor fasciae latae

    b. internal obturator

    c. external obturator

    d. biceps femoris

    e. deep gluteal

25. *If the common calcanean tendon of an animal is torn (separated), the animal loses most of its ability to:*

    a. extend the stifle

    b. extend the hip

    c. extend the hock

    d. flex the hock

    e. flex the digits

26. *Removing the anconeus muscle would most expose the:*

    a. tendon of the biceps brachii muscle

    b. medial collateral ligament of the elbow

    c. lateral collateral ligament of the elbow

    d. caudolateral aspect of the elbow

    e. supinator muscle

27. *Movement of the proximal portion of the tibia caudally, relative to the femur, is an indication of a torn:*

    a. long digital extensor
    b. popliteus
    c. cranial cruciate ligament
    d. caudal cruciate ligament
    e. collateral ligament

28. *If the distal physis of the ulna is destroyed in a 6-month-old dog,:*

    a. the antebrachium of the limb would cease to lengthen
    b. the distal end of the limb (manus) would deviate medially
    c. the distal end of the limb (manus) would deviate laterally
    d. the limb would continue to lengthen at the same rate as the unaffected liimb
    e. lengthening of the antebrachium would be unaffected, as the limb is mature by this age

29. *In the midcervical region, lateral reflection of the left sternohyoideus muscle would most reveal the adjacent but deeper:*

    a. trachea
    b. esophagus
    c. left common carotid artery
    d. left sternocephalicus muscle
    e. left sternothyroideus muscle

30. *Double dewclaws are a desirable trait in which dog breed?*

    a. German Shepherd
    b. Boston Terrier
    c. Collie
    d. Briard
    e. Golden Retriever

31. *The ligamentum nuchae:*

    a. assists in extension of the cervical vertebrae
    b. is present in cats
    c. attaches to the nuchal crest of the skull in dogs
    d. arises, in dogs and cats, from the last 5 cervical and first thoracic vertebrae
    e. is in contact, in dogs and cats, with all cervical vertebrae

32. *Which bone or portion of bone in the thoracic limb is **least** stressed by the weight of the animal during the support phase of locomotion?*

    a. ulna
    b. lateral humeral epicondyle
    c. radius
    d. radial carpal bone
    e. humeral diaphysis

33. *An intervertebral disk is **least** likely to rupture:*

    a. dorsally
    b. between vertebrae in the 11th thoracic to 4th lumbar area
    c. where it contacts an intercapital ligament
    d. into the vertebral canal
    e. at vertebral levels with adjacent longus colli muscles

34. *Section through the vertebral arch and removal of the lamina of the most cranial lumbar vertebra requires detachment and retraction of the:*

    a. multifidus
    b. iliocostalis
    c. longissimus
    d. rhomboideus
    e. serratus dorsalis

35. *Which structure does **not** cross the stifle articulation from the femur to the crus?*

    a. tendon of the long digital extensor
    b. cranial cruciate ligament
    c. caudal cruciate ligament
    d. lateral collateral ligament
    e. meniscofemoral ligament

Correct answers are on pages 89-99.

Dogs and Cats, continued

36. *Which joint has the **least** developed collateral ligaments?*

    a. shoulder
    b. elbow
    c. antebrachiocarpal joint
    d. stifle
    e. proximal interphalangeal joint

37. *Tearing and separation of the tendon of insertion of which muscle would most impair an animal's ability to stand on the affected limb?*

    a. biceps brachii
    b. common digital extensor
    c. deep digital flexor
    d. gastrocnemius
    e. quadriceps femoris

38. *The patella normally is:*

    a. within the tendon of the gastrocnemius muscle
    b. within the tendon of the cranial tibial muscle
    c. attached to the medial meniscus
    d. attached to the lateral meniscus
    e. positioned proximal to the femorotibial joint space

39. *A standing dog that lifts its left foreleg to lick the metacarpal pad would **least** likely have near-maximal contraction of its:*

    a. right triceps brachii
    b. left pronator teres
    c. left deep digital flexor
    d. left biceps brachii
    e. left suppinator

40. *Reflection of the tensor fasciae latae and sartorius cranially, middle and deep gluteus dorsally, and vastus lateralis distocaudally would reveal the:*

    a. long adductor muscle
    b. cranial surface of the hip joint capsule
    c. pectineus muscle

    d. femoral triangle
    e. internal obturator

41. *A deep laceration directed dorsoventrally across the zygomatic and masseteric regions of the head would most likely damage the:*

    a. nasolacrimal duct
    b. parotid salivary duct
    c. mandibular salivary duct
    d. monostomatic sublingual salivary duct
    e. zygomatic salivary duct

42. *The duodenocolic fold connects mesentery of which structures?*

    a. ascending duodenum and ascending colon
    b. ascending duodenum and descending colon
    c. descending duodenum and ascending colon
    d. descending duodenum and descending colon
    e. caudal duodenal flexure and transverse colon

43. *An incision through the skin and superficial fascia over the ventral portion of the 11th intercostal space would first reveal which subcutaneous skeletal muscle?*

    a. thoracic diaphragm
    b. latissimus dorsi
    c. quadratus lumborum
    d. external abdominal oblique
    e. external intercostal

44. *Which structures are **not** normally adjacent to each other?*

    a. caudate process of the caudate liver lobe and right kidney
    b. papillary process of the caudate liver lobe and lesser curvature of the stomach
    c. prostate gland and urethra
    d. left lobe of the pancreas and caudal duodenal flexure
    e. caudal margin of the greater omentum and dorsal surface of the urinary bladder

45. *Which structure is normally located in the right half of a dog's body?*

a. descending duodenum
b. descending colon
c. spleen
d. gastric fundus
e. mid-cervical portion of the esophagus

a. rectococcygeus
b. coccygeus
c. levator ani
d. external anal sphincter
e. superficial gluteus

46. *In a normal dog or cat, an incision through the ventral abdominal wall into the peritoneal cavity, between the umbilicus and urinary bladder, would first reveal the:*

a. jejunum
b. descending colon
c. ureter
d. greater omentum
e. transverse colon

47. *If you make a 4-centimeter craniocaudal incision in the linea alba of the abdomen, you will cut parallel to and between the fibers of the right and left:*

a. rectus abdominis
b. internal abdominal oblique
c. external abdominal oblique
d. transversus abdominis
e. transversus thoracis

48. *The pelvic diaphragm is composed of fascia and the:*

a. constrictor vulvae and vestibuli
b. levator ani and coccygeus
c. internal and external obturators
d. rectococcygeus and retractor penis
e. internal and external anal sphincters

49. *In dogs, which tooth has the most roots?*

a. 4th upper premolar
b. 2nd upper premolar
c. canine
d. 2nd lower premolar
e. 1st lower premolar

50. *Which muscle would most require reflection or incision to provide surgical access to the anal sacs?*

51. *Paralysis of which muscle would most interfere with opening of the mouth?*

a. lateral pterygoid
b. medial pterygoid
c. digastricus
d. masseter
e. temporalis

52. *A segment of bowel with blood vessels coursing along both its mesenteric and antimesenteric borders is the:*

a. ascending duodenum
b. terminal portion of the ileum
c. transverse colon
d. descending colon
e. rectum

53. *Anal sacs:*

a. do not occur in cats
b. occupy the space between coccygeus and levator ani muscles
c. empty their secretions into the rectum
d. are situated between the external and internal anal sphincters
e. are encased in fat and fascia of the ischiorectal fossae

54. *As the stomach distends and changes position in the abdominal cavity, the organ that consequently moves caudally due to a common mesenteric attachment with the stomach is the:*

a. duodenum
b. right kidney
c. right lobe of the pancreas
d. liver
e. spleen

Correct answers are on pages 89-99.

Dogs and Cats, continued

55. When inserted through the omental (epiploic) foramen, one's finger lies between the:

    a. portal vein and bile duct
    b. portal vein and caudal vena cava
    c. caudal vena cava and abdominal aorta
    d. bile duct and pancreatic duct
    e. hepatic artery and bile duct

56. An abnormal mass within the base of the lingual frenulum would most likely interfere with discharge of secretions from the:

    a. mandibular salivary gland
    b. zygomatic salivary gland
    c. parotid salivary gland
    d. vomeronasal gland
    e. lacrimal gland

57. A dog swallows a sharp bone. If the bone subsequently penetrates the parietal portion of the stomach, it would also most likely:

    a. enter the omental bursa
    b. puncture the gallbladder
    c. pierce the left ventricle of the heart
    d. pierce the liver
    e. tear through the greater omentum

58. A visceral serous membrane is **not** present on the surface of the:

    a. right accessory lobe of the lung
    b. liver
    c. stomach
    d. spleen
    e. cervical esophagus

59. The fourth upper premolar (shearing tooth or carnassial tooth) in dogs has how many roots?

    a. the number varies with the individual dog
    b. 2 lateral and 2 medial
    c. 2 lateral and 1 medial
    d. 1 medial and 2 lateral
    e. 1 medial and 1 lateral

60. If a hernia of the thoracic diaphragm develops so slowly that no serous membranes rupture while the gastric fundus moves into the thoracic cavity, how many layers of serous membrane would be present between the pleural cavity and the smooth muscle of the stomach?

    a. 5
    b. 4
    c. 3
    d. 2
    e. 1

61. Which segment of gut has the longest supportive attachment, from the abdominal wall to the gut segment?

    a. descending duodenum
    b. jejunum
    c. esophagus
    d. descending colon
    e. transverse colon

62. In a dog that has not eaten recently, which structure is situated caudal to the root of the mesentery?

    a. cecum
    b. transverse colon
    c. body of the pancreas
    d. spleen
    e. right kidney

63. The tracheal carina is positioned:

    a. dorsal to the esophagus
    b. between the base of the heart and the esophagus
    c. caudal to the base of the heart
    d. to the left of the pulmonary trunk
    e. to the left of the ascending aorta

64. The middle ear cavity normally drains into the:

    a. frontal sinus
    b. external auditory meatus
    c. nasopharynx

d. laryngopharynx

e. nasal cavity

65. *Not including the tiny interarytenoid cartilage, the larynx of dogs and cats consists of:*

a. 2 paired and 3 unpaired cartilages

b. 1 paired and 2 unpaired cartilages

c. 3 unpaired cartilages

d. 1 paired and 3 unpaired cartilages

e. 4 unpaired cartilages

66. *Which bone forms the ventral portion of the nasal septum and part of the dorsal wall of the nasopharynx?*

a. sphenoid

b. maxillary

c. palatine

d. pterygoid

e. vomer

67. *When the lungs are fully inflated, their caudolateral margins extend caudally to about the transverse level of the:*

a. 6th thoracic vertebra

b. 8th thoracic vertebra

c. 10th thoracic vertebra

d. 12th thoracic vertebra

e. 2nd lumbar vertebra

68. *The accessory lobe of the right lung is curled around the:*

a. esophagus

b. aorta

c. caudal vena cava

d. trachea

e. right azygos vein

69. *The cricoarytenoideus dorsalis functions in:*

a. constricting the pharynx

b. constricting the esophagus

c. tightening the cricothyroid ligament

d. closing the rima glottidis

e. opening the rima glottidis

70. *A tear or rip in a dog's thoracic diaphragm, between the diaphragmatic openings of the esophagus and caudal vena cava, would most likely permit:*

a. lung tissue to collapse

b. lung tissue to enter the abdominal cavity

c. abdominal viscera to enter the pericardial cavity

d. liver lobes to enter the right pleural cavity

e. liver lobes to enter the left pleural cavity

71. *Passing a nasogastric tube through the nasal cavity is difficult in carnivores because the:*

a. epiglottis occludes the nasopharyngeal lumen

b. vomer divides the nasopharyngeal meatus into 2 channels

c. ethmoid conchae project into the ventral nasal meatus

d. dorsal conchae end caudally in a cul de sac

e. ventral conchae are highly branched

72. *A dog is brought to your clinic with a puncture wound in the left thoracic wall, and you diagnose a collapsed lung. What is the least number of serous membranes (layers) that could have been punctured?*

a. none

b. 1

c. 2

d. 3

e. 4

73. *In a resting dog that is not panting or swallowing, the apex or tip of the epiglottis is normally positioned in the:*

a. laryngopharynx

b. oropharynx

c. intrapharyngeal ostium

d. piriform recess

e. laryngeal vestibule

Correct answers are on pages 89-99.

Dogs and Cats, continued

74. *Which cartilage of the larynx is most responsible for preventing collapse or constriction of the laryngeal airway?*

    a. cricoid
    b. arytenoid
    c. thyroid
    d. epiglottis
    e. interarytenoid

75. *Fracture of the right 5th rib, with severe damage to lung tissue directly deep to the rib, would most likely result in:*

    a. puncture and collapse of only the right cranial lobe
    b. puncture and collapse of only the right middle lobe
    c. puncture of the right middle lobe and collapse of the right lung
    d. puncture and collapse of only the right caudal lobe
    e. puncture of the right caudal lobe and collapse of the right lung

76. *The urinary bladder is supported by:*

    a. 1 ligament or mesentery
    b. 2 ligaments or mesenteries
    c. 3 ligaments or mesenteries
    d. 4 ligaments or mesenteries
    e. 5 ligaments or mesenteries

77. *The ureters open into the urinary bladder through its:*

    a. apex
    b. dorsocranial surface
    c. dorsocaudal surgace
    d. ventrocranial surface
    e. ventrocaudal surface

78. *Which structure projects into the renal pelvis?*

    a. renal cortex
    b. renal papilla
    c. renal sinus
    d. renal calyx
    e. urachus

79. *The portion of the ureter that receives urine from the renal crest is the:*

    a. renal hilus
    b. renal pelvis
    c. renal sinus
    d. renal trigone
    e. renal papilla

80. *Concerning the urethra of dogs and cats, which statement is most accurate?*

    a. The preprostatic portion of the feline urethra is relatively longer than that of the dog.
    b. The urethralis muscle is composed of smooth (nonstriated) muscle.
    c. The urethralis muscle is not present in cats.
    d. The pelvic portion of the male urethra is contained within connective tissue caudal to the most caudal extent of the peritoneal cavity.
    e. The ductus deferens enters the postprostatic portion of the male urethra.

81. *In male dogs, the erectile tissue at the proximal end of the glans penis that is an integral part of the "tie" during copulation is the:*

    a. bulbus glandis
    b. penile frenulum
    c. corpus spongiosum penis
    d. corpus cavernosum penis
    e. ischiocavernosus

82. *The portion of the penis that is in direct contact with and surrounds the urethra is the:*

    a. os penis
    b. bulbus glandis
    c. corpus cavernosum penis
    d. corpus spongiosum penis
    e. pars longa glandis

83. In female dogs, the vaginal fornix is:

   a. located cranioventral to the external uterine ostium
   b. located caudodorsal to the external uterine ostium
   c. the most caudal portion of the vagina
   d. a reflection of the vaginal wall away from the urethral tubercle
   e. divided into 2 compartments by a median septum

84. The fossa clitoridis:

   a. is cranial to the urethral tubercle
   b. is in the dorsal wall of the vagina
   c. is outside (external to) the rima pudendi
   d. contains the external urethral opening
   e. is in the caudoventral portion of the vaginal wall

85. Concerning the genital anatomy of male dogs and cats, which statement is **least** accurate?

   a. Within the scrotum, the ductus deferens is medial to the epididymis.
   b. The ductus deferens arises from the epididymis at the cranial margin of the testis.
   c. The cremaster muscle is external to the parietal vaginal tunic.
   d. The spermatic cord is synonymous with the visceral layer of the vaginal tunic and its contents.
   e. During development, the testis descends into the scrotum through the inguinal canal while remaining outside the vaginal canal.

86. The round ligament of the uterus:

   a. is a remnant of the umbilical artery
   b. is a remnant of the umbilical vein
   c. spans the distance from the uterine horn to the inguinal canal
   d. attaches the ovary to the uterus
   e. contains the uterine branch of the ovarian artery

87. The vagina is positioned:

   a. directly dorsal to the rectum
   b. directly ventral to the urethra
   c. within the pubovesicular excavation
   d. within the rectogenital excavation
   e. ventral to the perineal body

88. Over most of the penile body, the dorsal artery and nerve of the penis are in contact with the:

   a. bulbospongiosus
   b. ischiocavernosus
   c. corpus cavernosum
   d. corpus spongiosum
   e. retractor penis

89. Which structure curves or loops around the caudal portion of the ureter?

   a. round ligament of the uterus
   b. suspensory ligament of the ovary
   c. median ligament of the bladder
   d. ductus deferens
   e. testicular artery

90. From dorsal to ventral, pelvic structures are arranged in the order of:

   a. vagina, rectum, urethra
   b. vagina, urethra, rectum
   c. rectum, urethra, vagina
   d. rectum, vagina, urethra
   e. urethra, rectum, vagina

91. The ovarian bursa:

   a. is a membranous sac totally separating the ovary from the peritoneal cavity
   b. is composed of membranes within which most of the uterine tube is located
   c. contains the round ligament of the uterus
   d. contains the suspensory ligament of the ovary
   e. is not present in cats

Correct answers are on pages 89-99.

Dogs and Cats, continued

92. *A loop of intestine passes through (within) the vaginal canal, reaching the level of the testis and without tearing of any serosal layer. What is the minimum number of serous layers between the smooth muscle of the intestinal wall and the lumen of the ductus deferens?*

   a. none
   b. 1
   c. 2
   d. 3
   e. 4

93. *Which of the following is a direct indication of long-standing pulmonary hypertension (constricted pulmonary vessels)?*

   a. enlarged right atrium
   b. enlarged left atrium
   c. dilated aortic bulb
   d. tracheal collapse
   e. left ventricular hypertrophy

94. *Which vessel carries the **least** amount of blood to an organ, such as the heart, lungs, gut, liver, pancreas, urinary bladder or uterus?*

   a. internal thoracic artery
   b. celiac artery
   c. cranial mesenteric artery
   d. caudal mesenteric artery
   e. portal vein

95. *If absorbed into the venous system, a substance injected into the peritoneal cavity would most likely be carried through the:*

   a. omental veins to the external pudendal vien
   b. deep epigastric veins to the portal vein
   c. omental veins to the phrenicoabdominal veins
   d. cranial deep epigastric veins to the caudal vena cava
   e. cranial mesenteric veins to the portal vein

96. *If you make a ventral midline incision through the skin and sternum into the thoracic cavity, you would be cutting between and parallel to which vessels?*

   a. internal thoracic
   b. lateral thoracic
   c. external thoracic
   d. mediastinal
   e. phrenic

97. *Sharp bony fragments in a fractured temporomandibular joint would most likely damage the adjacent:*

   a. internal carotid artery
   b. lingual artery
   c. external ophthalmic artery
   d. caudal auricular artery
   e. maxillary artery

98. *In adult animals, remnants of the arterial blood supply to the fetal placenta supply blood to the:*

   a. liver
   b. duodenum
   c. jejunoileum
   d. linea alba
   e. urinary bladder

99. *Incomplete occlusion of the cephalic vein during venipucture allows venous blood to continue flowing from the cranial surface of the antebrachium toward the heart, through the:*

   a. axillobrachial vein
   b. omobrachial vein
   c. median vein
   d. median cubital vein
   e. accessory cephalic vein

100. *Concerning the vascular system in dogs and cats, which statement is **least** accurate?*

   a. Two left renal arteries often supply the left kidney.
   b. The cranial margin of the left kidney in dogs is caudal to that of the right kidney.
   c. The left testicular vein drains into the left renal vein.
   d. The right renal vein drains into the portal vein.

e. The origin of the right testicular artery from the dorsal aorta is cranial to that of the left testicular artery.

101. Which vein does **not** normally drain directly into the right atrium?

a. right pulmonary vein
b. cranial vena cava
c. caudal vena cava
d. great cardiac vein
e. right azygos vein

102. If the celiac artery is severed, which organ would be **least** deprived of arterial blood?

a. stomach
b. gallbladder
c. spleen
d. liver
e. pancreas

103. The coronary arteries are branches of the:

a. pulmonary trunk
b. aorta
c. right atrium
d. left atrium
e. brachiocephalic trunk

104. Esophageal dilatation or megaesophagus and regurgitation of solid foods in a young puppy may indicate a vascular ring anomaly. In affected puppies, the esophagus is constricted by a ring formed by the:

a. longus colli and right and left costocervial trunks
b. left aortic arch, base of the heart, and left ligamentum arteriosum
c. right aortic arch, base of the heart, and right ligamentum arteriosum
d. right aortic arch, base of the heart, and left ligamentum arteriosum
e. right and left pulmonary arteries, and right ligamentum arteriosum

105. In cats, which artery passes through an osseous foramen?

a. brachial artery
b. median artery
c. common interosseous artery
d. femoral artery
e. cranial tibial artery

106. In an angiographic study, contrast medium injected into the cranial mesenteric artery would **least** likely appear in the:

a. duodenum
b. jejunum
c. ileum
d. cecum
e. spleen

107. You accidentally sever the right and left prostatic arteries during prostatic surgery in a dog. This will now deprive all of the following tissues of much of their normal blood supply **except** for the:

a. urinary bladder
b. ductus deferens
c. urethra
d. ureter
e. testicle

108. Pulsating blood spurting from a laceration across the ventral cervical region would most likely be from the:

a. external jugular vein
b. internal jugular vein
c. subclavian artery
d. common carotid artery
e. vertebral artery

109. A piece of debris that is larger than the diameter of a large capillary breaks away from a blood clot in the femoral vein. This debris would most likely first be trapped in the vascular bed of the:

a. liver
b. lung
c. brain
d. spleen
e. kidneys

Correct answers are on pages 89-99.

Dogs and Cats, continued

110. *In a normal animal, a substance injected into the left external jugular vein would pass sequentially through the:*

a. left atrium, left ventricle, lung, right atrium and right ventricle

b. left atrium, left ventricle, aorta, left coronary artery, heart muscle and great cardiac vein

c. right atrium, right ventricle, aorta, liver, caudal vena cava and left atrium

d. right atrium, right ventricle, pulmonary trunk, lung, pulmonary veins and left atrium

e. linguofacial vein, facial vein and deep facial vein

111. *In a surgical procedure on the thoracic cavity, you incise the thoracic wall at the 6th intercostal space. If you ligate and then sever the dorsal 6th intercostal artery and vein, the most likely result would be:*

a. bloodless surgery

b. bleeding from branches of the costocervical trunk

c. bleeding from branches of the phrenico-abdominal vessels

d. bleeding from branches of the vertebral vessels

e. bleeding from branches of the internal thoracic vessels

112. *If you wished to place a long intravascular cannula into the pulmonary trunk without surgically entering the pleural or peritoneal cavities, the most appropriate vascular approach would be via the:*

a. left femoral artery

b. left femoral vein

c. left common carotid artery

d. left brachial artery

e. right azygos vein

113. *Which portion of the heart is most closely adjacent to the dome of the thoracic diaphragm?*

a. left ventricle

b. right ventricle

c. apex of the ventricles

d. right atrium

e. left atrium

114. *Venous blood from which structure does **not** first drain into the liver before passing into the heart?*

a. pancreas

b. spleen

c. adrenal gland

d. descending colon

e. stomach

115. *The pelvic organs receive most of their blood supply via the:*

a. caudal mesenteric artery

b. umbilical artery

c. vaginal or prostatic artery

d. caudal gluteal artery

e. external iliac artery

116. *Excluding the ovaries, uterus, testes and kidneys, all abdominal organs that are suspended from the abdominal wall by mesentery receive blood from the abdominal aorta through:*

a. 2 unpaired arteries

b. 2 unpaired and 1 paired arteries

c. 3 unpaired arteries

d. 3 paired arteries

e. 5 vessels

117. *Fats that are digested and absorbed into lacteals are then carried most directly into the:*

a. hepatic vein

b. portal vein

c. right azygos vein

d. cisterna chyli

e. lumbar trunk

118. *If a medial iliac lymph node is greatly enlarged but the caudal mesenteric, superficial inguinal and popliteal lymph nodes are of*

normal size, you would most likely observe an
infection in the:

a. tail
b. descending colon
c. cranial rectum
d. prepuce
e. metatarsal pad

119. *Which structures are* ***least*** *closely associated
with each other in location?*

a. tibial nerve and popliteal lymph node
b. axillary nerve and proper axillary lymph node
c. internal thoracic artery and sternal lymph
    node
d. right azygos vein and right tracheobronchial
    lymph node
e. mandibular nerve and mandibular lymph
    node

120. *A dog has a malignant growth on its
prepuce. On cytologic examination, you detect
malignant cells in the superficial inguinal
lymph nodes. Which lymph nodes should you
next examine to see if the neoplasm has spread
along a lymphatic drainage route?*

a. axillary proper
b. accessory axillary
c. popliteal
d. medial iliac
e. jejunal

121. *The thoracic duct:*

a. drains into the cisterna chyli
b. drains lymph from the pelvic limbs, tail and
    intestines
c. drains the pulmonary and tracheobronchial
    lymph nodes
d. crosses the lateral surface of the pericardium
e. enters the right azygos vein

122. *Concerning the cisterna chyli, which
statement is* ***least*** *accurate?*

a. The thoracic duct drains the cisterna chyli.

b. Both the intestinal and lumbar lymphatic
    trunks drain into the cisterna chyli.
c. The cisterna chyli is situated between the
    crura of the thoracic diaphragm.
d. The vessels draining the cisterna chyli pass
    through the esophageal hiatus of the
    thoracic diaphragm.
e. The cisterna chyli is a thin-walled structure
    that is not easily observed grossly.

123. *A dog with enlarged superficial inguinal
and axillary lymph nodes and normal
superficial cervical and popliteal lymph nodes
most likely has an infection in its:*

a. thoracic limb
b. pelvic limb
c. thoracic and pelvic limbs
d. thoracic and pelvic organs
e. mammary glands

124. *Which structure is* ***not*** *contained within the
mediastinum?*

a. thymus
b. thoracic portion of the esophagus
c. thoracic portion of the trachea
d. heart
e. thoracic portion of the caudal vena cava

125. *A needle inserted through the skin rostro-
medial to the temporomandibular joint would
most likely penetrate the:*

a. medial pterygoid muscle
b. digastricus muscle
c. masseter muscle
d. temporalis muscle
e. geniohyoideus muscle

126. *Which structure is found in both cats and
dogs?*

a. soleus muscles
b. sacrotuberous ligaments
c. anconeus muscles
d. nuchal ligament
e. supracondylar foramina

Correct answers are on pages 89-99.

Dogs and Cats, continued

127. *Concerning positional relationships, which statement is **least** accurate?*

  a. The esophagus is dorsal to the tracheal carina.
  b. In the midcervical region, the esophagus is dorsolateral to the trachea and on the left.
  c. The trachealis muscle is located within the dorsal portion of the trachea.
  d. The pylorus of the stomach and cranial portion of the duodenum are located toward the left side of the abdominal cavity.
  e. The prostate gland is ventral to the rectum.

128. *Dorsocranial displacement of the proximal femur indicates that:*

  a. the femoral nerve is damaged
  b. the obturator nerve is damaged
  c. the tuber ischiadicum is fractured
  d. an intracapsular ligament is ruptured
  e. the sacrotuberous ligament is torn

129. *The lacrimal gland:*

  a. is ventral to the eyeball
  b. is lateral to the eyeball
  c. secretes fluid that enters the conjunctival sac through the caudal surface of the third eyelid
  d. secretes fluid that enters the anterior chamber of the eye
  e. secretes fluid that drains from the orbital region into the nasal vestibule

130. *Enlarging the cartilaginous external auditory meatus by cutting ventrally through the pretragic incisure would most likely damage the:*

  a. scutiform cartilage
  b. accessory nerve
  c. facial vein
  d. parotid salivary gland
  e. mandibular salivary gland

131. *Considering anatomic position, which surgical approach to an organ or structure is **least** appropriate?*

  a. left abdominal wall approach to the spleen
  b. right abdominal wall approach to the descending portion of the duodenum
  c. left abdominal wall approach to the descending colon
  d. right thoracic wall approach to the pulmonary arterial trunk
  e. right thoracic wall approach to the intrathoracic caudal vena cava

132. *Cats do **not** have a:*

  a. clavicle
  b. lateral laryngeal ventricle
  c. gastrocnemius muscle
  d. supracondylar foramen in the distal portion of the humerus
  e. gallbladder

133. *Which structure does **not** pass through all or part of the inguinal canal?*

  a. cremaster muscle
  b. deep femoral artery
  c. external pudendal artery
  d. testicular artery
  e. ductus deferens

134. *A thistle in the medial aspect of the 3rd digit, on the surface facing the 2nd digit, is in the:*

  a. axial surface of the 1st interdigital space
  b. abaxial surface of the 1st interdigital space
  c. axial surface of the 2nd interdigital space
  d. abaxial surface of the 2nd interdigital space
  e. axial surface of the 3rd interdigital space

135. *Which of the following does **not** pass into or out of the tympanooccipital fissure?*

  a. hypoglossal nerve
  b. internal carotid artery
  c. vagus nerve
  d. accessory nerve
  e. glossopharyngeal nerve

*136. During surgical repair of a ruptured crus of the thoracic diaphragm via an abdominal approach, you are **least** likely to encounter the:*

a. phrenic nerve
b. major splanchnic nerve
c. cisterna chyli
d. adrenal gland
e. phrenicoabdominal vein

137. The vitreous body of the canine eye:

a. is formed by the ciliary body
b. is located within the posterior chamber of the eye
c. is firmly attached to the caudal aspect of the lens capsule
d. contains blood vessels in the adult animal
e. forms the tapetum lucidum

*138. Which muscle is composed of smooth muscle and, as such, is **not** under voluntary control?*

a. trachealis
b. cricoarytenoideus dorsalis
c. urethralis
d. bulbospongiosus
e. ischiocavernosus

*139. Which structure evidences the **least** difference in fetal and adult positions?*

a. testis
b. thoracic diaphragm
c. thyroid gland
d. trapezius
e. cranial preputial muscle

140. While you retract the biceps femoris caudally, separating and lifting the major trochanter of the femur and the muscles that insert upon it would most reveal the:

a. pudendal nerve
b. external pudendal artery
c. femoral nerve

d. obturator nerve
e. ischiatic nerve

*141. "Sinking" of the manus, with more of the palmar surface coming in contact with the ground, would **least** likely result from damage to the:*

a. medial humeral epicondyle
b. elbow articulation
c. median nerve
d. ulnar nerve
e. radial nerve

142. In a dog with a severed common calcanean tendon, an adjacent structure that should be examined for damage is the:

a. saphenous nerve
b. common fibular nerve
c. tibial nerve
d. cranial tibial artery
e. fibula

143. A fracture through the distomedial portion of a cat's humerus would most likely involve direct injury to the:

a. cephalic vein
b. radial nerve
c. median nerve
d. ulnar nerve
e. head of the radius

*144. If a bone tumor spreads from the vertebral column via a venous pathway, neoplastic cells are **least** likely to be carried by the:*

a. vertebral veins
b. costocervical vein
c. right azygos vein
d. subclavian vein
e. caudal vena cava

Correct answers are on pages 89-99.

Dogs and Cats, continued

*145. During surgical correction of an inguinal hernia, one must avoid damaging stuctures passing through the inguinal canal. These include all of the following **except** the:*

a. external pudendal artery
b. ductus deferens
c. genitofemoral nerve
d. pudendal nerve
e. testicular artery

*146. Concerning positional relationships, which statement is **least** accurate?*

a. Part of the thoracic diaphragm is dorsocaudal to the right kidney.
b. The caudal extent of the lung is caudolateral to much of the liver.
c. Lung tissue extends craniomedially, past the first ribs.
d. The right kidney of dogs is cranial to the left kidney.
e. The left lung occupies more space in the thoracic cavity than does the right lung.

147. The space between the plica venae cavae and the mediastinum is occupied by the:

a. accessory lobe of the right lung
b. cranial vena cava
c. caudal vena cava
d. pleural cupula
e. thymus

148. Most intrinsic striated muscles of the larynx attach to the:

a. epiglottis
b. arytenoid cartilage
c. thyroid cartilage
d. cricoid cartilage
e. hyoid bones

149. A transverse incision through the skin of the plantar surface of the calcaneus, distal to the insertion of the common calcanean tendon, would most likely damage the:

a. gastrocnemius tendon
b. deep digital flexor tendon
c. superficial digital flexor tendon
d. cranial tibial artery
e. superficial fibular nerve

150. In a surgical approach to the thoracic cavity from the left side, you would most likely first observe the:

a. ascending aorta
b. pulmonary trunk
c. caudal vena cava
d. nonauricular portion of the right atrium
e. middle tracheobronchial lymph node

151. A common characteristic of the humeral, cubital, coxal and genual articulations is that each has:

a. well-developed collateral ligaments
b. at least one intracapsular ligament
c. at least one sesamoid bone associated with it
d. only one joint cavity filled with synovial fluid
e. opposing articular surfaces covered by synovial membrane

152. Caudal to the anticlinal vertebra of carnivores,:

a. no costotransverse articulations are present
b. multifidus muscles are absent
c. accessory processes of the vertebrae are absent
d. intervertebral articular surfaces are oriented in the sagittal plane
e. the ventral longitudinal ligament of the vertebral column is absent

153. In an adult dog or cat, the thymus is located in the:

a. cervical region
b. pleural cavity
c. cranial mediastinum
d. fibrous pericardium
e. pericardial cavity

Horses

N.G. Ghoshal

154. *The fetlock joint capsule can be entered through its dorsal, lateral, palmar or plantar aspects. If you elect to puncture this joint capsule by adopting a palmar or plantar approach, what anatomic landmark is **not** used to execute the procedure?*

   a. distal ends of the "splint" bones
   b. distal sesamoid bone
   c. third metacarpal or metatarsal bone
   d. suspensory ligament or interosseous muscle
   e. proximal sesamoid bones

155. *The podotrochlear or navicular bursa is often involved in "navicular disease." This structure is located adjacent to the:*

   a. distal sesamoid bone and deep digital flexor tendon
   b. proximal sesamoid bone and suspensory ligament
   c. superficial digital flexor tendon
   d. interosseous muscle
   e. third metatarsal bone and splint bone

156. *In racing horses, fractures of the distal phalanx (PIII) of the thoracic limb usually involve the articular surface of the distal interphalangeal joint. These conditions are said to happen during counterclockwise turns on parts of the bone carrying the most weight. Which parts of the distal phalanx of the thoracic limb are commonly fractured?*

   a. medial side of left PIII and lateral side of right PIII
   b. lateral side of left PIII and medial side of right PIII
   c. solear surface of left PIII and semilunar line of right PIII
   d. semilunar line of left PIII and solear surface of right PIII
   e. medial side of left PIII and semilunar line of right PIII

157. *Arthritic lesions are sometimes seen in the equine hock, usually on its medial side, though this process may later spread to other sites. Which tarsal bone is the **primary** site of arthritis?*

   a. third tarsal bone and central tarsal bone
   b. central tarsal bone and talus
   c. talus and calcaneus
   d. calcaneus and third tarsal bone
   e. third tarsal bone and talus

158. *Distal to the fetlock joint, which of the following represents the normal dorsal-palmar or dorsal-plantar relationship of the digital vessels and nerve on the medial and lateral aspects of the proximal phalanx?*

   a. digital vein, artery and nerve
   b. digital artery, vein and nerve
   c. digital nerve, artery and vein
   d. digital artery, nerve and vein
   e. digital vein, nerve and artery

159. *Among the following joints of the vertebral column, which has the most movement?*

   a. intercentral joint or intervertebral symphysis
   b. lumbar intertransverse joint
   c. lumbosacral intertransverse joint
   d. lumbosacral joint
   e. sacroiliac joint

160. *Fibrotic and ossifying myopathy does **not** involve which of the following muscles?*

   a. biceps femoris
   b. semitendinosus
   c. gluteus medius
   d. semimembranosus
   e. gracilis

Correct answers are on pages 89-99.

Horses, continued

161. *Which of the following sites is used for cerebrospinal fluid collection in the horse?*

    a. lumbosacral joint
    b. first intercaudal joint
    c. sacrocaudal joint
    d. sacroiliac joint
    e. intersacral joint

162. *To aspirate cerebrospinal fluid from the subarachnoid space of horses, which anatomic landmark is usually used?*

    a. a transverse line across the caudal aspects of the coxal tubers intersecting the midline, or a transverse line across the cranial aspects of the sacral tubers intersecting the midline
    b. a transverse line connecting the cranial aspects of the coxal tubers intersecting the midline, or a transverse line connecting the caudal aspects of the sacral tubers intersecting the midline
    c. a transverse line connecting the cranial aspects of the coxal tubers intersecting a transverse line connecting the caudal aspects of the sacral tubers
    d. a transverse line connecting the caudal aspects of the coxal tubers intersecting a transverse line connecting the cranial aspects of the sacral tubers
    e. a transverse line connecting the midline 10 cm cranial to the base of the tail

163. *Horses with back problems are **least** likely to manifest which of the following signs?*

    a. resentment and discomfort on palpation, saddling or grooming of the affected side
    b. change in temperament
    c. stiff gait or restricted activity
    d. opisthotonus
    e. poor performance

164. *Inflammation of which of the following bursae would likely cause lameness and elicit pain?*

    a. subligamentous bursae
    b. subtendinous bursae
    c. subfascial bursae
    d. subcutaneous bursae
    e. submuscular bursae

165. *Reciprocal apparatus dysfunction can lead to acute, severe pelvic limb lameness. Which of the following structures is **not** a part of the reciprocal apparatus in horses?*

    a. fibrous band embedded in the lateral head of the gastrocnemius muscle
    b. semitendinosus muscle
    c. peroneus (fibularis) tertius muscle
    d. superficial digital flexor muscle
    e. none of these are part of the reciprocal apparatus

166. *A horse was tied to a large wooden post and left unattended for 2 days. When the owner returned, the animal could not bear weight on the left pelvic limb and had no signs of trauma. On examination, you note a diffuse soft tissue swelling caudal to the stifle joint, but radiographs reveal that the joint is normal. The affected limb can be protracted, but while bearing minimum weight the hock hyperflexes and drops toward the ground. On further examination, the hock can be flexed or extended without influencing the position of the stifle, and the fetlock and pastern joints can be extended while the hock is maintained in flexion. The above findings suggest functional loss of which component of the reciprocal apparatus in this horse?*

    a. superficial digital flexor muscle
    b. gastrocnemius muscle
    c. peroneus (fibularis) tertius muscle
    d. biceps femoris muscle
    e. semitendinosus muscle

167. *Abdominal pain (colic) has numerous causes. Recent findings indicate that damage to the nerves supplying the gastrointestinal tract is responsible for this condition. Which of the following changes is **not** involved in colic of horses?*

    a. damage to the myenteric (Auerbach) plexus of autonomic nerves

b. injury to the submucous (Meissner) plexus of autonomic nerves

c. interruption of movement of food through the ascending (great) colon due to lack of contraction of its smooth muscle wall

d. disruption of both absorbing and secreting activities that occur during digestion

e. hypersecretion of bile and pancreatic enzymes from vagal stimulation

168. In a standing horse, which part of the hoof wall bears the most support?

a. stratum externum
b. stratum internum
c. stratum medium
d. laminar corium
e. sole

169. The hoof receives its nutrient blood supply via the:

a. corium
b. horny laminae
c. collateral cartilages of the distal phalanx
d. digital cushion
e. white line or zone

170. Occlusion or stenosis of which of the following is most likely to cause an immediate backflow of blood into the liver of a horse?

a. aortic valve
b. mitral or bicuspid (left atrioventricular) valve
c. pulmonic valve
d. tricuspid (right atrioventricular) valve
e. common bile duct

171. Sialoliths usually involve the duct of the parotid salivary gland, causing considerable increase in size due to obstruction. A sialolith can be confirmed radiographically and treated by surgical removal. While coursing along the rostral border of the masseter muscle, which rostral-caudal relationship of the parotid duct in the horse is correct?

a. duct, facial vein, facial artery
b. facial artery, facial vein, duct

c. facial vein, duct, facial artery
d. facial artery, duct, facial vein
e. duct, facial artery, facial vein

172. In chronic pulmonary emphysema (heaves), which of the following becomes distinct due to forced expiration, giving rise to a "heave line" extending from the cartilage of the 12th or 13th rib to the tuber coxae? (This line is greatly exaggerated in animals showing marked expiratory abdominal breathing.)

a. latissimus dorsi muscle
b. external abdominal oblique muscle
c. ascending pectoral muscle
d. serratus ventralis thoracis muscle
e. cutaneous trunci muscle

173. Horses are less likely to develop coxofemoral (hip joint) luxations or dislocations because of the:

a. ligament of the head of the femur
b. prepubic tendon
c. transverse acetabular ligament
d. accessory ligament of the head of the femur
e. symphysial (subpelvic) tendon

174. Which of the following is a permanent tooth evident along with deciduous dentition in horses?

a. fourth premolar
b. second premolar
c. first premolar
d. third premolar
e. canine

175. A horse has a "full mouth," that is, all of its incisors are in wear. The upper corner incisors have a "hook." There is an indication of a faint dental star on the central incisor. What is the approximate age of this horse?

a. 5 years
b. 6 years
c. 8 years
d. 7 years
e. 18 years

Correct answers are on pages 89-99.

Horses, continued

176. *Infection of the diverticulum of the auditory tube (guttural pouch) may result in extension to involve related blood vessels and nerves, manifesting characteristic clinical signs. Involvement of which of the following can cause colic from intestinal stasis concurrent with guttural pouch infection?*

    a. glossopharyngeal nerve
    b. facial nerve
    c. vagus nerve
    d. hypoglossal nerve
    e. accessory nerve

177. *In many diseases of the upper respiratory tract, the deglutition or swallowing reflex is often impaired. Which of the following muscles is **not** a pharyngeal constrictor?*

    a. pterygopharyngeus muscle
    b. palatopharyngeus muscle
    c. hyopharyngeus muscle
    d. thyropharyngeus and cricopharyngeus muscles
    e. stylopharyngeus caudalis muscle

178. *The skeleton of the larynx is formed by a set of cartilages held together by muscles and ligaments. The laryngeal cartilage that is paired is the:*

    a. epiglottic
    b. arytenoid
    c. cricoid
    d. thyroid
    e. styloid

179. *During endoscopic examination of the upper respiratory tract, which laryngeal cartilages are normally visible protruding into the pharynx?*

    a. cricoid and styloid
    b. thyroid and cricoid
    c. arytenoid and thyroid
    d. epiglottic and styloid
    e. arytenoid and epiglottic

180. *Concerning the gubernaculum, which statement is **least** accurate?*

    a. It is present in both male and female animals.
    b. After birth it consists of the proper ligament of the testis and ligament of the tail of the epididymis.
    c. The ligament of the tail of the epididymis is homologous to the scrotal ligament.
    d. The proper ligament of the testis is homologous to the proper ligament of the ovary.
    e. The round ligament of the uterus is represented by the ligament of the tail of the epididymis in males.

181. *In closed castration of stallions, the incision does **not** involve the:*

    a. skin
    b. cremaster fascia
    c. internal spermatic fascia
    d. parietal layer of the vaginal tunic
    e. external spermatic fascia

182. *Concerning the ovaries of mares, which statement is **least** accurate?*

    a. They are located in the sublumbar region.
    b. They are large and bean shaped.
    c. Ovulation usually occurs at the ovarian fossa.
    d. They are suspended by the mesovarium.
    e. Ruptured follicles can ovulate from any surface of the ovary.

183. *The dorsal surface of which carpal bones is most likely to be involved in chip fractures?*

    a. radiocarpal, third carpal, intermediate carpal
    b. ulnar carpal, second carpal
    c. radiocarpal, second carpal, fourth carpal
    d. carpal, ulnar carpal, second carpal
    e. intermediate carpal, fourth carpal

184. *Concerning laryngeal hemiplegia, which statement is **least** accurate?*

    a. The condition is usually due to left recurrent laryngeal nerve paralysis.

b. The clinical sign most evident is inspiratory dyspnea.
c. Laryngoscopic examination reveals an abducted arytenoid cartilage on the affected side.
d. Chronically affected horses demonstrate atrophy of the cricoarytenoideus dorsalis muscle on the affected side.
e. One surgical approach for correction of the condition involves exposure of the laryngeal ventricles by incising the cricothyroid ligament (membrane).

185. Which of the following would lead to a "blue baby" condition, or mixture of relatively unoxygenated blood in the somatic arterial circulation?

a. patent ductus venosus or persistent right aortic arch
b. patent foramen ovale or left vena cava
c. persistent right aortic arch or persistent ductus arteriosus
d. persistent ductus arteriosus or patent foramen ovale
e. left vena cava or patent ductus venosus

186. A horse is kicked on the side of the rib cage, rupturing a vein coursing along the ventral border of the latissimus dorsi muscle. Which vein was most likely ruptured?

a. cranial superficial epigastric vein
b. internal thoracic vein
c. azygous vein
d. superficial thoracic of the thoracodorsal vein
e. external thoracic vein

187. A surgical approach to a chip fracture at the distal dorsomedial aspect of the radial carpal bone requires an incision over the dorsal aspect of the carpus:

a. just medial to the tendon of the extensor carpi radialis muscle
b. between the extensor carpi radialis and common digital extensor tendons
c. between the common digital extensor and lateral digital extensor tendons
d. between the lateral digital extensor and ulnaris lateralis (extensor carpi ulnaris) tendons
e. between the flexor carpi radialis and superficial digital flexor tendons

188. Fracture of the extensor process of the distal phalanx results in pyramidal disease if left untreated. In such cases, which of the following continues to exert tension on the fractured bony fragment in the thoracic limb?

a. lateral digital extensor tendon
b. flexor carpi radialis tendon
c. interosseus medius tendon (suspensory ligament)
d. extensor carpi ulnaris (ulnaris lateralis) tendon
e. superficial digital flexor tendon

189. Drooping of the superior eyelid (ptosis) is **not** associated with damage to the:

a. nasociliary nerve
b. facial nerve
c. oculomotor nerve
d. sympathetic supply to the head
e. ophthalmic nerve

190. Surgical approach to the opening of the maxillary paranasal sinus should avoid the:

a. orbit rostrally
b. osseous infraorbital canal medially
c. dorsal buccal branch dorsally
d. osseous nasolacrimal duct ventrally
e. sinus of the deep facial vein dorsally

191. An obstruction of the left atrioventricular (mitral) valve would first be manifested as retrograde accumulation of blood in the:

a. liver
b. right ventricle
c. left ventricle
d. lungs
e. cervical and cephalic regions

Correct answers are on pages 89-99.

Horses, continued

192. *The first permanent tooth to erupt in horses is the:*

    a. first (central) incisor tooth
    b. first cheek tooth
    c. first molar tooth
    d. canine tooth
    e. first upper premolar tooth

193. *"Floating" is a procedure in which the sharp edges of the cheek teeth are filed off. On the superior dental arcade, the sharp edge is found on what surface of the teeth?*

    a. labial surface
    b. vestibular (buccal) surface
    c. vestibular border of the masticatory surface
    d. contact surface
    e. rostral surface

194. *The cranial border of the area of thoracic percussion and auscultation is formed by the:*

    a. long head of the triceps brachii muscle
    b. costal arch
    c. first rib
    d. pectoralis transversus muscle
    e. latissimus dorsi muscle

195. *A sudden inability to retract the upper lip to the left side or to dilate the left nostril, even though perception of pin pricks is preserved over the entire head region, would most likely result from injury of the:*

    a. maxillary nerve of the trigeminal
    b. glossopharyngeal nerve
    c. mandibular branch of cranial nerve V
    d. dorsal buccal branch of the facial nerve
    e. sympathetic innervation to the facial region

196. *Which of the following ganglia are **not** generally considered part of the peripheral nervous system?*

    a. dorsal root ganglia
    b. basal ganglia
    c. sympathetic chain glanglia
    d. collateral ganglia
    e. terminal glanglia

197. *Considering the autonomic nervous system, which statement is **least** accurate?*

    a. Chromaffin cells in the adrenal medulla, which migrate from the developing neural crest, act as postsynaptic neurons.
    b. Splanchnic nerves are considered presynaptic fibers.
    c. Presynaptic fibers have relatively less myelin than postsynaptic fibers.
    d. Parasympathetic presynaptic fibers are relatively longer than sympathetic presynaptic fibers.
    e. The parasympathetic origin of presynaptic neurons is generally considered craniosacral.

198. *To reach the abdominal viscera, the major (greater) splanchnic nerve courses through the:*

    a. aortic hiatus
    b. caval foramen
    c. esophageal hiatus
    d. lumbocostal arch
    e. vertebral canal

199. *Innervation to the palmar aspect of the digit of the equine thoracic limb is supplied directly and/or indirectly via the:*

    a. palmar branch of the scapular nerve and caudal cutaneous branch of the ulnar nerve
    b. superficial branch of the median nerve and palmar branch of the radial nerve
    c. caudal cutaneous scapular nerve and palmar branch of the median nerve
    d. continuation of the median nerve and palmar branch of the ulnar nerve
    e. superficial branch of the radial nerve and caudal cutaneous antebrachial nerve

200. *Most of the postganglionic sympathetic fibers that innervate structures in the head region have synapses at the:*

a. caudal cervical ganglion
b. middle cervical (vertebral) ganglion
c. cranial cervical ganglion
d. cervicothoracic (stellate) ganglion
e. collateral myenteric ganglion

201. *To focus on near objects,:*

a. lens curvature increases and the ciliary muscles relax
b. tension on the suspensory ligaments of the lens decreases and the ciliary muscles relax
c. tension on the suspensory ligaments of the lens increases and the ciliary muscles contract
d. lens curvature increases and tension on the suspensory ligaments of the lens increases
e. the ciliary muscles contract and lens curvature increases

202. *Each auditory tube diverticulum (guttural pouch) is subdivided into a small lateral and a large medial compartment by the:*

a. rectus capitis ventralis muscle
b. longus capitis muscle
c. pterygoideus lateralis muscle
d. medial retropharyngeal lymph node
e. stylohyoid bone (great cornu)

203. *Concerning the thyroid gland, which statement is **least** accurate?*

a. It consists of 2 lateral lobes and a slender isthmus.
b. It is situated on the cranial part of the trachea.
c. It is a ductless or endocrine gland.
d. It receives most of its blood supply from the cranial thyroid artery off the common carotid.
e. The larger dorsal lobe receives blood from the cranial thyroid artery, while the smaller ventral lobe receives blood from the dorsal thyroid branch of the brachiocephalic artery.

204. *The cranial laryngeal nerve innervates the:*

a. thyroarytenoideus muscle
b. cricoarytenoideus dorsalis muscle
c. thyrohyoideus muscle
d. cricothyroideus muscle
e. cricoarytenoideus lateralis muscle

205. *On the skull, the infraorbital foramen is located:*

a. midway and 1 inch caudally on a line drawn from the rostral end of the facial crest to the nasoincisive notch
b. superficial to the levator labii superioris muscle
c. in the area 2 inches caudal to the middle of the facial crest
d. 2 inches cranial to a line drawn from the caudal aspect of the nasoincisive notch to the facial crest
e. 3 inches cranial to a line drawn between the auditory meati

206. *Concerning the cheek teeth, which statement is most accurate?*

a. They number 6 on the upper arcade on each side (3 premolars and 3 molars).
b. All of them have roots that are vertical in respect to the alveolar border of the maxilla.
c. The molars are present in deciduous dentition.
d. They have roots that project into the maxillary paranasal sinus, with the exception of the first and second cheek teeth.
e. They should not be floated in young animals.

207. *The tympanic cavity, which houses the auditory ossicles and communicates with the nasopharynx by means of the auditory (eustachian) tube, is a part of the:*

a. external ear
b. middle ear
c. internal ear
d. auditory vesicles
e. guttural pouch

Correct answers are on pages 89-99.

Horses, continued

208. *All of the following are muscles that do not have a synovial sheath surrounding its tendon as the tendon passes the carpus to reach the metacarpal region* **except** *the:*

   a. flexor carpi radialis muscle
   b. extensor carpi radialis muscle
   c. common digital extensor muscle
   d. medial carpal extensor muscle
   e. lateral digital extensor muscle

209. *On flexion of the equine carpus, which synovial sac (joint space) opens the* **least** *amount on its dorsal surface?*

   a. carpometacarpal joint
   b. midcarpal joint
   c. antebrachiocarpal joint
   d. proximal radioulnar joint
   e. metacarpophalangeal joint

210. *The interosseus medius muscle (suspensory ligament) contains a variable amount of skeletal muscle fibers and therefore fatigues upon prolonged exertion. Which nerves innervate this structure in horses?*

   a. radial and musculocutaneous nerves
   b. median and radial nerves
   c. ulnar and median nerves
   d. musculocutaneous and ulnar nerves
   e. radial and ulnar nerves

211. *Which supporting structure of the fetlock joint arises from the proximal palmar sesamoids and inserts on the proximal palmar surface of the middle phalanx?*

   a. superficial (straight) distal sesamoidean ligament
   b. middle (oblique) distal sesamoidean ligament
   c. deep (cruciate) distal sesamoidean ligament
   d. short sesamoidean ligaments
   e. collateral sesamoidean ligaments

212. *Concerning the distal phalanx of horses, which statement is most accurate?*

   a. It furnishes attachment for the superficial (straight) distal sesamoidean ligament.
   b. It articulates with the proximal palmar sesamoid bones.
   c. It has a joint capsule that communicates with the podotrochlear (navicular) bursa.
   d. It has an extensor process on its proximodorsal aspect.
   e. In horses with chronic laminitis, the crena at the solear border rotates dorsally, while the palmar or plantar processes rotate ventrally.

213. *The teres major tuberosity of the humerus is the point of insertion of the:*

   a. teres major and deltoideus muscles
   b. teres major and latissimus dorsi muscles
   c. teres minor and latissimus dorsi muscles
   d. deltoideus and teres minor muscles
   e. latissimus dorsi and deltoideus muscles

214. *The accessory carpal bone serves as a point of attachment for the:*

   a. deep digital flexor and flexor carpi ulnaris muscles
   b. ulnaris lateralis (extensor carpi ulnaris) and deep digital flexor muscles
   c. flexor carpi ulnaris and superficial digital flexor muscles
   d. deep digital flexor and superficial digital flexor muscles
   e. flexor carpi ulnaris and ulnaris lateralis (extensor carpi ulnaris) muscles

215. *The flexors of the carpus and digit (considering the ulnaris lateralis muscle as a flexor) are innervated by the:*

   a. median, antebrachial and scapular nerves
   b. ulnar, volar and antebrachial nerves
   c. radial, scapular and pedal nerves
   d. median, ulnar and radial nerves
   e. radial, humeral and postbrachial nerves

216. *Cutting the thoracodorsal nerve near its origin results in dysfunction of the:*

   a. latissimus dorsi muscle

b. cranial preputial muscles

c. trapezius muscle

d. cutaneous trunci muscle

e. subscapularis muscle

217. *The largest blood vessel that directly or indirectly supplies the structures distal to the equine carpus is the:*

a. collateral ulnar artery

b. common interosseous artery

c. radial artery

d. median artery

e. cranial superficial antebrachial artery

218. *The craniolateral group of muscles of the forearm (antebrachium) receives its primary blood supply and nerve supply by way of the:*

a. transverse cubital artery and radial nerve

b. deep brachial artery and musculocutaneous nerve

c. collateral radial artery and ulnar nerve

d. transverse cubital artery and ulnar nerve

e. common interosseous artery and median nerve

219. *Which actions exert pressure on the intertuberal (bicipital) bursa and elicit pain if the bursa is inflamed?*

a. flexion of the elbow, flexion of the shoulder

b. extension of the elbow, flexion of the shoulder

c. flexion of the elbow, extension of the shoulder

d. extension of the elbow, extension of the shoulder

e. extension of the elbow only

220. *A horse with a laceration in the skin overlying the accessory carpal bone requires local anesthesia of which nerve to suture the wound?*

a. radial nerve

b. ulnar nerve

c. median nerve

d. musculocutaneous nerve

e. axillary nerve

221. *The collateral radial artery, which is an important source of nutrients for the radial nerve in the brachial region, arises from which vessel?*

a. caudal circumflex humeral artery

b. brachial artery

c. deep brachial artery

d. collateral ulnar artery

e. axillary artery

222. *The lacertus fibrosus is a tendon of insertion of the:*

a. extensor carpi radialis muscle

b. coracobrachialis muscle

c. brachialis muscle

d. biceps brachii muscle

e. triceps brachii muscle

223. *The suprascapular nerve is most easily injured by crushing against the:*

a. acromion process

b. tuber spinae

c. cranial border of the scapula

d. caudal border of the scapula

e. major tuberosity of the humerus

224. *Transection of the axillary nerve near its origin results in dysfunction of all of the following **except** the:*

a. deltoideus muscle

b. teres minor muscle

c. supraspinatus muscle

d. caudal belly of the subscapularis muscle

e. teres major muscle

225. *The oval window of the inner ear is covered by the:*

a. base of the stapes

b. head of the incus

c. long crus of the incus

d. tensor tympani muscle

e. tympanic membrane

Correct answers are on pages 89-99.

Horses, continued

226. *The stylomastoid foramen provides passage for the:*

   a. chorda tympani nerve
   b. mental artery
   c. mandibular nerve
   d. facial nerve
   e. middle meningeal artery

227. *Jugular venipuncture is more safely performed in the cranial half of the neck because the external jugular vein is separated from the common carotid artery by the:*

   a. sternocephalicus muscle
   b. omohyoideus muscle
   c. sternothyroideus muscle
   d. omotransversarius muscle
   e. longus capitis muscle

228. *The cranial subligamentous nuchal bursa (atlantal bursa) is situated between the funicular portion of the nuchal ligament and the neural arch of the atlas. Greatest pressure on this bursa results from contraction of the:*

   a. rhomboideus muscle
   b. longissimus cervicis muscle
   c. serratus ventralis cervicis muscle
   d. longissimus capitis et altantis muscle
   e. longus capitis muscle

229. *Concerning the mandibular lymph nodes of horses, which statement is **least** accurate?*

   a. They lie in the intermandibular space.
   b. They lie along each side of the omohyoideus muscle.
   c. They are covered only by the skin and a thin layer of fascia and cutaneous muscle.
   d. They drain lymph from the structures of the caudal cervical and cranial thoracic regions.
   e. They are readily palpable, even when not enlarged.

230. *Viborg's triangle is bounded by the:*

   a. linguofacial vein, mandibular ramus and tendon of the sternomandibularis muscle
   b. facial vein, maxillary vein and mandibular ramus
   c. linguofacial vein, omohyoideus muscle and caudal border of the mandibular ramus
   d. facial vein, mandibular ramus and omohyoideus muscle
   e. tendon of the sternomandibularis muscle, maxillary vein and cranial border of the mandibular ramus

231. *The extrinsic muscles of the tongue are the:*

   a. styloglossus, hyoglossus and geniohyoideus
   b. genioglossus, styloglossus and mylohyoideus
   c. hyoglossus, styloglossus and genioglossus
   d. genioglossus, geniohyoideus and sternohyoideus
   e. styloglossus, longus capitis and thryohyoideus

232. *Concerning the palatoglossal arch of horses, which statement is **least** accurate?*

   a. It is frequently referred to as the rostral pillar of the soft palate.
   b. It is a short, thick fold on each side, passing from the oral surface of the soft palate to the lateral border of the tongue.
   c. It forms the rostral boundary of the tonsillar sinus (fossa) containing the palatine tonsil.
   d. It partially obstructs the upper airway to cause "roaring" in horses with recurrent laryngeal nerve damage.
   e. It forms the lateral boundary of the pharyngeal opening.

233. *The dorsal oblique muscle of the eyeball is innervated by:*

   a. cranial nerve III
   b. cranial nerve IV
   c. cranial nerve V
   d. cranial nerve VI
   e. cranial nerve VII

234. *Light passes from outside of the eye through the structures and media of the eye in which sequence?*

a. cornea, aqueous humor, lens, vitreous humor and retina
b. cornea, aqueous humor, anterior chamber, lens, posterior chamber and retina
c. cornea, anterior chamber, iris, aqueous humor, lens and retina
d. cornea, pupil, iris, lens, vitreous humor and retina
e. cornea, anterior chamber, aqueous humor, lens, posterior chamber and retina

235. *The perilymph (exolymph) of the inner ear is continuous with the cerebrospinal fluid through the:*

a. facial canal
b. endolymphatic duct
c. scala vestibuli
d. cochlear duct
e. eustachian duct

236. *A nasogastric tube can be conveniently passed through the:*

a. dorsal nasal meatus
b. middle nasal meatus
c. ventral nasal meatus
d. common nasal meatus
e. frontal nasal meatus

237. *The transverse diameter of the cranial pelvic aperture (pelvic inlet) is measured between the:*

a. sacral promontory and cranial border of the pubis
b. two psoas minor tubercles near the middle of the body (shaft) of the ilium
c. auricular surfaces between 2 ilia
d. third sacral vertebra and pelvic symphysis
e. points of the ischium

238. *The caudal extension of the peritoneal cavity between the rectum and reproductive organs is termed the:*

a. rectogenital pouch or excavation
b. vesicogenital pouch or excavation
c. pararectal fossa
d. pubovesical pouch or excavation
e. genitoperitoneal evagination

239. *The testis is covered by a thick capsule of dense white connective tissue called the:*

a. dartos
b. parietal layer of the vaginal tunic
c. visceral layer of the vaginal tunic
d. tunica albuginea
e. internal spermatic fascia

240. *The ejaculatory duct of horses is formed by the conjoined:*

a. ductus deferens and prostate gland duct
b. prostate gland and vesicular gland (seminal vesicle) ducts
c. ductus deferens and bulbourethral gland openings
d. prostate gland openings and urethral crest
e. ductus deferens and duct of the vesicular gland (seminal vesicle)

241. *The main blood supply to the equine penis is via the:*

a. external pudendal artery
b. perineal artery
c. internal pudendal artery
d. testicular artery
e. obturator artery

242. *The "tail setting" operation in horses involves transection of the:*

a. sacrocaudalis ventralis lateralis muscle
b. sacrocaudalis ventralis medialis muscle
c. sacrocaudalis dorsalis lateralis and medialis muscles
d. coccygeus muscle
e. sacrocaudalis ventralis lateralis and medialis muscles

Correct answers are on pages 89-99.

Horses, continued

243. *The tendon of the accessory gluteal muscle is most commonly damaged due to stretching in harness racing horses. The action on the coxofemoral (hip) joint that places the greatest tension on this muscle (tension is applied during the relaxed phase of the stride for this muscle) is:*

   a. flexion
   b. extension
   c. abduction
   d. adduction
   e. inward rotation

244. *The external and internal parts of the internal lamina of the prepuce of the horse are continuous at the level of the:*

   a. preputial frenulum
   b. preputial orifice
   c. preputial ring
   d. attachment of the retractor penis muscle
   e. junction of the glans penis with the prepuce

245. *Which arteries are found in the broad ligament?*

   a. ovarian, middle uterine and deep caudal epigastric arteries
   b. uterine, ovarian and uterine branch of the vaginal (urogenital) arteries
   c. ovarian, deep cranial epigastric and uterine branch of the pudendal arteries
   d. middle uterine, deep cranial epigastric and ovarian branch of the cystic arteries
   e. cranial uterine, ovarian and superficial caudal epigastric arteries

246. *Which muscle most aids in voiding urine or semen from the penis?*

   a. ischiocavernous muscle
   b. ischiourethralis muscle
   c. retractor penis muscle
   d. bulbospongiosus muscle
   e. urethralis muscle

247. *Immediately following defecation, the caudally displaced anus is repositioned by action of the:*

   a. coccygeus muscle
   b. rectococcygeus muscle
   c. levator ani muscle
   d. sacrocaudalis dorsalis lateralis muscle
   e. sacrocaudalis ventralis medialis muscle

248. *The tunica albuginea is a layer of white fibrous connective tissue covering the:*

   a. abdominal tunic and penis
   b. testis and dartos muscle
   c. penis and testis
   d. dartos muscle and prepuce
   e. prepuce and abdominal tunic

249. *The terminal branches of the internal iliac artery are the:*

   a. cranial gluteal and internal pudendal arteries
   b. caudal gluteal and internal pudendal arteries
   c. caudal gluteal and external pudendal arteries
   d. dorsal and ventral perineal arteries
   e. external pudendal and dorsal perineal muscles

250. *In horses, which of the following is **not** required to maintain the pelvic limb in the extended position?*

   a. patellar fibrocartilage
   b. medial patellar ligament
   c. peroneus (fibularis) tertius muscle
   d. superficial digital flexor muscle
   e. interosseus medius muscle

251. *In horses, the pudendoepigastric trunk:*

   a. arises from the external iliac artery
   b. arises usually from the femoral artery
   c. gives off the caudal deep epigastric artery just before passing through the superficial inguinal ring
   d. passes through the vaginal ring

e. terminates as the caudal superficial epigastric and external pudendal arteries

252. *The femoral ring and the superficial inguinal ring are separated by the:*

a. pectineus muscle
b. prepubic tendon
c. inguinal ligament
d. symphysial tendon
e. body (shaft) of the ilium

253. *Which synovial joint capsule is the largest and most distensible?*

a. tarsometatarsal joint
b. proximal intertarsal joint
c. distal intertarsal joint
d. middle intertarsal joint
e. tibiotarsal or tarsocrural joint

254. *Which hoof structure does* **not** *contain nerve fibers?*

a. white line or zone (junction of epidermal and dermal lamellae)
b. clinical white line (junction of the sole and wall)
c. coronary corium
d. digital cushion
e. corium of the frog

255. *Which of the following supplies the germinal epithelium that produces the stratum medium of the hoof wall?*

a. perioplic corium
b. coronary corium
c. lamellar corium
d. corium of the sole
e. corium of the frog

256. *The main arterial supply in the metatarsal region is positioned on the:*

a. dorsolateral surface between metatarsal bones III and IV

b. dorsomedial surface between metatarsal bones II and III
c. plantar surface between metatarsal bone III and the interosseus medius muscle
d. plantar lateral surface between the flexor tendons and the interosseus medius muscle
e. plantar medial surface between the flexor tendons and the interosseus medius muscle

257. *Concerning colloquial terms for musculoskeletal conditions, which statement is* **least** *accurate?*

a. Capped hock describes inflammation of the subcutaneous calcaneal bursa.
b. Curb describes inflammation and thickening of the long plantar ligament.
c. Thoroughpin describes inflammation of the tarsal sheath of the deep digital flexor tendon.
d. Bog spavin describes synovitis of the femoropatellar joint capsule.
e. Quittor describes necrotic infection of the collateral cartilages of the distal phalanx.

258. *Femoral nerve paralysis (crural paralysis) affects the:*

a. obturatorius externus muscle
b. gemellus muscle
c. quadriceps femoris muscle
d. sartorius muscle
e. adductor muscle

259. *In repairing a mid-body fracture of tibia, which approach to the tibia would disturb the* **fewest** *muscles, nerves and vessels?*

a. lateral
b. caudal
c. caudomedial
d. craniomedial
e. caudolateral

Correct answers are on pages 89-99.

Horses, continued

260. *The primary anatomic structure involved with surgery to relieve the pain associated with bone spavin is the:*

   a. lateral digital extensor tendon
   b. peroneus (fibularis) tertius muscle
   c. metatarsal bones II and IV
   d. medial ridge of the femoral trochlea
   e. medial (cunean) tendon of the cranialis tibialis

261. *In the pelvic limb of horses, the accessory ligament (inferior check ligament) is a part of which muscle?*

   a. long digital extensor
   b. deep digital flexor
   c. tibialis cranialis
   d. peroneus (fibularis) tertius
   e. superficial digital flexor

262. *The visceral layer of the serous pericardium is:*

   a. firmly fused to the fibrous pericardium
   b. also known as the serocardium and is loosely attached to the fibrous pericardium
   c. also known as the epicardium and is firmly attached to the heart muscle
   d. covered on its outer surface with pericardial mediastinal pleura
   e. also known as the endopericardium and is covered on its outer surface with pericardial serous pleura

263. *The equine lung has relatively fewer visible external fissures as compared with the lung of other species. In horses, the lobes have fused to provide more functional pulmonary tissue. Because of this fusion, which lobe is considered **absent** in horses?*

   a. right cranial lobe
   b. right middle lobe
   c. right caudal lobe
   d. accessory lobe
   e. left caudal lobe

264. *What structure lies in the mediastinal recess of horses?*

   a. caudal vena cava
   b. right phrenic nerve
   c. thymus in young animals
   d. accessory lobe of the right lung
   e. cranial vena cava

265. *At the approximate level of the seventh intercostal space, the correct dorsoventral sequence of the thoracic visceral structures listed below is:*

   a. thoracic aorta, caudal vena cava, esophagus
   b. caudal vena cava, thoracic aorta, esophagus
   c. esophagus, caudal vena cava, thoracic aorta
   d. esophagus, thoracic aorta, caudal vena cava
   e. thoracic aorta, esophagus, caudal vena cava

266. *An abdominal incision in the xiphoid region would most likely expose the:*

   a. stomach
   b. liver
   c. apex of the cecum
   d. spleen
   e. greater omentum

267. *Concerning the inguinal ligament of horses, which statement is most accurate?*

   a. It is an aponeurotic thickening and not a true ligament.
   b. It passes across the cranial surface of the pubis, connecting both iliopubic emenences.
   c. It passes through the inguinal canal.
   d. It is the origin of the retractor costae muscle.
   e. It forms a part of the pelvic diaphragm.

268. *The structure located immediately deep to the right paralumbar fossa is the:*

   a. base of the cecum
   b. descending (small) colon
   c. major portion of the small intestine
   d. pelvic flexure of the ascending (great) colon
   e. duodenal flexure of the ascending (great) colon

269. The equine large intestine is characterized by:

    a. a distinct ileocolic orifice
    b. a descending colon divided into right, left, dorsal and ventral parts
    c. an ascending colon with sacculations (haustra) and 2 bands (taeniae) throughout its length
    d. a descending colon with sacculations (haustra) and 3 bands (taeniae) along its most caudal portion
    e. a pelvic flexure

270. The stomach of normal horses is:

    a. situated mostly in the left half of the abdominal cavity
    b. always covered by the rib cage
    c. located caudal to the major portion of the liver
    d. all of the above
    e. none of the above

271. Concerning the cranial mesenteric artery, which statement is **least** accurate?

    a. It is a paired vessel whose branches supply blood to the kidneys.
    b. It vascularizes mainly the small intestine, cecum and major portion of the colon.
    c. This vessel and some of its branches are sometimes the site of aneurysm.
    d. It courses within the root of the mesentery.
    e. Migrating larvae of *Strongylus vulgaris* may damage it, causing endarteritis.

272. The equine kidney is characterized by:

    a. a multilobulated external appearance
    b. 2 terminal recesses into which excretory ducts of the cranial and caudal poles empty
    c. adrenal (suprarenal) glands lying along the kidney's lateral borders
    d. absence of a renal pelvis
    e. a gray-green medulla and bright red cortex on cut section

273. If a line is drawn between the tuber coxae and the point of the shoulder on the right side of a horse and a biopsy needle is inserted at the twelfth intercostal space along this line, which structure would be punctured first?

    a. spleen
    b. gallbladder
    c. stomach
    d. liver
    e. descending duodenum

Pigs

N.G. Ghoshal

274. The mammalian liver has, in general, 4 basic lobes that are partially or completely separated by external fissures. In some species, the lateral and medial lobes are further subdivided incompletely by secondary fissures. What structures are **absent** in pigs?

    a. gallbladder and common bile duct
    b. divided cranial and caudal lobes
    c. papillary process of the caudate lobe and caudate ligament
    d. divided medial and lateral lobes
    e. mamillary process of the lateral lobe and gallbladder

Correct answers are on pages 89-99.

Pigs, continued

275. In the literature, it is claimed that the ischiatic tuber does not fuse with the body of the ischium for a variable time. In young pigs, sometimes the ischiatic tuber is detached by the traction of the powerful "hamstring" muscles, which include the:

   a. semimembranous and adductor muscles
   b. semitendinosus and gluteobiceps muscles
   c. adductor and gracilis muscles
   d. gastrocnemius and gluteobiceps muscles
   e. biceps femoris and semimembranous muscles

276. In pigs, the epiphyseal plate between the supraglenoid tuber (tubercle) and the scapula is said to close/ossify at about 1 year of age. Before that time, if the epiphyseal plate becomes separated by injury, the animal shows a change in gait and posture. Which muscles are most likely to be involved?

   a. supraspinatus and subscapularis muscles
   b. triceps brachii and suprascapularis muscles
   c. coracobrachialis and infraspinatus muscles
   d. biceps brachii and coracobrachialis muscles
   e. subscapularis and infraspinatus muscles

277. In suckling newborn pigs, occasionally the "needle teeth" are clipped to prevent injury to the sow's nipples. In this process, which tooth is **not** clipped?

   a. deciduous "corner" incisor of the upper dental arcade
   b. deciduous canine of the upper dental arcade
   c. deciduous "corner" incisor of the lower dental arcade
   d. deciduous canine of the lower dental arcade
   e. deciduous first incisor of the upper dental arcade

278. In boars, which teeth are used as defensive weapons?

   a. incisors
   b. canines
   c. premolars
   d. molars
   e. wolf teeth

279. The teeth of the upper dental arcade are innervated by the:

   a. infraorbital nerve
   b. ophthalmic nerve
   c. mandibular nerve
   d. lingual nerve
   e. hypoglossal nerve

280. Which artery supplies blood to the teeth of the lower dental arcade?

   a. infraorbital artery
   b. facial artery
   c. inferior alveolar artery
   d. transverse facial artery
   e. lingual artery

281. Arrangements and configurations of the nasal conchae are frequently examined at necropsy of young pigs with atrophic rhinitis. In reference to the teeth, where is the nasal cavity sectioned for evaluation or scoring the degree of involvement and/or damage?

   a. third premolar
   b. first molar
   c. third upper incisor
   d. interdental space between second premolar and canine tooth
   e. canine tooth

282. In domestic animals, lymphatic tissue accumulations are found in several locations in the pharyngeal mucosa, called the tonsils. In pigs, which tonsillar structure is **absent**?

   a. paraepiglottic tonsil
   b. lingual tonsil
   c. palatine tonsil
   d. tonsil of the soft palate
   e. pharyngeal tonsil

283. During collection of blood from the cranial vena cava, the right side is preferred so as to avoid injury to the:

a. thyroid gland, left brachiocephalic artery and thymus

b. left phrenic nerve, thymus and heart

c. thoracic duct, thyroid gland and left phrenic nerve

d. heart, left phrenic nerve and thymus

e. left brachiocephalic artery, thymus and thyroid gland

284. *Which site is commonly used for thoracentesis (paracentesis of the thoracic cavity) in pigs?*

a. 6th intercostal space on either side, slightly dorsal to the costochondral joint

b. 7th intercostal space on either side, slightly dorsal to the costochrondral joint

c. 3rd intercostal space on the left side, about 1 cm ventral to the olecranon

d. 4th intercostal space on the right side, about 5 cm dorsal to the olecranon

e. 8th intercostal space on either side, about 2 cm ventral to the olecranon

285. *Which nerve provides parasympathetic innervation to the stomach of pigs?*

a. dorsal and ventral vagal trunks

b. minor splanchnic and phrenic nerves

c. major splanchnic and epigastric nerves

d. phrenic nerve and lateral vagal trunk

e. medial vagal trunk and epigastric nerve

286. *Among the cardiac valves in pigs, which lies most cranially?*

a. pulmonary valve

b. aortic valve

c. right atrioventricular valve

d. left atrioventricular valve

e. pulmonoaortic valve

287. *Irrespective of its size and shape, the porcine heart can be readily distinguished from the heart of other species because:*

a. only the brachiocephalic artery (trunk) arises separately from the aortic arch

b. the right subclavian and brachiocephalic arteries arise separately from the aortic arch

c. the brachiocephalic artery and the bicarotid trunk separate independently from the aortic arch

d. the left subclavian and brachiocephalic arteries arise separately from the aortic arch

e. only the right subclavian artery arises separately from the aortic arch

288. *The liver is firmly attached to the abdominal surface of the diaphragm by several ligaments. Which hepatic ligament is* **absent** *in pigs?*

a. right triangular ligament

b. left triangular ligament

c. caudate ligament

d. coronary ligament

e. falciform ligament

289. *Concerning the location of the intestines in pigs, which statement is* **least** *accurate?*

a. The descending duodenum and ascending colon lie on the right side of the abdomen.

b. The transverse colon passes from right to left, cranial to the mesenteric root.

c. The ascending duodenum and descending colon are on the left side of the abdominal cavity.

d. The caudal flexure of the duodenum courses from right to left, caudal to the mesenteric root.

e. The caudal flexure of the colon courses from right to left, cranial to the mesenteric root.

290. *The ascending colon in pigs receives its blood supply from the:*

a. left and right colic arteries

b. right and middle colic arteries

c. right colic artery and colic branches of the cranial mesenteric artery

d. middle and left colic arteries

e. cranial mesenteric branches of the left colic artery

Correct answers are on pages 89-99.

Pigs, continued

291. *In pigs, which of the following does **not** drain into the portal vein?*

    a. pancreas
    b. liver
    c. stomach
    d. small intestine
    e. spleen

292. *The gallbladder of pigs is located between the:*

    a. left and right lobes of the liver
    b. quadrate and caudate lobes of the liver
    c. quadrate and right medial lobes of the liver
    d. papillary and caudate processes of the liver
    e. quadrate and left medial lobes of the liver

293. *In pigs, epidural anesthesia is administered at:*

    a. the sacrocaudal joint
    b. the 1st intercaudal joint
    c. a site 1 inch cranial to a transverse line drawn between the tubera coxae
    d. the lumbosacral joint
    e. the joint between the last 2 lumbar vertebrae

294. *Which nerve does **not** exit through the orbitorotundum foramen in pigs?*

    a. optic nerve
    b. adducent nerve
    c. ophthalmic nerve
    d. oculomotor nerve
    e. trochlear nerve

295. *Damage to the lateral thoracic nerve would result in motor dysfunction of which muscle?*

    a. rectus abdominis, rectus femoris, cutaneus trunci
    b. caudal preputial (when present), rectus abdominis, external intercostal
    c. external intercostal, cranial preputial, rectus abdominis

    d. cranial preputial, caudal preputial (when present), cutaneus trunci
    e. external intercostal, internal intercostal, cutaneus trunci

296. *Which of the following is **not** a natural orifice in the wall of the abdomen?*

    a. esophageal hiatus
    b. umbilicus
    c. epiploic (omental) foramen
    d. deep inguinal ring
    e. cranial pelvic aperture (pelvic inlet)

297. *The ischiatic (sciatic) nerve leaves the confines of the pelvic cavity via the:*

    a. obturator foramen
    b. major (greater) ischiatic foramen
    c. minor (lesser) ischiatic foramen
    d. caudal pelvic aperture (pelvic outlet)
    e. cranial pelvic aperture (pelvic inlet)

298. *The scrotum develops as a diverticulum from the caudoventral wall of the trunk; therefore, most of the structures of the abdominal wall have extensions into the scrotal wall. In "open" castration, the last layer incised would correspond to which layer of the abdominal wall?*

    a. fascia on the external abdominal oblique muscle
    b. internal abdominal oblique muscle
    c. transversalis fascia
    d. parietal layer of the abdominal peritoneum
    e. skin

299. *Concerning the penis of boars, which statement is **least** accurate?*

    a. Both cranial and caudal preputial muscles are usually present.
    b. The penis forms a sigmoid flexure that is prescrotal.
    c. The os penis is located cranial to the sigmoid flexure.

d. Parasympathetic stimulation causes erection, whereas sympathetic stimulation results in ejaculation.

e. The major blood supply of the penis comes from the artery of the penis near the ischiatic arch.

300. Scrotal hernia is most accurately described as a loop of the intestine that has passed through the:

a. superficial inguinal ring
b. vaginal ring and is found between the vaginal tunic and dartos muscle
c. deep inguinal ring to the outside of the vaginal ring
d. vaginal ring and is found between the visceral and parietal layers of the vaginal tunic (inside the vaginal cavity)
e. deep inguinal ring and is found between the vaginal tunic and dartos muscle

301. Concerning the kidneys of pigs, which statement is **least** accurate?

a. They are smooth externally but lobated internally.
b. A hilus is present.
c. A renal pelvis is absent.
d. Renal calices are present.

e. They are bean shaped, flattened and covered by a capsule.

302. The proximal end of the ulna (olecranon) in pigs is said to fuse with the body of the ulna at 3 to 3 1/2 years of age. If the epiphyseal (growth) plate between them is separated by injury, which muscle group is affected?

a. flexor muscles of the shoulder joint
b. extensor muscles of the elbow joint
c. extensor muscles of the carpal joint
d. flexor muscles of the elbow joint
e. extensor muscles of the shoulder joint

303. In domestic quadrupeds, the "pelvic diaphragm" is not well developed because most of the pelvic viscera are supported by the bony floor of the pelvic cavity. Which muscles are part of the pelvic diaphragm?

a. rectococcygeus and levator ani muscles
b. coccygeus and sacrocaudalis medialis muscles
c. levator ani and coccygeus muscles
d. sacrocaudalis ventralis medialis and lateralis muscles
e. sacrocaudalis lateralis and rectococcygeus muscles

Ruminants

N.G. Ghoshal

304. In ruminants, which bones contain alveoli in which teeth develop?

a. incisive and frontal bones
b. mandible and incisive bone
c. maxilla and mandible
d. frontal bone and maxilla
e. stylohyoid and incisive bones

305. In estimating the age of an animal, various characteristics of teeth are considered, such as form, number, type, structure and periods of eruption. Which surface of the teeth is frequently used in determining age in ruminants?

a. labial surface
b. lingual surface
c. buccal surface
d. contact surface
e. occlusal surface

Correct answers are on pages 89-99.

Ruminants, continued

306. *Which blood vessel supplies the teeth of the lower (inferior) dental arcade in ruminants?*

    a. infraorbital artery
    b. inferior alveolar artery
    c. superficial temporal artery
    d. facial artery
    e. minor palatine artery

307. *Which blood vessel supplies the teeth of the upper (superior) dental arcade in ruminants?*

    a. inferior alveolar artery
    b. transverse facial artery
    c. major palatine artery
    d. infraorbital artery
    e. rostral deep temporal artery

308. *Which nerve supplies the teeth of the upper (superior) dental arcade in ruminants?*

    a. infraorbital nerve
    b. inferior alveolar nerve
    c. lingual nerve
    d. supraorbital nerve
    e. dorsal buccal branch of the facial nerve

309. *Which nerve supplies the teeth of the lower (inferior) dental arcade in ruminants?*

    a. infraorbital nerve
    b. ventral buccal branch of the facial nerve
    c. inferior alveolar nerve
    d. lingual nerve
    e. buccal nerve

310. *The blood vessels and nerves that supply the upper cheek teeth in ruminants traverse the:*

    a. palatine canal
    b. supraorbital canal
    c. mandibular canal
    d. sphenopalatine foramen
    e. infraorbital canal

311. *The blood vessels and nerves that supply the lower cheek teeth in ruminants traverse the:*

    a. mandibular canal
    b. infraorbital canal
    c. optic canal
    d. nasolacrimal canal
    e. hypoglossal canal

312. *Which paranasal sinus is present in the ox but* **absent** *in small ruminants?*

    a. frontal sinus
    b. maxillary sinus
    c. palatine sinus
    d. sphenoid sinus
    e. lacrimal sinus

313. *In ruminant breeds with horns, which paranasal sinus is characterized by postorbital, nuchal and cornual diverticula?*

    a. maxillary sinus
    b. caudal frontal sinus
    c. palatine sinus
    d. ethmoid sinus
    e. dorsal and ventral conchal sinuses

314. *To avoid invading the frontal paranasal sinus, calves should be dehorned:*

    a. before 4 months of age
    b. at about 6 months of age
    c. at about 8 months of age
    d. before 1 year of age
    e. after 18 months of age

315. *In ruminants, the paranasal sinuses drain into or communicate with the:*

    a. dorsal nasal meatus
    b. middle nasal meatus
    c. ventral nasal meatus
    d. ethmoid meatus
    e. middle nasal and ethmoid meati

316. *It is important to know the boundaries of the caudal frontal sinus of oxen for trephining and drainage. Which of the following represents the rostral limit of the caudal frontal sinus?*

a. region of the poll (intercornual protuberance)

b. temporal line

c. interfrontal suture

d. an oblique septum that runs caudomedially from the middle of the orbit to the midline (at the transverse plane of the caudal margin of the orbit)

e. a transverse line connecting the rostral margins of the orbits

317. *Which diverticulum poses difficulty while draining the caudal frontal sinus in oxen?*

a. nuchal diverticulum

b. cornual diverticulum

c. postorbital diverticulum

d. preorbital diverticulum

e. temporal diverticulum

318. *The temporal line is an important landmark for anesthetizing the bovine horn, which is a part of the:*

a. occipital bone

b. parietal bone

c. temporal bone

d. zygomatic bone

e. frontal bone

319. *Many nerves innervate the horn in oxen. The major nerve supplying the bovine horn is derived from the:*

a. frontal sinus branch

b. cornual nerve

c. infratrochlear nerve

d. branch of the second cervical spinal nerve

e. supraorbital nerve

320. *The major blood supply to the bovine horn is via the cornual artery, which is a branch of the:*

a. superficial temporal artery

b. caudal auricular artery

c. supraorbital artery

d. caudal deep temporal artery

e. external carotid artery

321. *Because bovine horn is innervated by several nerves, some veterinarians prefer to administer a ring block while dehorning cattle. Despite this procedure, complete desensitization of the horn is **not** accomplished because:*

a. the cornual nerve is difficult to anesthetize

b. a branch of the second cervical spinal nerve courses deep to caudal auricular muscles

c. blocking the infratrochlear nerve is not alway successful

d. the frontal sinus branch courses within the frontal paranasal sinus

e. the supraorbital nerve does not reach the base of the horn in all instances

322. *To anesthetize the cornual nerve in oxen, the anesthetic should be deposited subcutaneously:*

a. midway between the eye and the horn

b. between the medial canthus of the eye and the base of the horn

c. between the base of the ear and base of the horn

d. midway between the lateral canthus of the eye and the auditory meatus

e. 1-2 cm dorsal to the medial canthus of the eye

323. *If not removed completely during dehorning, the modified skin around the base of the bovine horn can continue to generate horny growth. This patch of skin is called the:*

a. glabrous skin

b. glossy skin

c. epikeras

d. scruff

e. deciduous skin

324. *The scent glands of goats are modified sebaceous glands that, unless resected or cauterized, produce a repulsive musky odor in milk and meat. Which site contains an abundance of these scent glands?*

a. chin region

b. dorsum of the trunk

c. interdigital space

d. inguinal region

e. caudomedial to the base of the horn

Correct answers are on pages 89-99.

Ruminants, continued

325. *In Peterson's eye block in oxen, anesthetic is deposited around which foramen?*

    a. optic foramen
    b. ethmoid foramen
    c. orbitorotundum foramen
    d. maxillary foramen
    e. sphenopalatine foramen

326. *Which cranial nerve does **not** emerge through the orbitorotundum foramen and innervate the bulbar (ocular) muscles and adnexa of the eyeball?*

    a. trochlear nerve
    b. abducent nerve
    c. ophthalmic nerve
    d. oculomotor nerve
    e. optic nerve

327. *In Peterson's eye block in cattle, the teeth of the upper (superior) dental arcade and the horns (when present) are simultaneously desensitized because the nerves supplying both of these structures are derived from the:*

    a. ophthalmic nerve
    b. maxillary nerve
    c. mandibular nerve
    d. oculomotor nerve
    e. abducent nerve

328. *In Peterson's eye block, which bony landmarks are used to locate the site for insertion of the needle?*

    a. frontal process of the mandible, coronoid process of the zygomatic bone, temporal process of the parietal bone
    b. temporal process of the mandible, frontal process of the parietal bone, coronoid process of the zygomatic bone
    c. styloid process of the temporal bone, temporal process of the parietal bone, frontal process of the zygomatic bone
    d. frontal process of the zygomatic bone, temporal process of the zygomatic bone, coronoid process of the mandible

    e. temporal process of the mandible, styloid process of the mandible, zygomatic process of the frontal bone

329. *In Peterson's eye block, which of the following might pose some difficulties while inserting the needle to arrive at the desired site?*

    a. zygomatic process of the mandible
    b. frontal crest of the basisphenoid bone
    c. lacrimal bulla and zygomatic arch
    d. pterygoid crest of the basisphenoid bone and coronoid process of the mandible
    e. zygomatic arch and coronoid process of the frontal bone

330. *If Peterson's eye block is not executed properly in cattle, the animal may die. Which of the following may cause such accidental death?*

    a. anesthetic reaching the brain via the ophthalmic artery
    b. exsanguination from laceration of the ophthalmic artery
    c. anesthetic reaching the brain via the subarachnoid space or via the emissary veins of the orbitorotundum foramen connected with the dural sinuses
    d. exsanguination from laceration of the cornual artery
    e. anesthetic reaching the brain via the internal carotid artery or via the cerebral arterial circle (of Willis)

331. *Which artery is present in the ox but **absent** in small ruminants?*

    a. facial artery
    b. transverse facial artery
    c. superficial temporal artery
    d. caudal auricular artery
    e. external ophthalmic artery

332. *Because jugular venipuncture is a common procedure in domestic animals, it is important to know the boundary of the jugular furrow (groove) among different species. A well-defined cranioventral boundary of the jugular*

*furrow in sheep is lacking because of **absence** of the:*

a. sternohyoideus muscle
b. sternothyroideus muscle
c. sternomandibularis muscle
d. omohyoideus muscle
e. omotransversarius muscle

333. *In small ruminants, which of the following is **absent** within the carotid sheath, including the pretracheal lamina?*

a. vagosympathetic trunk
b. common carotid artery
c. tracheal lymph duct
d. internal jugular vein
e. recurrent laryngeal nerve

334. *Bone marrow is sometimes aspirated from the ribs or sternum in oxen. Which ribs are widest and most accessible for this procedure?*

a. 4th and 5th ribs
b. 6th to 8th ribs
c. 1st to 3rd ribs
d. 9th and 10th ribs
e. 11th to 13th ribs

335. *Which site is frequently used for thoracentesis (thoracic paracentesis) in oxen?*

a. 6th or 7th intercostal space on the left or right side, slightly dorsal to the costochondral junction
b. 7th intercostal space on the right side, 3 cm ventral to the costochondral junction
c. 5th intercostal space on the left side, somewhat dorsal to the olecranon
d. 4th intercostal space on the right side, somewhat dorsal to the olecranon
e. 4th intercostal space on the left side, 3 cm ventral to the costochondral junction

336. *In cattle, local anesthesia of the paralumbar fossa involves anesthesia of all of the following **except** the:*

a. costoabdominal nerve
b. iliohypogastric nerve
c. ilioepigastric nerve
d. lateral thoracic nerve (sometimes)
e. ilioinguinal nerve

337. *Knowledge concerning the direction of fibers of the muscles of the lateral abdominal wall is very important in abdominal surgery. While making a paralumbar incision, you find a muscle layer whose fibers course cranioventrally or caudodorsally. This muscle is the:*

a. external abdominal oblique muscle
b. transversus abdominis muscle
c. internal abdominal oblique muscle
d. rectus abdominis muscle
e. costal part of the diaphragm

338. *In removing foreign bodies from the reticulum, the rumen is entered via the dorsal sac in the left paralumbar fossa. As the surgeon's hand advances cranially toward the reticulum, it passes over the:*

a. cranial and caudal ruminal pillars
b. cranial ruminal pillar and ruminoreticular fold
c. ruminoreticular fold and right longitudinal pillar
d. left longitudinal pillar and caudal ruminal pillar
e. ruminoreticular fold and left longitudinal pillar

339. *Parasympathetic innervation of the ruminant stomach is responsible for gastric motility and secretory activity. Any interruption of nervous stimuli to the tunica muscularis is likely to interfere with gastric function. Which nerves provide parasympathetic innervation to the ruminant stomach?*

a. major and minor splanchnic nerves
b. ventral and dorsal vagal trunks
c. medial vagal trunk and ramus parasympatheticus
d. ramus communicans and lateral vagal trunk
e. minor splanchnic nerve and medial vagal trunk

Correct answers are on pages 89-99.

Ruminants, continued

340. *Which structure in the thoracic cavity of ruminants, when enlarged or involved, could interfere with escape of gas from the rumen (belching or eructation) and/or gastric motility?*

  a. caudal mediastinal lymph node
  b. thoracic duct
  c. left tracheobronchial lymph node
  d. thoracic aorta
  e. left ventricle

341. *The peritoneum is a serous membrane that lines the abdominal cavity and part of the pelvic cavity, leaving a retroperitoneal part of the pelvic cavity caudally. When damaged, the peritoneum becomes inflamed more readily than other tissues. In males, the peritoneal cavity is a closed sac, but in females it communicates with the exterior of the body, increasing the chances of spreading infection (peritonitis) via the:*

  a. ovarian bursa
  b. abdominal openings of the uterine tubes
  c. deep inguinal rings
  d. caudal abdominal aperture or pelvic inlet
  e. openings on the diaphragm

342. *During rectal palpation, the peritoneal folds inside the pelvic cavity often serve as important landmarks for locating organs and/or structures in both sexes. The peritoneal reflection (excavation/pouch) located between the urinary bladder and the reproductive organs in either sex is called the:*

  a. pararectal fossa
  b. rectogenital excavation
  c. vesicogenital excavation
  d. pubovesical excavation
  e. pubic fossa

343. *Of the cardiac valves in ruminants, which is located most cranially?*

  a. pulmonary valve
  b. aortic valve
  c. right atrioventricular valve
  d. left atrioventricular valve
  e. pulmonoaortic valve

344. *Of the cardiac valves in ruminants, which lies most caudally and somewhat dorsally, at about the level of the left shoulder joint?*

  a. left atrioventricular valve
  b. pulmonary valve
  c. right atrioventricular valve
  d. aortic valve
  e. pulmonoaortic valve

345. *In oxen, only a relatively small surface area of the lung is accessible to auscultation and/or percussion because a greater part of the cranial thoracic wall lies deep to the large mass of the:*

  a. serratus ventralis thoracis muscle
  b. latissimus dorsi muscle
  c. long head of the triceps brachii muscle
  d. external abdominal oblique muscle
  e. ascending pectoral muscle

346. *In cattle, attempted passage of a stomach tube through the oral cavity is sometimes obstructed by the:*

  a. enlarged caudal extension of the soft palate
  b. large lingual tonsil
  c. constricted piriform recess of the laryngopharynx
  d. constricted palatopharyngeal arch
  e. torus linguae

347. *In congestive heart failure in cows, abnormal distention and pulsation are often seen in the external jugular vein, as well as in the "milk veins" (conjoined cranial superficial and caudal superficial epigastric veins), associated with ventral subcutaneous edema. Insufficiency and/or stenosis of which cardiac valve would manifest this condition?*

  a. aortic valve
  b. right atrioventricular valve
  c. pulmonary valve
  d. left atrioventricular valve
  e. pulmonoaortic valve

348. Twisting of the neck and head in calves (wryneck, torticollis) is occasionally caused by sprain or injury to the brachiocephalicus muscle during parturition. Which nerve innervates this muscle?

a. facial nerve
b. cervical spinal nerve
c. suprascapular nerve
d. accessory nerve
e. axillary nerve

349. In domestic ruminants, the relative size of the omasum varies. Concerning the size of the omasum and reticulum, which statement is most accurate?

a. The omasum is larger than the reticulum in cattle but smaller than the reticulum in sheep and goats.
b. The omasum is slightly smaller than the reticulum in cattle.
c. The omasum is much larger than the reticulum sheep and goats.
d. The omasum is approximately half as large as the reticulum in cattle.
e. The omasum and reticulum are of relatively equal size in all ruminants.

350. The omasum is usually located in the ventral half on the right side of the abdomen, underlying the area approximately between the 7th and 12th ribs, and is separated from the right abdominal wall by the:

a. greater omentum
b. lesser omentum
c. mesoduodenum
d. hepatic ligaments
e. epigastric ligaments

351. Which of the following is the "true" or "glandular" stomach in ruminants and does **not** form a part of the forestomach?

a. rumen
b. reticulum
c. omasum
d. abomasum

e. ruminoreticular complex

352. Abomasal displacement is common in some breeds of cattle. The condition is corrected by surgically fixing which structure to the dorsal part of the right flank?

a. greater omentum
b. lesser omentum
c. mesoduodenum
d. omental bursa
e. greater mesentery

353. Accumulation of gas in the abomasum produces a distinctive "ping" on simultaneous auscultation-percussion over the distended viscus. When auscultating and percussing the area between the right 7th and 13th ribs in a cow, how would you differentiate the "ping" produced by a right-displaced abomasum from that produced by a gas-distended cecum?

a. in both instances, the "ping" is located at the right paralumbar fossa
b. the "ping" produced by a distended cecum does not extend cranially, to the rib cage
c. the "ping" associated with a right-displaced abomasum is confined to an area within the rib cage
d. all of the above
e. the "ping" produced by a distended cecum is of a higher pitch than that associated with a right-displaced abomasum

354. Concerning the blood supply of the abomasum, which statement is **least** accurate?

a. The lesser curvature is supplied by the left gastric artery, as well as the right gastric branch of the hepatic artery.
b. The left gastroepiploic artery is a branch of the left gastric artery in ruminants and supplies a part of the greater curvature.
c. The left gastroepiploic artery is a branch of the splenic artery.
d. The right gastroepiploic artery is a branch of the hepatic artery.
e. The right gastroepiploic artery vascularizes part of the greater curvature.

Correct answers are on pages 89-99.

Ruminants, continued

355. *The ascending colon of ruminants receives its blood supply from the:*

  a. right colic artery and colic branches of the cranial mesenteric artery

  b. left colic artery and epigastric branches of the caudal duodenal artery

  c. middle colic artery and colic branches of the caudal mesenteric artery

  d. caudal colic artery

  e. colic branches of the left epigastric artery

356. *Concerning the general position of the intestines in ruminants, which statement is* ***least*** *accurate?*

  a. The ascending duodenum and the descending colon are on the left side of the abdominal cavity.

  b. The descending duodenum and the ascending colon lie on the right side of the abdomen.

  c. The caudal flexure of the duodenum courses from the right to the left side caudal to the mesenteric root.

  d. The ascending colon and cranial flexure of the duodenum lie close to the midline.

  e. The transverse colon passes from the right to the left cranial to the mesenteric root.

357. *For a paravertebral lumbar nerve block in cattle, the Cakala and Farquharson techniques are used. In the Farquharson method, the last thoracic and first 2 or 3 lumbar spinal nerves are anesthetized as they exit through the intervertebral foramina. In the Cakala method, these nerves are anesthetized as they cross the tips of transverse processes of some lumbar vertebrae. Which sites are used to block the ventral branches of T_{13}, L_1 and L_2 spinal nerves in the Cakala method?*

  a. to anesthetize T_{13}, anesthetic is deposited at the tip of the transverse process of the 11th thoracic vertebra

  b. to anesthetize L_1, anesthetic is deposited at the tip of the transverse process of the 2nd lumbar vertebra

  c. to anesthetize L_2, anesthetic is deposited at the tip of the transverse process of the 6th lumbar vertebra

  d. to anesthetize T_{13}, anesthetic is deposited at the tip of the transverse process of the 3rd lumbar vertebra

  e. to anesthetize T_{13}, L_1 and L_2, anesthetic is deposited at the tip of the transverse process of the 11th and 12th thoracic vertebrae

358. *At necropsy, the liver is always examined for gross lesions and inflammatory changes. Normally the borders of the liver are thin and sharp, except for the "rounded border," which is thick and located:*

  a. between the esophageal notch and the caudal vena cava

  b. between the caudate and quadrate lobes

  c. between the caudal vena cava and the right lobe

  d. adjacent to the caudate lobe and the gallbladder

  e. between the gallbladder and the esophageal notch

359. *Blood from which organ does* ***not*** *drain into the caudal vena cava?*

  a. liver

  b. stomach

  c. testis

  d. kidney

  e. adrenal (suprarenal) gland

360. *Blood from which organ does* ***not*** *drain into the portal vein?*

  a. pancreas

  b. small intestine

  c. spleen

  d. rectum

  e. cecum

361. *The gallbladder of ruminants is located between the:*

  a. left and right lobes of the liver

b. quadrate and right lobes of the liver

c. quadrate and caudate lobes of the liver

d. caudate and papillary processes of the caudate lobe of the liver

e. left medial and quadrate lobes of the liver

362. *In liver biopsy of the ox, the biopsy needle is inserted:*

a. at the 10th or 11th intercostal space on the right side, one-fourth of the length of the bony rib ventral to the vertebra

b. along a line drawn from the center of the left paralumbar fossa to the 13th intercostal space

c. at the 10th or 11th intercostal space on the left side, slightly dorsal to the costochondral junction

d. at the 13th intercostal space on the left side, slightly ventral to the costochondral junction

e. along a line drawn from the center of the left tuber coxae to the left olecranon, at the point of intersection with the last rib

363. *In a 3-year-old cow, which dental findings are most likely to be observed?*

a. a visible "neck" at the gum line on the permanent inferior (lower) central incisors (I_1)

b. inferior (lower) deciduous canine (DC/I_4) teeth still present, with recent eruption of the third permanent inferior incisors (I_3)

c. only the permanent inferior (lower) central incisors (I_3) present and in wear, with all other incisors deciduous

d. all incisor teeth still firmly anchored into their alveoli, allowing no movement of the teeth on digital manipulation

e. recent eruption of the superior (upper) corner incisors

364. *The largest blood vessel that directly or indirectly supplies the structures distal to the carpus in ruminants is the:*

a. common interosseous artery

b. radial artery

c. cranial superficial antebrachial artery

d. collateral ulnar artery

e. median artery

365. *The longest artery that supplies the distal regions of the pelvic limb of ruminants arises from the:*

a. femoral artery

b. popliteal artery

c. caudal femoral artery

d. external pudendal artery

e. caudal gluteal artery

366. *Damage to the suprascapular nerve near the neck of the scapula would result in motor dysfunction of the:*

a. biceps brachii and infraspinatus muscles

b. deltoideus and infraspinatus muscles

c. supraspinatus and biceps brachii muscles

d. supraspinatus and infraspinatus muscles

e. deltoideus and supraspinatus muscles

367. *The spinal nerve exiting the intervertebral foramen between the last cervical and first thoracic vertebrae is the:*

a. 7th cervical nerve

b. 1st thoracic nerve

c. 8th cervical nerve

d. 1st intercostal nerve

e. 6th cervical nerve

368. *Concerning the ninth rib of ruminants, which statement is **least** accurate?*

a. Morphologically it has a bony and a cartilaginous part.

b. Dorsally it articulates with the body of the 8th and 9th thoracic vertebrae.

c. It forms a synovial joint between its bony and cartilaginous parts, allowing lateral expansion of the rib cage during inspiration.

d. It is the longest of all of the ribs.

e. Dorsally it articulates with the 9th thoracic vertebra only.

Correct answers are on pages 89-99.

Ruminants, continued

369. *In which species is unilateral pleuritis **least** likely to spread to the opposite pleural hemicavity to cause generalized pleuritis?*

    a. both small and large ruminants
    b. ox and goat
    c. sheep and goat
    d. ox and sheep
    e. sheep only

370. *Reverse peristalsis, as in regurgitation of food for remastication, is easily accomplished in ruminants because:*

    a. the tunica muscularis is entirely striated (voluntary) throughout its course, and an abdominal segment of the esophagus is lacking
    b. the tunica muscularis consists entirely of smooth muscle that is very responsive to the increased vagal tone of ruminants
    c. the cranial two-thirds of the esophagus contains striated muscle, while the caudal one-third contains smooth muscle
    d. the esophagus has cervical, thoracic and short abdominal parts
    e. the abdominal segment consists of hypertrophied striated muscle with exceptional tone

371. *When an endotracheal tube is inserted beyond the level of the third intercostal space in the ox, it is most likely to cause atelectasis (collapse) of the:*

    a. middle lobe of the right lung
    b. caudal lobe of the left lung
    c. accessory lobe of the right lung
    d. cranial lobe of the right lung
    e. caudal lobe of the right lung

372. *In aspiration biopsy of the superficial cervical lymph nodes of cattle, the biopsy needle must pass through the:*

    a. cervical part of the trapezius muscle
    b. subclavius muscle
    c. omotransversarius and cleidocephalicus muscles

    d. deltoideus muscle
    e. supraspinatus muscle

373. *In cattle, which structures are visible after incision into the right paralumbar fossa?*

    a. jejunum and ascending duodenum
    b. descending duodenum and cecum
    c. greater omentum and descending duodenum
    d. cecum and jejunum
    e. lesser omentum and ascending duodenum

374. *Penile paralysis and prolapse in bulls can be associated with paralysis of the:*

    a. caudal preputial muscle
    b. retractor penis muscle
    c. ischiocavernosus muscle
    d. bulbospongiosus muscle
    e. external anal sphincter muscle

375. *Concerning uterine caruncles, which statement is **least** accurate?*

    a. They are endometrial sites for the attachment of fetal membranes.
    b. They are present in ruminants.
    c. They form placentomes for fetal-maternal interface, in conjunction with fetal cotyledons.
    d. They remain constant in position but enlarge greatly during pregnancy.
    e. They tend to change position but remain the same size during pregnancy.

376. *You are called upon to treat a cow whose mammary gland is sagging along the midline (intermammary groove), with the teats pointing laterally. This condition is most likely the result of:*

    a. rupture of the medial suspensory ligament of the udder and the cow's not being milked for 2 days
    b. rupture of the lateral suspensory ligament of the udder
    c. rupture of both medial and lateral suspensory ligaments of the udder

---

d. obstruction of the lactiferous sinus, resulting in accumulated milk in the udder

e. rupture of the prepubic tendon

377. *An enlargement in the area just cranial to the base of the scrotum in a bull is most likely caused by:*

a. blockage of the urethra due to urinary calculi

b. laceration of the prepuce

c. a scrotal hernia

d. hematoma of the penis

e. an umbilical hernia

378. *Concerning the median caudal (coccygeal) artery of the ox, which statement is **least** accurate?*

a. The median caudal artery is commonly used for evaluating the pulse.

b. The median caudal artery is the caudal extension of the median sacral artery, which, in turn, is the continuation of the abdominal aorta.

c. The median caudal artery courses within the hemal arch of the ventral crest of the caudal vertebrae, which are sometimes fused, enclosing the artery.

d. The median caudal artery is too deep for pulse evaluation but can be used for collection of arterial blood for blood gas analysis.

e. Blood samples are frequently taken from the median caudal vessels.

379. *A problem in dairy cows is frostbite of the teats, resulting in a "hard milker." This condition involves the:*

a. lactiferous duct

b. lactiferous sinus

c. papillary duct

d. annular fold between the glandular and the teat (papillary) parts of the lactiferous sinus

e. teat (papillary) part of the lactiferous sinus

380. *On rectal palpation in a bull, you detect a signet ring-like structure (transverse band) surrounding the pelvic urethra. This structure is the:*

a. bulbourethral (Cowper's) gland

b. body of the prostate gland

c. portion of the vesicular gland

d. ampulla of the ductus deferens

e. thickening of the urethralis muscle

381. *Paralysis of the fibular (common peroneal) nerve in the vicinity of the lateral tibial condyle of the ox would most likely result in impaired:*

a. extension of the digits and flexion of the hock

b. flexion of the digits and extension of the hock

c. extension of the hock and stifle

d. flexion of the hock and coxofemoral joints

e. flexion of the digits only

382. *Stenosis (occlusion) of which heart valve is most likely to cause an immediate backflow of blood into the lungs in ruminants?*

a. aortic valve

b. pulmonary valve

c. left atrioventricular valve

d. right atrioventricular valve

e. pulmonoaortic valve

383. *For amputation of the third (medial) digit of the pelvic limb of an unanesthetized ox, local anesthesia is used to block the:*

a. medial plantar, and superficial and deep fibular (peroneal) nerves

b. medial plantar and superficial fibular (peroneal) nerves only

c. lateral plantar, and superficial and deep fibular (peroneal) nerves

d. medial plantar, plantar metatarsals, and deep fibular (peroneal) nerves

e. medial plantar, lateral plantar, and superficial and deep fibular (peroneal) nerves

Correct answers are on pages 89-99.

Ruminants, continued

384. Concerning the kidneys, which statement is least accurate?

 a. A hilus is present in all ruminants.
 b. Their external morphology is smooth in small ruminants.
 c. In the ox, externally the kidneys are lobulated.
 d. A renal pelvis is absent in the ox, sheep and goat.
 e. Renal calices are present in the ox.

385. Which muscle is affected in femoral nerve paralysis?

 a. adductor muscle
 b. gemellus muscle
 c. quadriceps femoris muscle
 d. pectineus muscle
 e. intrapelvic portion of the external obturator muscle

386. The conjugate diameter of the cranial pelvic aperture (pelvic inlet) is measured between the:

 a. 2 psoas minor tubercles near the middle of the ilial body
 b. 2 iliopubic eminences
 c. sacral promontory and cranial border of the pubis
 d. 3rd caudal vertebra and pelvic floor
 e. auricular surfaces between both ilia

387. During incision of a bull's penis for removal of urinary calculi, excessive hemorrhage may be avoided if one does not incise the:

 a. dorsal artery of the penis
 b. artery of the bulb of the penis
 c. dorsal perineal artery
 d. deep artery of the penis
 e. preputial branch of the caudal superficial epigastric artery

388. On rectal palpation in a cow, fremitus can be felt in the (middle) uterine artery in advanced pregnancy. One can be sure that it is the uterine artery and not the external iliac artery because of all of the following except:

 a. the uterine artery can be followed proximally to the umbilical artery, which courses along the lateral ligament of the urinary bladder
 b. the freely movable nature of the uterine artery
 c. the relatively fixed position of the external iliac artery
 d. the more lateral position of the external iliac artery close to the body of the ilium
 e. the freely movable nature of the external iliac artery

389. The proximal end of the ulna (olecranon) of the ox is said to fuse with the body of the ulna from 3 1/2 to 4 years of age. Following injury, if the epiphyseal (growth) plate between them is separated, which muscle group would be affected?

 a. extensor muscles of the shoulder joint
 b. flexor muscles of the shoulder joint
 c. flexor muscles of the elbow joint
 d. extensor muscles of the elbow joint
 e. extensor muscles of the carpal joint

390. The paralumbar fossa is a distinct, almost triangular area on the caudodorsal abdominal wall of ruminants. Its caudoventral boundary is formed by the:

 a. last or 13th rib
 b. lateral borders of the iliocostalis and longissimus lumborum muscles
 c. free ends or tips of the lumbar transverse processes
 d. fold (costocoxal crus) of the internal abdominal oblique muscle
 e. lateral borders of the longissimus trunci and costoabdominal muscles

391. In which species does the bile duct join the pancreatic duct before emptying into the duodenum at the major duodenal papilla?

 a. ox
 b. ox and sheep
 c. ox and goat

---

d. both large and small ruminants

e. small ruminants only

392. *Which muscle most aids in voiding of urine or semen from the penis?*

a. bulbospongiosus muscle

b. ischiocavernosus muscle

c. urethralis muscle

d. retractor penis muscle

e. ischiourethralis muscle

393. *The ejaculatory duct in ruminants is formed by joining of the:*

a. ductus deferens and prostate gland duct

b. ductus deferens and vesicular gland duct

c. prostate gland and vesicular gland ducts

d. ductus deferens and bulbourethral gland openings

e. prostate gland openings and urethral crest

394. *The annular fold (site of "high spider") is located immediately distal to which portion of the udder of the cow?*

a. gland sinus

b. teat sinus

c. lactiferous duct

d. papillary duct (teat canal)

e. teat orifice

395. *"Udder" is a collective term used to designate the bovine mammary gland complex, each representing a mammary gland and its teat. In which region of the body is the udder of female ruminants located?*

a. perineal region

b. umbilical region

c. between the thighs

d. abdominal region

e. inguinal region

396. *Distended lymphatics on the surface of the udder, as observed with severe mastitis, can be distinguished from the superficial veins of a high-producing dairy cow:*

a. by the craniodorsal course of the lymphatics to the proper axillary lymph node

b. by the caudodorsal course of the lymphatics to the superficial inguinal (mammary) lymph node

c. by the direct course of the lymphatics toward the superficial inguinal ring

d. only by aspirating a sample of the contents of the vessel with a needle and syringe

e. by palpation for a bounding pulse in the distended veins

397. *Which nerves should be anesthetized for amputation of a cow's udder?*

a. dorsal branches of nerves L_1 and L_2

b. genitofemoral and pudendal epigastric nerves

c. hypogastric nerves and supramammary

d. pelvic nerves

e. genitofemoral, pudendal and ventral branches of nerves L_1 and L_2

398. *In cows, metritis can lead to mastitis because part of the venous drainage from the reproductive tract is said to drain into the venous circle at the base of the udder by way of the:*

a. external pudendal vein

b. internal iliac vein

c. ventral perineal vein

d. subcutaneous abdominal or milk vein

e. external iliac vein

399. *For epidural anesthesia in the ox, local anesthetic is injected into the epidural space at the sacrocaudal space or the first intercaudal space, with the needle perforating the ligamentum flavum. The space filled by the ligament is the:*

a. interarcual space

b. intervertebral foramen

c. lateral vertebral foramen

d. interspinous space

e. intertransverse space

Correct answers are on pages 89-99.

Ruminants, continued

400. *Amputation of the bovine digit at the level of a fetlock joint with "footrot" (infectious pododermatitis) is best avoided for all of the following reasons* **except***:*

   a. the 2 synovial sacs communicate on the palmar/plantar surface, and both joints would be opened

   b. cattle treated in this manner typically develop a painful neuroma

   c. the exposed synovial membrane of the joint would continue to secrete synovial fluid

   d. the digital synovial sheaths would be opened and exposed to infection

   e. there would be very little support to prevent splaying of the remaining digit because both proximal and distal interdigital ligaments would be transected

401. *In old, multiparous ruminants, the ischiorectal (ischioanal) fossa is visible as a triangular depression along the lateral aspect of the anus. This space is normally occupied by fat and connective tissue. In certain surgical procedures, nerve blocks are applied through this space. Which of the following does* **not** *course through this area?*

   a. internal pudendal artery

   b. deep perineal nerve

   c. obturator nerve

   d. ventral perineal vessels

   e. pudendal nerve

402. *Concerning the ruminant stomach, which statement is* **least** *accurate?*

   a. The rumen, reticulum and omasum do not develop from the esophagus but from the nonglandular portion of the developing stomach.

   b. The ruminoreticular groove allows liquids to bypass the rumen.

   c. The coronary pillars are only associated with the caudal ruminal pillar.

   d. The atrium ruminis is bounded by the ruminoretricular fold and the cranial ruminal pillar.

   e. The ruminal recess is not a typical blind sac because it develops from a flexure in the tube-like rumen primordium and lacks circular muscle.

403. *Among domestic ruminants, the infraorbital sinus is only present in sheep and lies rostral to the medial angle of the eye. This cutaneous pouch forms a shallow external depression in:*

   a. the frontal bone

   b. the zygomatic bone

   c. the sphenoid bone

   d. the lacrimal bone

   e. the nasal bone

Birds

N.G. Ghoshal

404. *Though there are many types of feathers and their intermediate forms, which type covers predominantly the entire body of birds?*

   a. contour feather

   b. down feather

   c. filoplume feather

   d. bristle feather

   e. powder feather

405. *To some extent, all birds have a "kinetic skull," permitting extreme opening of the mouth by upward and downward movements of the upper jaw. Which bone is part of the nasofrontal hinge?*

   a. occipital bone

   b. nasal conchae

   c. quadrate bone

   d. maxilla

e. parietal bone

406. *Which muscle contributes to the upward stroke of the wings of birds in flight?*

a. supracoracoid
b. biceps femoris
c. complexus
d. triceps brachii
e. biceps brachii

407. *In the wing, the humerus is usually pneumatized (air filled). If it is fractured, it could become a site of infection that could spread to the:*

a. caudal thoracic air sac
b. abdominal air sac
c. clavicular air sac
d. cranial thoracic air sac
e. vertebral air sac

408. *Which air sac is filled with relatively fresh air during inspiration via the lateroventral secondary bronchi?*

a. clavicular air sac
b. cranial inguinal air sac
c. caudal thoracic air sac
d. cranial thoracic air sac
e. caudal inguinal air sac

409. *Concerning the notarium, which statement is most accurate?*

a. It is formed by fusion of a number of cervical vertebrae.
b. It is present in pigeons, doves, turkeys, chickens and quail.
c. It is present in swans, ducks and geese.
d. It is formed by fusion of all of the thoracic vertebrae.
e. It is formed by fusion of some cervical, all thoracic and all lumbar vertebrae.

410. *Concerning the crop or ingluvies, which statement is most accurate?*

a. It is a diverticulum of the air sac at the thoracic inlet.
b. It lies on the left side of the neck in chickens, on the right side in parakeets, and on both sides in pigeons.
c. In hoatzin, it consists of a thoracic and an abdominal part.
d. In pigeons and doves, it produces "crop milk" during incubation, under the influence of prolactin.
e. It is extremely muscular and not very distensible.

411. *Which structure is **absent** from the large intestine of birds?*

a. cecum
b. colon
c. rectum
d. colorectum
e. coprodeum

412. *Concerning the cecum of birds, which statement is **least** accurate?*

a. There are 2 ceca that arise at the junction of the ileum and colon.
b. Each cecum opens separately into the rectum.
c. Cecal tonsils are present in the proximal parts of the ceca.
d. A single cecum is present in herons and grebes.
e. In parrots, parakeets and some pigeons, the cecum is absent.

413. *Concerning the liver and gallbladder in birds, which statement is **least** accurate?*

a. The liver usually has 2 lobes.
b. A gallbladder is normally present in all birds.
c. In domestic fowl, both lobes are drained separately by the right and left hepatic ducts.
d. Both pancreatic ducts and hepatic ducts empty at the duodenal papilla.
e. For biopsy, the liver is approached by a transabdominal percutaneous needle with the bird in right lateral recumbency.

Correct answers are on pages 89-99.

Birds, continued

414. *Concerning the infraorbital sinus in birds, which statement is **least** accurate?*

  a. It is a small, triangular space lying along the rostroventral margin of the eye.
  b. It is located subcutaneously and lacks a complete bony wall.
  c. It communicates with the caudal nasal concha and the nasal cavity via 2 openings.
  d. The cavity of the infraorbital sinus is connected to the rostral and middle nasal conchae.
  e. In many respiratory diseases, it becomes obstructed with exudate.

415. *Concerning the syrinx, which statement is most accurate?*

  a. It is located at the caudal end of the trachea and is responsible for production of sound.
  b. It is surrounded by the cranial thoracic air sac.
  c. It lies at the cranial end of the trachea in the cranial neck region.
  d. It is present between the primary bronchi and the lungs.
  e. It is present as an asymmetric dilatation on the right side in female ducks.

416. *Which air sac is single (unpaired)?*

  a. abdominal air sac
  b. cervical air sac
  c. caudal thoracic air sac
  d. clavicular air sac
  e. cranial thoracic air sac

417. *Concerning the testes in birds, which statement is **least** accurate?*

  a. They are surrounded by the abdominal air sac.
  b. In most birds, the rete testis lies on the dorsomedial surface of the testis.
  c. The mediastinal testis and testicular septa or lobules are absent.
  d. The tunica albuginea surrounds each testis.

  e. After the nuptial phase in birds with distinct breeding cycles, the testis undergoes dissolution.

418. *Concerning the epididymis, which statement is **least** accurate?*

  a. It is rudimentary.
  b. It is concealed by a short mesentery, suspending the testis.
  c. The efferent ductules arise throughout the entire length of the epididymis.
  d. It consists of a head, body and tail.
  e. The epididymal duct continues as the ductus deferens.

419. *Which of the following is **absent** from male birds?*

  a. epididymis
  b. testis
  c. ductus deferens
  d. accessory sex glands (except in Japanese quail)
  e. phallus

420. *Concerning the reproductive system in birds, which statement is **least** accurate?*

  a. Males are heterogametic and determine the sex of offspring.
  b. The left reproductive organs in adult females are only functional in most birds.
  c. The rudiments of the right ovary and oviduct persist and remain nonfunctional.
  d. Usually the right ovary remains in an ambisexual or bisexual state.
  e. If disease renders the left ovary nonfunctional, the right ovary may compensate for this loss of function.

421. *Which segment of the oviduct produces the albumen of birds' eggs?*

  a. vagina
  b. isthmus
  c. folliculorum
  d. caudal infundibulum
  e. stapus

422. *During passage of an ovum through the reproductive tract in birds, in which segment does it stay for the longest period?*

   a. infundibulum

   b. magnum

   c. isthmus

   d. uterus

   e. vagina

423. *Concerning the kidneys in birds, which statement is **least** accurate?*

   a. They are lobulated.

   b. They are divided by the external iliac and ischiatic arteries, characteristic of birds in general.

   c. On section, they show a distinct cortex, medulla and pelvis.

   d. They lie inside the renal or iliac fossa.

   e. They are located midway between the lungs cranially and the synsacrum caudally.

424. *Concerning the kidneys in birds, which statement is **least** accurate?*

   a. In most birds, they are divided externally into cranial, middle and caudal lobes.

   b. In passerines, the middle lobe is largely fused with the other 2 lobes.

   c. In many birds (except chickens), both caudal lobes are fused along the midline.

   d. Spinal nerves of the lumbosacral plexus pass through the substance of the kidneys.

   e. In renal biopsy of a potential breeding female, the left kidney should be sampled because the right reproductive organs are functional in most adult females.

425. *The cloaca of birds is the common passageway for the digestive and urogenital systems and is divided internally by mucosal folds into 3 compartments. Which represents the cranial compartment and receives the rectum?*

   a. urodeum

   b. proctodeum

   c. coprodeum

   d. genodeum

   e. synprodeum

426. *The cloacal bursa (of Fabricius) is associated with which compartment of the cloaca?*

   a. coprodeum

   b. proctodeum

   c. urodeum

   d. synprodeum

   e. genodeum

427. *Concerning the heart and adjacent vessels in birds, which statement is **least** accurate?*

   a. The heart is slightly deflected to the right of the midline.

   b. The aorta curves to the right as it leaves the heart.

   c. The left jugular vein is usually larger than the corresponding right vein.

   d. The aorta divides into the right and left brachiocephalic arteries.

   e. Before entering the heart, the right and left pulmonary veins in chickens join to form a common trunk.

428. *Concerning the spinal cord in birds, which statement is **least** accurate?*

   a. In birds adapted for flying, the cervical enlargement is larger than the lumbosacral enlargement.

   b. In flightless birds, the lumbosacral enlargement is larger than the cervical enlargement.

   c. The spinal cord has almost the same length as the vertebral column.

   d. In the lumbar region, the spinal cord presents the "gelatinous or glycogen body" of unknown function.

   e. The dorsal portion of the "gelatinous or glycogen body" encloses the central canal of the spinal cord.

Correct answers are on pages 89-99.

Birds, continued

429. *In cage birds, which structure requires professional care (trimming) to maintain normal function?*

   a. sternal bursa
   b. spurs or calcars
   c. claws
   d. semiplume feathers
   e. ceres

430. *In the "de-flight" operation in birds, which structure is **not** transected or clipped?*

   a. contour feathers
   b. tendon of the triceps brachii muscle
   c. tendon of the extensor carpi radialis muscle
   d. ventral metacarpal artery
   e. tendon of the sternotrachealis muscle

431. *Cosmetic "pinioning" is occasionally performed in adult birds to prevent flight. Which type of feather is clipped in this procedure?*

   a. down feather
   b. primary contour feather
   c. secondary contour feather
   d. semiplume feather
   e. filoplume feather

432. *Concerning the pecten of the eye in birds, which statement is **least** accurate?*

   a. It is present in the retina, near the optic disk.
   b. Its size and complexity vary between species.
   c. It is better developed in diurnal birds than in nocturnal birds.
   d. It provides nutrients to the retina by diffusion.
   e. It screens out bright sunlight and reflects an image onto the retina.

433. *Concerning the pancreas of birds, which statement is **least** accurate?*

   a. It is cream colored and located in the duodenal loop in most species.
   b. It consists of dorsal, ventral and splenic lobes.
   c. The light-colored beta cells are present in all pancreatic lobes.
   d. The dark-colored alpha cells are present in all pancreatic lobes.
   e. The number of pancreatic ducts varies between 1 and 3, and they empty on the duodenal papilla along the bile duct.

Reptiles

F.L. Frye

434. *Male lizards and snakes have paired copulatory organs called:*

   a. claspers
   b. paracloacal spurs
   c. hemipenes
   d. cloacal vents
   e. vasa deferentia

435. *Most reptiles are unable to generate internal warmth, as do birds and mammals. This characteristic of "cold-bloodedness" is called:*

   a. hypothermia
   b. poikilothermy
   c. hyperthermia
   d. hypospadias
   e. endothermy

436. *Many reptiles can survive very low oxygen tension in their inspired air. They accomplish this by a process called:*

   a. hypoxia
   b. hyperpnea

c. aerobic respiration

d. hypermetria

e. anaerobic respiration

437. *An important characteristic of the blood of fish, amphibians, reptiles and birds is that all formed elements of the blood retain their:*

a. flagella

b. cilia

c. nuclei

d. mantles

e. follicles

438. *The characteristic, often colorful pigmentation of reptilian skin is associated with:*

a. chromatophores

b. zoospores

c. retinoblasts

d. ceroid pigment

e. lipofucsin

439. *Which reptiles have a hard palate that divides the oral cavity from the nasal cavity?*

a. chelonians (turtles, tortoises, terrapins)

b. serpents (snakes)

c. crocodilians (alligators, crocodiles, caimans, gharials)

d. monotremes (spiny echidna, platypus)

e. saurians (lizards)

440. *Which reptiles are characterized by their functional 4-chambered heart?*

a. crocodilians

b. lizards

c. tuatara (a primitive "living fossil" from New Zealand)

d. turtles, tortoises and terrapins

e. snakes

441. *The vascular system of reptiles differs markedly from that of mammals because it includes:*

a. a hepatic portal vein

b. a renal portal vein

c. a celiac vein

d. paired pulmonary arteries

e. paired pulmonary veins

442. *When handling reptiles, one must not apply excessive force to the cervical and cephalic parts of the skeleton because reptiles:*

a. have paired occipital condyles supporting the skull

b. have a single occipital condyle supporting the skull

c. do not have mineralized cervical spines

d. do not have carotid arteries

e. do not have jugular veins

443. *Reptiles generally have paired lungs, with a single exception. Which reptiles usually have only a solitary lung?*

a. crocodilians (alligators, crocodiles, caiman, gharials)

b. snakes

c. chelonians (turtles, tortoises, terrapins)

d. lizards

e. tuatara

444. *Snakes can swallow whole prey animals of relatively enormous size because of the osseous features of their:*

a. premaxilla

b. maxilla

c. quadrate apparatus

d. hyoid apparatus

e. vomer bone

445. *Which body system serves a secondary function as a hydrostatic organ in diving reptiles?*

a. reticuloendothelial system

b. lungs

c. liver

d. kidneys

e. heart

Correct answers are on pages 89-99.

Reptiles, continued

446. Which type of bone is **not** a feature of the typical reptilian skeleton?

   a. compact bone
   b. pneumatized bone
   c. cancellous bone
   d. diaphyseal bone
   e. metaphyseal bone

447. Of the major classifications of brain organization, which best describes the reptilian brain?

   a. mostly neocortex
   b. mostly paleocortex
   c. lacking a cerebellum
   d. lacking cerebral hemispheres
   e. lacking olfactory bulbs or lobes

448. Though reptiles, like fish and amphibians, are thought of as "cold-blooded," some reptiles can produce internal body warmth without having to bask in the sun. These are the:

   a. crocodilians
   b. lizards
   c. tortoises
   d. brooding female pythons and large sea turtles
   e. water snakes

449. Synthesis of vitamin D3 involves the:

   a. skin, liver, lung, spleen, adrenal and pancreas
   b. skin, liver, kidney, spleen and pancreas
   c. skin, liver, kidney, parathyroid gland, thyroid and bone
   d. skin, testis or ovary, and vas deferens or oviducts
   e. skin, spleen, adrenal gland and pancreas

450. In reptiles, spermatozoa mature in the:

   a. seminiferous tubules
   b. interstitial cells
   c. prostate gland
   d. epididymis
   e. bulbourethral gland

451. When injecting reptiles with aminoglycoside antibiotics, which can be nephrotoxic, the preferred site is the cranial half of the body. This is because the reptilian vascular system includes a:

   a. splanchnic venous system
   b. renal portal system
   c. hepatic portal system
   d. coronary artery system
   e. pulmonary artery system

452. Which structure in snakes, lizards, turtles and the tuatara is unpaired?

   a. testis or ovary
   b. atrium
   c. ventricle
   d. kidney
   e. adrenal gland

453. In reptiles, the feces pass from the colon and rectum into the:

   a. antrum
   b. vestibule
   c. coprodeum
   d. urodeum
   e. cecum

454. In some lizards and the tuatara, the paired lateral eyes are augmented by an accessory visual structure called the:

   a. labial pit
   b. nasal pit organ
   c. parietal eye
   d. vomeronasal (Jacobson's) organ
   e. pecten

455. In which reptile is the gallbladder separated by a considerable distance from the liver and located closer to the pancreas and spleen?

   a. chelonia (turtles, tortoises, terrapins)
   b. snakes
   c. lizards
   d. crocodilians (alligators, crocodiles, caiman, gharial)

e. tuatara

456. *Some pythons and boas, and all pit vipers have labial or facial pit organs as part of their sensory apparatus. These structures are sensitive to:*

a. light
b. touch
c. atmospheric pressure
d. sound
e. heat

457. *Rod cells predominate in the retina of some reptiles. One would expect these animals to:*

a. differentiate colors with great fidelity
b. have better vision at night or in dim light
c. withstand cold better than other reptiles
d. hear high-frequency sound waves
e. better balance themselves in a variety of postures

458. *The organ of Corti in reptiles is found in the:*

a. pancreas
b. urinary bladder
c. retina
d. inner ear
e. ethmoid sinus

Answers

1. **e** The common calcanean tendon inserts on the tuber calcaneus. Separation of the tuber would result in a decrease in function of the gastrocnemius muscle and other components of the common calcanean tendon. Flexion of the digits would be little affected, as the digital flexor tendons would still be functional (particularly those of the deep digital flexor, as the deep digital flexor tendon passes through the tarsal canal medial to the calcaneus).

2. **d** The serratus ventralis muscle attaches the serrated face of the scapula dorsally to the rib cage ventrally. Thus, the trunk is suspended from the scapula by the serratus ventralis muscle. The trapezius muscle attaches the scapular spine dorsolaterally to the trunk dorsally; paralysis of the trapezius would decrease the animal's ability to maintain the dorsal portion of the scapula tightly against the trunk. Fracture of the scapular neck might also permit some elevation of the scapula relative to the trunk due to pain and concurrent relaxation of the serratus ventralis muscle.

3. **e** The internal obdurator, external obdurator and gemellus muscles arise from the dorsal, ventral and lateral surfaces of the bony pelvis, respectively. They all insert in or adjacent to the trochanteric fossa of the femoral bone. Though these muscles may have some extensor action on the hip joint, their major function is to rotate the cranial surface of the limb laterally.

4. **d** One head of the triceps brachii arises from the caudal surface of the scapula and would have flexor action on the shoulder. All 4 heads of the triceps brachii insert by means of a common tendon on the olecranon and have a primary role in extension of the elbow joint.

5. **c** The digastricus is composed of a caudal and a rostral portion, each having separate cranial innervation. The digastricus, which extends from the base of the skull to the caudoventral surface of the mandible, acts to open the lower jaw. The masseter, temporalis and pterygoid muscles all elevate (close) the lower jaw, while the buccinator tightens the cheek pouch.

6. **a** Both the gastrocnemius and superficial digital flexor tendons attach to the calcanean tuberosity; however, the tendon of the superficial digital flexor continues on distally to the plantar surface of the digits.

7. **e** Transecting the patellar ligament and associated fascia would permit the stifle to flex, as the extensor muscles of the stifle joint would be deprived of their insertion on the tibial tuberosity. The long digital extensor tendon arises from the craniolateral surface of

the femoral bone, crosses the stifle joint, and passes down the craniolateral surface of the crus to reach the dorsal surface of the pes. Flexion of the stifle joint results in increased tension on this digital extensor muscle.

8. **a** A single articular space occurs between the patella, femoral bone, tibia and fibula of the stifle in dogs and cats.

9. **c** The proximal two-thirds of the femur is covered laterally by the vastus lateralis portion of the quadriceps femoris. Fibers of the biceps femoris muscle, which is positioned largely caudolateral to the femoral bone, fan out into the patellar region, as well as into the proximocranial crural region and onto the common calcanean tendon.

10. **e**

11. **a** Primary ossification centers are established in the diaphyses of long bones before birth. Secondary centers of ossification are initiated in the epiphyses and in some osseous prominences during the first several months of postnatal life. The epiphyseal plate, or physis, is the zone of tissue between the epiphysis and diaphysis. It consist of several regions: nonproliferating cartilage zone, proliferating cartilage zone, zone of hypertrophy and maturation, and a zone of calcification. When the physis ceases to proliferate, the epiphyseal plate becomes calcified and bone lengthening ceases.

12. **a** Muscles of the ciliary body cause stretching or relaxation of the lens of the eye.

13. **d** The ventral surface of the cervical vertebrae is covered by longus capitis and longus colli muscles, with the longus capitis located more laterally than the longus colli. Fascicles of the longus colli muscle arise from the ventral surface of the transverse processes, cross one intervertebral space, and insert on the ventral surface of the body of the next cervical vertebra. Thus, the bodies of the right and left longus colli muscles completely cover the ventral surface of the cervical intervertebral disks.

14. **d** The 1st cervical vertebra, or atlas, has very large, undivided transverse processes. The 6th cervical vertebra, with dorsal and ventral subdivisions of each transverse process, is easy to identify on radiographs. Novices may mistake the ventral subdivision in radiographs for a foreign body.

15. **e** The tendon of origin of the deep digital flexor arises from the caudal surface of bones in the crus (tibia and fibula).

16. **d**

17. **c**

18. **d** Tendons of the deep digital flexor attach to the flexor tubercle of each distal phalanx in the thoracic and pelvic limbs. The common digital extensor in the thoracic limb and the long digital extensor in the pelvic limb attach to the extensor process of each distal phalanx. The lateral digital extensor contributes tendons to the extensor processes of the distal phalanx of some digits.

19. **e** The flexor carpi ulnaris and, to some extent, the extensor carpi ulnaris insert on the accessory carpal bone. Partial loss of function in these muscles would convey weight in the standing dog to the superficial and deep digital flexor muscles; some sinking of the carpus would likely occur. The lateral epicondyle of the humerus is the point of attachment for many extensor muscles of the carpus and digits.

20. **d**

21. **c** The deltoideus muscle spans the distance from the scapular spine to the deltoid tuberosity of the humerus. It covers the lateral aspect of the shoulder joint and the tendons of insertion of the supraspinatus, infraspinatus and teres minor muscles.

22. **e**

23. **e**

24. **e** The tendons of insertion of the superficial gluteus, on the third trochanter, and the middle and deep gluteus, on the major trochanter, cover the dorsal aspect of the hip joint. The caudal belly of the tensor fasciae latae covers the cranial aspect of the hip joint.

25. **c** The common calcanean tendon, constituting a union of fibers from the gastrocnemius, superficial digital flexor, gracilis, semitendinosus and biceps femoris, is a powerful extensor of the hock joint. A severed common calcanean tendon eliminates function of the superficial digital flexor, but the very strong deep digital flexor muscle would still be functional.

26. **d**

27. **d** Because the caudal cruciate ligament extends from the cranial portion of the femoral intercondylar fossa to the caudal portion of the tibial intercondylar region, tearing of this ligament permits the tibia to slide caudally relative to the femoral bone ("caudal drawer movement").

28. **c** The limbs continue to lengthen until the dog is approximately 12-13 months of age. If growth in the distal radial physis continues to lengthen the radius while the distal end of the ulna remains the same size, the medial portion of the manus will be pushed distally, while the lateral portion remains relatively static.

29. **e**

30. **d** Double dewclaws are considered a desirable trait in Briards and Great Pyrenees.

31. **a** Epaxial muscles in the cervical region are responsible for extending or dorsally bending the cervical vertebrae. The ligamentum nuchae provides an elastic force that permits the lowered head to be raised relatively easily.

32. **a** The line of force set up through the thoracic limb in a standing dog passes through the radial side of the carpus, the radius, the lateral portion of the distal end of the humerus, and the humeral diaphysis.

33. **c** The heads of each pair of ribs 1 to 10 articulate against the intervertebral spaces between the 7th cervical and 10th thoracic vertebrae. An intercapital ligament passes from the head of the rib on one side, over the intervertebral disk, to the head of the rib on the opposite side. Caudal to the 10th thoracic vertebra, the heads of the ribs articulate progressively further caudally, coming to be positioned against the body of one vertebra rather than on an intervertebral disk and adjacent bodies. The heads of these caudal several ribs are not connected to those on the other side by intercapital ligaments.

34. **a** Both the more medial multifidus and the more lateral longissimus muscles may be retracted during the laminectomy procedures; however, the multifidus muscles are directly dorsal to the lamina.

35. **e**

36. **a** Collateral ligaments, right and left, develop in the fibrous capsule of hinge joints. The more flexible a joint is for rotation, circumduction and swiveling functions, the less well developed are the collateral ligaments.

37. **e** To remain upright on its antebrachium and crus, the animal must maintain extension of the elbow and stifle. If the triceps brachii in the thoracic limb and the quadriceps femoris in the pelvic limb are functional, the animal can stand on its manus and pes (whether or not the manus and pes are truly functional).

38. **e** The patella is more proximally located in the trochlear groove of the femoral bone than you may realize.

39. **b**

40. **b**

41. **b**

42. **b**

43. **d** The external abdominal oblique extends as far cranially as the 4th rib and attaches on the ribs near the origin of the serratus ventralis muscle.

44. **d** The right lobe of the pancreas, situated in the mesoduodenum, extends toward the caudal duodenal flexure. The left lobe of the pancreas is situated in the deep leaf of the greater omentum.

45. **a**

46. **d** The superficial leaf of the greater omentum normally extends caudally, from the greater curvature of the stomach all the way to the urinary bladder before reflecting cranially as the deep leaf of the greater omentum. Before one can examine the jejunoileum or transverse colon, the caudal end of the omentum must be lifted and retracted cranially.

47. **a**

48. **b**

49. **a**

50. **d**

51. **c**

52. **b** From an embryologic viewpoint, the stomach, terminal ileum and cecum are unusual in having vascularity on both the dorsal and ventral surfaces.

53. **d**

54. **e** The liver has a common mesenteric attachment (lesser omentum) with the stomach but is not free to move because of its coronary ligament to the thoracic diaphragm. The duodenum and right lobe of the pancreas are suspended from the dorsal body wall by the

mesoduodenum, while the spleen is encased in the greater omentum.

55. **b**

56. **a** Secretions of both the mandibular salivary gland and monostomatic sublingual salivary gland exit via ducts through the sublingual caruncle at the base of the lingual frenulum.

57. **d** The parietal area of the stomach is that portion lying adjacent to the liver. Though an ingested bone might penetrate the gallbladder, the greatest area of contact is with the liver.

58. **e** The thoracic cavity and abdominal/pelvic cavities and their organs are covered by pleura and peritoneum, respectively. The cervical esophagus is surrounded by connective tissue, as it does not lie within a serous cavity.

59. **c**

60. **c** If they did not rupture, the diaphragmatic pleura, diaphragmatic peritoneum and visceral peritoneum on the stomach would separate the pleural cavity from the smooth muscle of the stomach wall.

61. **b**

62. **a** The root of the mesentery gathers from the jejunoileum to the dorsal body wall at about the 2nd and 3rd lumbar vertebrae. The transverse colon is maintained cranial to the mesojejunoileum. The body of the pancreas is fixed by mesoduodenum and greater omentum near the pyloric portion of the stomach at the level of the right 10th rib. In dogs, the right kidney is located between transverse levels of the 1st and 3rd lumbar vertebrae. The spleen of a dog with an empty stomach would lie largely on the left side of the abdomen, adjacent to the last rib. The cecum would normally be on the right side of the root of the mesentery at about the 3rd to 4th lumbar vertebral levels.

63. **b** The tracheal carina is the cartilagious wedge between the openings into the right and left primary bronchi from the trachea.

64. **c**

65. **d** The laryngeal cartilages include the interarytenoid, the paired arytenoids, and the unpaired epiglottic, thyroid and cricoid cartilages.

66. **e**

67. **d** The caudal peripheral margin, or basal margin, of the caudal lobes of the right and left lungs extends into the acutely angled costo-diaphragmatic recess. This recess is immediately cranial and parallel to the costal arch.

68. **c** The plica vena cava extends to the right and dorsally from the mediastinum, forming the mediastinal recess as a subdivision of the right pleural cavity. The dorsal margin of the plica, containing the caudal vena cava and right phrenic nerve, indents the right accessory lobe of the lung.

69. **e** By abducting the vocal folds laterally, the cricoarytenoideus dorsalis widens the lumen between the vocal folds. When much of the intrinsic laryngeal musculature is paralyzed on one side due to recurrent laryngeal nerve damage, loss of abduction of the vocal folds results in the characteristic sound of laryngeal hemiplegia ("roaring").

70. **d** Intraabdominal pressure is normally much higher than intrathoracic pressure. As a result of this pressure differential, abdominal organs move into the thoracic compartment with herniation of the thoracic diaphragm. Because the right pleural space is much larger than the left, and the caudal mediastinum deflects to the left to line the diaphragm as diaphragmatic pleura, abdominal organs move into the right pleural space if they penetrate the central or right portion of the thoracic diaphragm.

71. **e**

72. **b** The costal (parietal) pleura may be punctured, admitting air into the left pleural cavity and permitting the left lung to collapse. If the punture wound is not deep enough to damage the costal pleura and the lung collapses anyway, then there must be damage to the lung tissue and its surrounding pulmonary pleura, which would permit air from the lung to enter the left pleural cavity, collapsing the left lung.

73. **c** Except for brachycephalic dogs, in which the soft palate projects caudally beyond the epiglottis, the normal position of the tip of the epiglottis during quiet respiration is dorsal to the caudal free edge of the soft palate.

74. **a** The large U-shaped thyroid cartilage maintains laterally directed forces on the laryngeal membranes; however, the ring-shaped cricoid cartilage prevents collapse of the caudal portion of the larynx.

75. **c** Puncture of either the thoracic wall or lung tissue allows air to enter the pleural space and causes the entire lung on that side to collapse or deflate. The mediastinum is complete in carnivores and maintains the integrity of the pleural space on the opposite side. However, labored breathing due to one atelectatic lung may cause the mediastinum to rupture and the other lung to also collapse.

76. **c** The urinary bladder is supported by the median umbilical ligament and 2 lateral umbilical ligaments.

77. **c**

78. **b**

79. **b**

80. **a** The preprostatic portion of the feline urethra is relatively longer than that of dogs.

81. **a**

82. **d**

83. **a**

84. **e**

85. **b** The ductus deferens arises from the tail of the epididymis at the caudal pole of the testis.

86. **c**

87. **e** The perineal body is the fibromuscular tissue, caudal to the pelvic cavity, that interconnects the ventral wall of the rectum/anal canal and the dorsal wall of the vagina.

88. **c**

89. **d**

90. **d**

91. **b**

92. **c** The 2 serous layers would be the one covering the outside of the intestine (visceral peritoneum) and the one covering the ductus deferens (visceral vaginal tunic).

93. **a** Increased pulmonary vascular resistance would necessitate more forceful contractions of the right ventricle as blood backed up in the right side of the heart. First the right ventricle and then the right atrium would enlarge.

94. **a**

95. **e**

96. **a**

97. **e** In dogs, the maxillary artery passes ventrally, lateral to the temporomandibular joint, curves medially past the ventral surface of the joint, and enters the alar canal in the skull. In its course, this artery is immediately adjacent to the temporomandibular articulation.

98. **e** The umbilical arteries that supply blood to the apex of the urinary bladder are the remnants of the fetal arterial blood supply from the placenta.

99. **d** The median cubital vein interconnects the cephalic and median veins. Because it contains no valves, the median cubital vein carries blood from the cephalic vein to the median vein unless the median cubital is occluded by applying traction caudally on the skin at the cranial surface of the elbow.

100. **d** The right renal vein does not drain into the portal vein.

101. **a** The pulmonary veins drain into the left atrium. The right azygos vein sometimes drains into the right atrium, though it usually enters the cranial vena cava.

102. **e** The caudal pancreaticoduodenal artery from the cranial mesenteric artery is an alternative source of blood for caudal portion of the duodenum and pancreas.

103. **b** The right and left coronary arteries arise from the initial portion of the ascending aorta.

104. **d**

105. **a** The median nerve and brachial artery of cats pass through the supracondylar foramen on the medial side of the humerus.

106. **e** The spleen is supplied by the splenic arterial branch of the celiac artery.

107. **e**

108. **d**

109. **b** All blood passes through the lung each time it goes through the heart. The first capillary bed through which venous blood, other than that of the portal vein and the coronary circulation, passes is in the lung.

110. **d**

111. **e**

112. **b** As one would want to thread the cannula into the pulmonary trunk via first the right atrium and then the right ventricle, the cannula must be inserted into a peripheral vein. The right azygos vein cannot be used for cannulation unless the abdomen is opened.

113. **a**

114. **c**

115. c

116. c

117. d

118. **a** With infection of the descending colon or cranial rectum, the caudal mesenteric lymph node would be enlarged. The superficial inguinal and popliteal lymph nodes would be enlarged with infection in the pelvic limb. The prepuce is drained directly by the superficial inguinal (scrotal) lymph node.

119. e

120. **d** Lymph drainage from the superficial inguinal lymph node follows the external pudendal vascular pathway through the inguinal canal and then to the medial iliac lymph node.

121. **b** Lymph from the pelvic limbs, tail and intestines is collected into the cisterna chyli and passed on through the thoracic duct to the venous system.

122. **d** The vessels draining the cisterna chyli pass through the thoracic diaphragm with the dorsal aorta.

123. **e** If the superficial cervical and popliteal lymph nodes are not enlarged, there is likely no infection in much of the thoracic and pelvic limbs. The axillary and superficial inguinal lymph nodes drain the mammary glands, and lymph nodes in the midabdominal region drain both cranially and caudally, so this region should be examined more carefully.

124. e

125. **a** The medial pterygoid muscle inserts on the medial surface of the mandible adjacent to the mandibular foramen, through which the inferior alveolar nerve enters to provide innervation to teeth of the mandible.

126. c

127. d

128. **d** Though a number of structures may be damaged, the description indicates that the head of the femoral bone has been displaced from the acetabulum. Such a displacement would involve tearing and separation of the ligament of the head of the femoral bone.

129. e

130. d

131. d

132. b

133. b

134. **d** The axis of the limb passes through the interdigital space between the 3rd and 4th digits. The surface of each digit that faces the axis is the axial surface of that digit. The surface of each digit that faces away from the axis is the abaxial surface of that digit.

135. a

136. a

137. c

138. a

139. c

140. e

141. e

142. c

143. **c** In cats, the median nerve and brachial artery pass through the supracondylar foramen on the medial side of the humerus. Any damage to this bone in this region could also damage the median nerve.

144. **d** The vertebral, costocervical and right azygos veins and caudal vena cava all drain structures associated with the vertebral column.

145. d

146. **e** The left lung occupies more space in the thoracic cavity than does the right lung.

147. a

148. b

149. **c** The tendon of the deep digital flexor is partially protected by the tarsal canal, but that of the superficial digital flexor is vulnerable on the plantar surface of the calcaneus.

150. b

151. d

152. **d** The prearticular and postarticular processes of adjacent vertebrae of the caudal thoracic and lumbar vertebrae are oriented sagitally, such that this portion of the vertebral column can flex or extend ventrally and dorsally more easily than bending laterally.

153. c

154. b

155. a

156. b

157. **a**	199. **d**
158. **a**	200. **c**
159. **d**	201. **e**
160. **c**	202. **e**
161. **a**	203. **e**
162. **a**	204. **d**
163. **d**	205. **a**
164. **b**	206. **d**
165. **b**	207. **b**
166. **a**	208. **d**
167. **e**	209. **a**
168. **c**	210. **c**
169. **a**	211. **a**
170. **d**	212. **d**
171. **e**	213. **b**
172. **b**	214. **e**
173. **d**	215. **d**
174. **c**	216. **a**
175. **d**	217. **d**
176. **c**	218. **a**
177. **e**	219. **b**
178. **b**	220. **b**
179. **e**	221. **c**
180. **c**	222. **d**
181. **d**	223. **c**
182. **e**	224. **c**
183. **a**	225. **a**
184. **c**	226. **d**
185. **d**	227. **b**
186. **d**	228. **e**
187. **a**	229. **d**
188. **c**	230. **a**
189. **e**	231. **c**
190. **b**	232. **d**
191. **d**	233. **b**
192. **e**	234. **a**
193. **c**	235. **d**
194. **a**	236. **c**
195. **d**	237. **b**
196. **b**	238. **a**
197. **c**	239. **d**
198. **d**	240. **e**

241. e		282. c	
242. e		283. c	
243. a		284. d	
244. c		285. a	
245. b		286. a	
246. e		287. d	
247. c		288. c	
248. c		289. e	
249. b		290. c	
250. c		291. b	
251. e		292. c	
252. c		293. d	
253. e		294. a	
254. b		295. d	
255. b		296. c	
256. a		297. b	
257. d		298. d	
258. c		299. c	
259. d		300. d	
260. e		301. c	
261. b		302. b	
262. c		303. c	
263. b		304. c	
264. d		305. e	
265. e		306. b	
266. c		307. d	
267. a		308. a	
268. a		309. c	
269. e		310. e	
270. d		311. a	
271. a		312. d	
272. b		313. b	
273. d		314. a	
274. c		315. e	
275. b		316. d	
276. d		317. c	
277. e		318. e	
278. b		319. b	
279. a		320. a	
280. c		321. d	
281. d		322. a	

323. c	365. a
324. e	366. d
325. c	367. c
326. e	368. e
327. b	369. b
328. d	370. a
329. d	371. d
330. c	372. c
331. a	373. c
332. c	374. b
333. d	375. e
334. b	376. a
335. a	377. d
336. c	378. d
337. c	379. c
338. b	380. b
339. b	381. a
340. a	382. c
341. b	383. a
342. c	384. d
343. a	385. c
344. d	386. c
345. c	387. a
346. e	388. e
347. b	389. d
348. d	390. d
349. a	391. e
350. b	392. c
351. d	393. b
352. a	394. a
353. d	395. e
354. c	396. b
355. a	397. e
356. d	398. c
357. b	399. a
358. a	400. b
359. b	401. c
360. d	402. b
361. b	403. d
362. a	404. a
363. b	405. c
364. e	406. a

407. **c**

408. **c**

409. **b**

410. **d**

411. **b**

412. **a**

413. **b**

414. **d**

415. **a**

416. **d**

417. **c**

418. **d**

419. **d**

420. **a**

421. **d**

422. **d**

423. **c**

424. **e**

425. **c**

426. **b**

427. **c**

428. **e**

429. **c**

430. **e**

431. **c**

432. **b**

433. **d**

434. **c** Hemipenes are the paired copulatory organs of male snakes and lizards.

435. **b** Poikilothermy is defined as inability to produce internal warmth, and having a body temperature that varies with environmental temperature.

436. **e** Reptiles can respire anaerobically for differing periods.

437. **c** All of the formed elements of fish, amphibian, reptilian and avian blood retain their nuclei.

438. **a** Chromatophores are pigment cells responsible for the color of reptilian skin.

439. **c** Only crocodilians have a complete hard palate that separates the oral and nasal cavities.

440. **a** Only crocodilians have a functional 4-chambered heart; all other reptiles have 2 atria and a solitary ventricle.

441. **b** Reptiles have a renal portal system that drains the caudal portions of the body.

442. **b** The skull of all reptiles is supported by a single occipital condyle.

443. **b** With a single exception, snakes have only 1 functional lung, the left one.

444. **c** The quadrate apparatus permits snakes to partially unhinge their jaws to swallow enormous meals.

445. **b** The lungs of many diving reptiles serve a secondary purpose as hydrostatic organs.

446. **b** Pneumatized bone is not found in present-day reptiles, as it is in birds.

447. **b** The reptilian brain is largely comprised of paleocortex.

448. **d** Brooding females pythons and large marine turtles are partially endothermic or "warm-blooded."

449. **c** Synthesis of vitamin D3 requires the integrated functioning of skin, liver, kidney, parathyroid, thyroid and bone.

450. **d** As in other vertebrates, spermatozoa in reptiles mature within the coiled epididymis.

451. **b** Because reptiles have a renal portal system that delivers blood (and any injected drugs drained from the caudal half of the body) from the renal portal vein to the kidneys before entering the hepatic and general vascular system, the caudal portion of the body should be avoided when injecting nephrotoxic drugs.

452. **c** Snakes, lizards, turtles, and the tuatara have a single cardiac ventricle.

453. **c** In reptiles, feces pass from the colon/rectum into the coprodeum.

454. **c** The parietal eye is an accessory visual organ in some lizards and the tuatara.

455. **b** In snakes, the gallbladder is located some distance from the liver and is adjacent to the pancreas and spleen.

456. **e** The facial or labial pit organs of some snakes are highly sensitive to temperature differences and are used to help locate food or predators.

457. **b** Retinal rod cells are sensitive to light, rather than to color; therefore, an animal with more rod cells than cone cells would be able to see well in poor light conditions.

458. **d** The organ of Corti is found within the inner ear of reptiles, just as it is in higher vertebrates.

Notes

Notes

Section

4

Microbiology

G.R. Carter, M. Ikram

Recommended Reading

Biberstein EL and Zee YC: *Review of Veterinary Microbiology.* Blackwell Scientific, Boston, 1990.

Carter GR and Chengappa MM: *Microbial Diseases: A Veterinarian's Guide to Laboratory Diagnosis.* 2nd ed. Iowa State University Press, Ames, IA, 1993.

Carter GR and Chengappa MM: *Essentials of Veterinary Bacteriology and Mycology.* 4th ed. Lea & Febiger, Malvern, PA, 1991.

Carter GR and Cole, Jr JR: *Diagnostic Procedures in Veterinary Bacteriology and Mycology.* 5th ed. Academic Press, San Diego, 1990.

Fraser CM: *The Merck Veterinary Manual.* 7th ed. Merck, Rahway, NJ, 1991.

Timoney JF *et al: Hagan and Bruner's Microbiology and Infectious Diseases of Domestic Animals.* 8th ed. Comstock Publishing, Ithaca, NY, 1988.

Practice answer sheets are on pages 259-260.

Questions

For Questions 1 through 5, match the fungal species with their respective fungal diseases.

a. *Mortierella wolfii*
b. *Absidia corymbifera*
c. *Rhinosporidium seeberi*
d. *Candida albicans*
e. *Pythium insidiosum* (formerly *Hyphomyces destruens*)

1. *Cause of crop mycosis.*

2. *Cause of polyps on the nasal and ocular mucous membranes.*

3. *Cause of mycotic placentitis.*

4. *Cause of mycotic swamp cancer in horses.*

5. *Cause of zygomycosis in pigs and cattle.*

6. *What is the preferred antimycotic agent for treatment of mucocutaneous candidiasis?*

a. nystatin
b. griseofulvin
c. flucytosine
d. amphotericin B
e. sodium iodide

Correct answers are on pages 127-130.

7. *Concerning* Aspergillus *species, which statement is **least** accurate?*

   a. Nonseptate hyphae are seen in sections of lesions.
   b. Septate hyphae are seen in sections of lesions.
   c. They cause nasal infections in dogs.
   d. They cause guttural pouch mycosis.
   e. Agar-gel immunodiffusion may be used in diagnosis.

8. *You suspect that a horse has sporotrichosis. Which is the most reliable procedure for diagnosis in most equine cases?*

   a. isolation and identification by culture
   b. intradermal testing
   c. demonstration of characteristic yeast forms in Giemsa-stained smears of discharging pus
   d. latex agglutination test
   e. complement-fixation test

9. *On histologic examination, the invasive lesions of candidiasis contain primarily:*

   a. broad-based budding yeasts
   b. chlamydospores
   c. pseudohyphae, as well as some yeast cells
   d. arthrospores
   e. numerous inflammatory cells, but few fungal elements.

10. *Concerning* Coccidioides immitis, *which statement is **least** accurate?*

    a. Overt disease is the exception in dogs and other animals.
    b. The thick-walled, barrel-shaped arthroconidia are found in lesions.
    c. Spherules containing endospores are found in lesions.
    d. The skin test is usually negative in disseminated infections.
    e. The complement-fixation test is used to monitor the effect of treatment.

11. *Concerning blastomycosis, which statement is **least** accurate?*

    a. Systemic blastomycosis usually develops from an initial respiratory infection.
    b. Blastomycosis in dogs is rarely transmitted to people.
    c. The causal agent grows relatively slowly on culture media.
    d. The causal agent is dimorphic.
    e. The causal agent has a large, protective capsule.

12. *Which fungus is most important as a cause of **both** respiratory disease in poultry and mycotic abortion in mammals?*

    a. *Candida albicans*
    b. *Mortierella wolfii*
    c. *Cryptococcus neoformans*
    d. *Aspergillus fumigatus*
    e. *Blastomyces dermatitidis*

13. *Which agent causing human infections is associated with pigeon feces?*

    a. *Candida albicans*
    b. *Histoplasma capsulatum*
    c. *Cryptococcus neoformans*
    d. *Aspergillus fumigatus*
    e. *Blastomyces dermatitidis*

14. *Which finding strongly suggests a diagnosis of blastomycosis in an animal from the central United States?*

    a. a positive intradermal test
    b. demonstration of brown microcolonies in cultures of discharging pus
    c. demonstration of thick-walled yeast cells in smears of material from discharging skin lesions
    d. a positive complement-fixation test
    e. a positive hemagglutination test

15. *In a mixed practice (small and large animals), you are most apt to encounter* Cryptococcus neoformans *causing:*

    a. keratitis
    b. skin lesions

c. pulmonary infections

d. paranasal infections

e. intestinal infections

16. *In cattle,* Cryptococcus neoformans *is mainly of concern as a cause of:*

a. mastitis

b. pneumonia in feedlot calves

c. meningitis

d. granulomatous nasal lesions

e. chronic footrot

17. *Which fungus has a particular predilection for the reticuloendothelial system?*

a. *Blastomyces dermatitidis*

b. *Coccidioides immitis*

c. *Histoplasma capsulatum*

d. *Aspergillus fumigatus*

e. *Candida albicans*

18. *A fungus associated with ear infections in dogs is:*

a. *Aspergillus fumigatus*

b. *Cryptococcus neoformans*

c. *Malassezia pachydermatis (Pityrosporum canis)*

d. *Rhinosporidium seeberi*

e. *Sporothrix schenckii*

19. *Clinical disease caused by* Sporothrix schenckii:

a. usually results in disseminated lesions throughout the liver and spleen

b. most often results in lymphocutaneous disease characterized by nodules along the lymphactics

c. nearly always is restricted to the initial site of inoculation

d. seldom responds favorably to chemotherapy

e. is restricted to the stratum corneum of the epidermis

20. *Which dimorphic fungus has a mycelial phase on blood agar incubated at 37 C?*

a. *Coccidioides immitis*

b. *Blastomyces dermatitidis*

c. *Histoplasma farciminosum*

d. *Sporothrix schenckii*

e. *Histoplasma capsulatum*

21. *Which fungus is* **not** *known to be dimorphic?*

a. *Histoplasma capsulatum*

b. *Coccidioides immitis*

c. *Rhinosporidium seeberi*

d. *Sporothrix schenckii*

e. *Blastomyces dermatitidis*

22. *Variously colored microcolonies are seen on culture of material from lesions of:*

a. eumycotic mycetoma

b. blastomycosis

c. coccidioidomycosis

d. sporotrichosis

e. chromoblastomycosis

23. *Which fungus is most frequently transmitted from animals to children?*

a. *Blastomyces dermatitidis*

b. *Coccidioides immitis*

c. *Histoplasma capsulatum*

d. *Microsporum canis*

e. *Trichophyton mentagrophytes*

24. *A Wood's lamp is most effective in demonstrating fluorescence in hair infected with:*

a. *Trichophyton verrucosum*

b. *Microsporum gypseum*

c. *Microsporum canis*

d. *Trichophyton mentagrophytes*

e. *Microsporum nanum*

Correct answers are on pages 127-130.

25. Which organism most commonly infects the lymphatics of the limbs?

   a. *Blastomyces dermatitidis*
   b. *Coccidioides immitis*
   c. *Cryptococcus neoformans*
   d. *Sporothrix schenckii*
   e. *Histoplasma capsulatum*

26. Which drug is most frequently used in treatment of sporotrichosis in animals?

   a. potassium iodide
   b. griseofulvin
   c. amphotericin B
   d. cycloheximide
   e. flucytosine

27. Which dermatophyte is most likely to cause ringworm in cattle?

   a. *Trichophyton gallinae*
   b. *Microsporum canis*
   c. *Trichophyton verrucosum*
   d. *Microsporum gypseum*
   e. *Microsporum nanum*

28. The best stain to use for wet mounts of mycelial fungal cultures is:

   a. Gram's stain
   b. India ink
   c. lactophenol cotton blue
   d. modified Ziehl-Neelsen
   e. silver nitrate

29. Concerning fungal infections, which statement is **least** accurate?

   a. Immunity is primarily humoral.
   b. Immunity is primarily cell mediated.
   c. Chronic granulomatous infections are common.
   d. Animals or people with immunosuppression are often infected.
   e. Infected animals may develop a hypersensitivity reaction.

30. Concerning molds and yeasts, which statement is **least** accurate?

   a. They are eucaryotic.
   b. They have unique, rigid cell walls.
   c. Their cytoplasmic membranes contain sterols.
   d. They are procaryotic.
   e. They do not contain muramic acid.

31. The fungus most likely to be associated with feces in starling roosts is:

   a. *Blastomyces dermatitidis*
   b. *Coccidioides immitis*
   c. *Histoplasma capsulatum*
   d. *Microsporum gypseum*
   e. *Sporothrix schenckii*

32. The electron beams of an electron microscope are brought into focus by:

   a. radiation fields
   b. glass lenses
   c. magnetic fields
   d. laser beams
   e. quartz lenses

33. Which of the following is found in the cell wall of both Gram-positive and Gram-negative bacteria?

   a. peptidoglycan
   b. teichoic acid
   c. lipopolysaccharide
   d. lipid
   e. lipoprotein

34. A deamination reaction in bacteria generally results in production of:

   a. an acidic pH
   b. a neutral pH
   c. an alkaline pH
   d. hydrogen sulfide
   e. carbon dioxide

35. All of the following functions/properties have been attributed to bacterial capsules **except**:

    a. slime layer
    b. inhibition of antibiotic uptake
    c. inhibition of phagocytosis
    d. O-antigens
    e. K-antigens

36. Transfer of DNA from one bacterium to another via a bacteriophage is called:

    a. conjugation
    b. transfection
    c. transduction
    d. transformation
    e. replication

37. All of the following are examples of autonomously replicating DNA structures **except**:

    a. plasmid
    b. F-factor
    c. transposon
    d. R-factor
    e. episome

38. An acidic reaction in the slant and butt portions of a triple sugar-iron agar medium indicates:

    a. carbohydrate utilization
    b. deamination
    c. desulfurylation
    d. fermentation
    e. anaerobic growth

39. Synthesis of proteins in a faculative bacterial species grown in the presence of oxygen with glucose as the primary carbon source involves all the following **except**:

    a. anabolism
    b. catabolism
    c. oxidative phosphorylation
    d. anaerobic respiration
    e. ATP production

40. Bacterial mycolic acid residues are responsible for:

    a. the Gram-positive reaction
    b. the Gram-negative reaction
    c. spore resistance to heat
    d. the acid-fast reaction
    e. susceptibility to lysozyme

41. A bactericidal disinfectant is one that:

    a. causes thymine dimerization
    b. inhibits DNA synthesis
    c. results in irreversible inhibition of growth
    d. results in reversible inhibition of growth
    e. disrupts cell membranes

42. A bacterial species exhibiting an optimal growth temperature of 58 C, a need for high carbon dioxide levels, and growth inhibition by oxygen could be classified as all of the following **except**:

    a. anaerobic
    b. autotrophic
    c. thermophilic
    d. heterotrophic
    e. procaryotic

43. By convention, the term "fermentation" is loosely used to describe carbohydrate utilization by bacteria. Technically, fermentation is:

    a. an aerobic process
    b. a facultative process
    c. the production of organic acids
    d. an anaerobic process
    e. an anabolic process

44. Uptake of naked DNA by a bacterium is termed:

    a. transduction
    b. transfection
    c. competence
    d. transformation
    e. conjugation

Correct answers are on pages 127-130.

45. Which method is most suitable for sterilization of an antiserum?

   a. irradiation
   b. autoclaving
   c. oven baking
   d. filtration
   e. sonication

46. Which bacterium **rarely** causes mastitis in cows?

   a. *Streptococcus pyogenes*
   b. *Streptococcus agalactiae*
   c. *Actinomyces pyogenes*
   d. *Streptococcus uberis*
   e. *Streptococcus dysgalactiae*

47. The enzyme released by potentially pathogenic strains of Staphylococcus aureus, *causing clotting of plasma, is called:*

   a. catalase
   b. coagulase
   c. hyaluronidase
   d. lecithinase
   e. staphylokinase

48. Staphylococcus hyicus *is most frequently involved in:*

   a. mastitis in cows
   b. mastitis in sows
   c. urinary tract infections in animals
   d. exudative epidermitis in pigs
   e. staphylococcal pyoderma

49. The Lancefield serologic grouping of streptococci is based upon differences in:

   a. component c
   b. M protein
   c. hyaluronic acid
   d. hemolysin
   e. streptokinase

50. The CAMP test is used for rapid presumptive identification of:

   a. *Staphylococcus aureus*
   b. *Streptococcus uberis*
   c. enteropathogenic *Escherichia coli*
   d. *Streptococcus dysgalactiae*
   e. *Streptococcus agalactiae*

51. Which pyogenic organism is encountered most commonly as a cause of suppurative pneumonia in calves and young pigs?

   a. *Streptococcus zooepidemicus*
   b. *Actinomyces (Corynebacterium) pyogenes*
   c. *Staphylococcus aureus*
   d. *Corynebacterium pseudotuberculosis*
   e. *Corynebacterium kutscheri*

52. Abscesses of the cervical lymph nodes ("jowl abscesses") of swine are caused principally by:

   a. *Streptococcus porcinus*
   b. *Streptococcus pyogenes*
   c. *Streptococcus uberis*
   d. *Streptococcus suis*
   e. *Viridans* streptococci

53. Concerning Eubacterium suis, *which statement is* **least** *accurate?*

   a. It is aerobic.
   b. It is anaerobic.
   c. It causes pyelonephritis in sows.
   d. It can be recovered from boar's semen occasionally.
   e. It was formerly called *Corynebacterium suis.*

54. Which is the preferred clinical specimen to submit for laboratory diagnosis of rhodococcal pneumonia in foals?

   a. tracheal wash
   b. cotton swab from the nasal passages, without immersion in transport medium
   c. cotton swab from the nasal passages, immersed in transport medium
   d. cotton swab from the nasopharynx

e. unclotted blood sample

55. *Staphylococcal infections in dogs are most commonly caused by:*

   a. *Staphylococcus intermedius*
   b. *Staphylococcus aureus*
   c. *Staphylococcus epidermidis*
   d. *Staphylococcus hyicus*
   e. *Staphylococcus saprophyticus*

56. Concerning Listeria, *which statement is **least** accurate?*

   a. The genus *Listeria* is comprised of more than one species.
   b. *Listeria monocytogenes* infection is usually exogenous.
   c. *Listeria monocytogenes* infection is highly contagious.
   d. *Listeria monocytogenes* is a facultative intracellular parasite.
   e. *Listeria monocytogenes* is an important pathogen of people.

57. *Which bacterium occurs as a usually harmless commensal of the bovine teat duct?*

   a. *Actinomyces pyogenes*
   b. *Corynebacterium pilosum*
   c. *Corynebacterium cystitidis*
   d. *Corynebacterium renale*
   e. *Corynebacterium bovis*

58. *Concerning immunity to swine erysipelas, which statement is **least** accurate?*

   a. Bacterins elicit adequate, though short-term, immunity.
   b. Hyperimmune serum is effective in preventing the disease in contact animals.
   c. Immunity is predominantly cell mediated.
   d. A live attenuated strain is used for immunization.
   e. Immune complexes are involved in production of the skin lesions.

59. *Concerning neural listeriosis, which statement is **least** accurate?*

   a. Silage is a common source of the causal agent.
   b. Silage with a pH below 5.5 allows multiplication of *Listeria monocytogenes*.
   c. Treatment of affected sheep may be ineffective because of brain damage.
   d. Treatment may be ineffective because of inadequate concentrations of antibiotic in the brain.
   e. Rodents may contaminate silage with *Listeria* organisms.

60. *Which bacterium produces arthritis in swine, characterized by marked periarticular fibrosis of the hip, stifle or hock joints?*

   a. *Erysipelothrix rhusiopathiae*
   b. *Actinomyces pyogenes*
   c. *Staphylococcus aureus*
   d. *Streptococcus zooepidemicus*
   e. *Mycoplasma hyorhinis*

61. *In the visceral form of listeriosis, the organism is thought to enter the body via:*

   a. branches of the trigeminal nerve
   b. wounds
   c. the alimentary tract
   d. the genital tract
   e. the conjunctiva

62. *Tetanus is generally diagnosed by:*

   a. clinical signs
   b. demonstration of organisms in a direct smear
   c. fluorescent antibody test
   d. demonstration of toxin
   e. detection of tetanus antitoxin

63. *Which bacterium can survive indefinitely and multiply in the soil?*

   a. *Streptococcus equi*
   b. *Corynebacterium renale*
   c. *Erysipelothrix rhusiopathiae*
   d. *Streptococcus agalactiae*
   e. *Listeria monocytogenes*

Correct answers are on pages 127-130.

64. *Sporulation of* Bacillus anthracis *is most likely to occur in:*

   a. an anaerobic atmosphere
   b. healthy tissue
   c. necrotic tissue
   d. an aerobic atmosphere
   e. the bloodstream

65. *The different types of* Clostridium botulinum *are identified on the basis of:*

   a. serologic or antigenic specificity of their neurotoxins
   b. clinical signs seen in laboratory animals
   c. serologic specificity of their endotoxins
   d. differential biochemical tests
   e. differences in metabolic end products, using gas chromatography

66. *Concerning Sterne's spore vaccine, which statement is most accurate?*

   a. The organisms are capsulated and nontoxigenic.
   b. The organisms are capsulated and toxigenic.
   c. The organisms are not capsulated but toxigenic.
   d. The organisms are nontoxigenic and not capsulated.
   e. The organisms have been killed with formalin.

67. *Liver infarcts due to liver flukes are most likely to be associated with:*

   a. bacillary hemoglobinuria
   b. *Clostridium sordellii* infection
   c. *Clostridium novyi* type A infection
   d. *Clostridium novyi* type B infection
   e. *Clostridium colinum* infection

68. *In which species does anthrax frequently result in acute pharyngitis and swelling of the throat region?*

   a. pigs
   b. cattle
   c. sheep
   d. dogs
   e. cats

69. *According to current information, which bacterium is the **least** important cause of disease in animal species?*

   a. *Bacteroides melaninogenicus*
   b. *Fusobacterium necrophorum*
   c. *Bacteroides nodosus*
   d. *Actinomyces pyogenes*
   e. *Bacteroides fragilis*

70. *Which type of* Clostridium perfringens *causes overeating enterotoxemia of feedlot lambs in the United States?*

   a. type A
   b. type B
   c. type C
   d. type D
   e. type E

71. *Fusobacterium necrophorum is associated with all of the following **except**:*

   a. necrotic laryngitis
   b. exudative epidermitis of pigs
   c. diphtheria in calves
   d. liver abscesses in cattle
   e. footrot in cattle

72. *Concerning Pseudomonas pseudomallei, which statement is **least** accurate?*

   a. It is found in tropical soil and water.
   b. It infects farm animals as well as people.
   c. It is found in Southeast Asia.
   d. The disease it causes is common in the southern United States.
   e. It produces both acute and chronic disease.

73. *Concerning blackleg and malignant edema in cattle, which statement is **least** accurate?*

   a. They are both caused by Gram-positive spore formers.
   b. They both have the same usual mode of infection.

c. They are both characterized by gas gangrene of skeletal muscles.

d. They are both characterized by exotoxin production.

e. The causal agents may occur in the intestine.

74. *How long can the causal agent of contagious footrot in sheep survive on pasture?*

a. 1 week
b. 2 weeks
c. 4 weeks
d. 6 weeks
e. 2 months

75. *Concerning salmonellosis in farm animals, which statement is* **least** *accurate?*

a. The carrier state can be readily eliminated.
b. Subclinical carriers are common.
c. In carriers, the organism may be found in Peyer's patches.
d. Some *Salmonella* species produce enterotoxins.
e. *Salmonella* species do not ferment lactose.

76. *The test used to detect glanders in horses is based upon:*

a. an agar-gel precipitin test
b. a delayed hypersensitivity reaction
c. an agglutination reaction
d. a hemagglutination reaction
e. enzyme-linked immunosorbent assay

77. *Which Gram-negative organism has been frequently associated with mastitis in cows bedded on sawdust or wood shavings?*

a. *Proteus mirabilis*
b. *Serratia*
c. *Klebsiella*
d. *Providencia*
e. *Yersinia enterocolitica*

78. *Which sample would you submit for laboratory diagnosis of type C clostridial enterotoxemia in pigs?*

a. fresh small intestinal content
b. intestinal content preserved with formalin
c. feces from the large bowel
d. a portion of liver
e. portions of liver and kidney

79. *What is the most important cause of death in recently hatched chicks?*

a. fowl typhoid
b. avian diphtheria
c. fowl cholera
d. pullorum disease
e. crop mycosis

80. *Concerning* Francisella tularensis, *which statement is* **least** *accurate?*

a. It is a facultative intracellular parasite.
b. It causes granulomatous lesions.
c. Protective immunity is mainly cell mediated.
d. It is highly infectious.
e. Protective immunity is mainly humoral.

81. *Which bacterium is the most common isolate from animal wounds in the United States?*

a. *Pseudomonas aeruginosa*
b. *Pseudomonas pseudomallei*
c. *Pseudomonas mallei*
d. *Pasteurella pneumotropica*
e. *Providencia* species

82. *Concerning type-D strains of* Pasteurella multocida, *which statement is* **least** *accurate?*

a. They may produce an exotoxin.
b. They may produce a dermonecrotoxin.
c. They are frequently recovered from swine.
d. They alone are considered the cause of atrophic rhinitis.
e. They may be recovered from pneumonic lungs of swine.

Correct answers are on pages 127-130.

83. *Concerning* Pasteurella haemolytica, *which statement is **least** accurate?*

    a. It produces a leukotoxin.
    b. It occurs in different capsular types.
    c. Infections are common in pigs.
    d. It occurs in 2 biotypes.
    e. It has an important role in pneumonic pasteurellosis in cattle.

84. *In cattle with actinobacillosis* (Actinobacillus lignieresii), *the granules seen in lesions contain colonies of:*

    a. Gram-negative bacilli
    b. Gram-positive cocci
    c. Gram-positive filamentous, branching organisms
    d. Gram-negative cocci
    e. spirochetes

85. *Which bacterium is **rarely** associated with arthritis in swine?*

    a. *Mycoplasma granularum*
    b. *Mycoplasma hyorhinis*
    c. *Actinomyces pyogenes*
    d. *Erysipelothrix rhusiopathiae*
    e. *Pasteurella multocida*

86. *Concerning* Actinobacillus equuli, *which statement is **least** accurate?*

    a. The organism is most commonly found in soil.
    b. Disease may be manifested within 24 hours after birth.
    c. Purulent nephritis is a possible sequela.
    d. Death may follow severe enteritis.
    e. The organism may be carried in the intestinal tract.

87. *In the severe form of pasteurellosis, referred to as hemorrhagic septicemia, many of the pathologic changes and clinical manifestations are thought to be caused by:*

    a. exotoxins
    b. obstruction of capillaries by many organisms

    c. capsular substances
    d. endotoxins
    e. immune complexes

88. *Concerning* Campylobacter fetus *subspecies* venerealis *and* Campylobacter fetus *subspecies* fetus, *which statement is **least** accurate?*

    a. They both cause abortion in sheep.
    b. They both cause abortion in cattle.
    c. They are both transmitted venereally.
    d. They are both microaerophilic.
    e. They are both nonfermentative.

89. *The diarrhea and dehydration seen in calves with colibacillosis are mainly attributable to the effects of:*

    a. enterotoxin
    b. endotoxin
    c. capsular antigen
    d. lipopolysaccharide
    e. verotoxin

90. *Concerning* Actinobacillus pleuropneumoniae, *which statement is **least** accurate?*

    a. It causes a hemorrhagic necrotizing process.
    b. It produces a heat-stable toxin.
    c. It was previously known as *Haemophilus pleuropneumoniae.*
    d. It has a number of different serotypes.
    e. It requires the V factor for growth.

91. *Concerning* Campylobacter jejuni, *which statement is **least** accurate?*

    a. It is found as a commensal in the intestine of many animals.
    b. It causes avian infectious hepatitis.
    c. It is not transmissible to people.
    d. It may cause febrile enteritis in dogs and cats.
    e. It may produce a heat-labile enterotoxin.

92. *In addition to isolation and identification of the causal agent, which of the following is a convenient and useful aid to diagnosis of contagious equine metritis?*

---

a. complement-fixation test
b. examination of endometrial smears
c. serum enzyme activities
d. differential blood count
e. agar-gel precipitin test

93. Which of the following is thought to be involved in proliferative enteritis in swine?

a. *Campylobacter mucosalis*
b. *Campylobacter jejuni*
c. *Campylobacter coli*
d. *Campylobacter pylori*
e. *Campylobacter fecalis*

94. Concerning contagious equine metritis, which statement is **least** accurate?

a. The causal agent is a Gram-positive spirochete.
b. Infected mares have a copious purulent vulvar discharge.
c. The disease is rare in the United States.
d. Diagnosis is based on isolation and identification of the causal agent.
e. No clinical signs are seen in infected stallions.

95. Concerning Haemophilus parasuis, which statement is **least** accurate?

a. It is the cause of Glasser's disease.
b. It is a commensal organism.
c. It is a small Gram-positive bacillus.
d. It is a frequent secondary invader in swine influenza.
e. It is an extracellular parasite.

96. Which of the following is most appropriate for definitive diagnosis of infectious keratoconjunctivitis in cattle?

a. diagnosis based on clinical signs
b. submission of a swab from affected tissue for culture and identification
c. examination of Gram-stained smears form the conjunctiva
d. enzyme-linked immunosorbent assay
e. agar-gel immunodiffusion test

97. Which bacterium causes infectious (fowl) coryza?

a. *Haemophilus paragallinarum*
b. *Pasteurella gallinarum*
c. *Pasteurella anatipestifer*
d. *Moraxella bovis*
e. *Bordetella avium*

98. Which organism is encountered most frequently in enzootic pneumonia of pigs?

a. *Haemophilus parasuis*
b. *Streptococcus zooepidemicus*
c. *Pasteurella multocida*
d. *Pasteurella haemolytica*
e. *Actinobacillus pleuropneumoniae*

99. What is one of the most common features of Campylobacter *infection in bulls?*

a. severe orchitis and epididymitis
b. absence of gross lesions
c. arthritis
d. granulomatous ulcerations on the external genitalia
e. febrile enteritis

100. Concerning Brucella ovis, which statement is **least** accurate?

a. The complement-fixation test is useful in diagnosis.
b. It contains the A antigen but not the M antigen.
c. Culling of infected rams is useful in control.
d. Rams are more susceptible than ewes.
e. It causes placentitis and abortion in ewes.

101. Suspected Salmonella colonies on a culture plate can be reliably identified by:

a. carbohydrate fermentation
b. mouse inoculation
c. guinea pig inoculation
d. morphologic characteristics
e. serologic tests

Correct answers are on pages 127-130.

102. *In pigs,* Bordetella bronchiseptica *and*
Pasteurella multocida *may be found as*
commensals on the mucosa of the:

   a. bronchi
   b. upper respiratory tract
   c. large bowel
   d. genital tract
   e. skin

103. *Which type of tuberculin test is used*
routinely in rhesus monkeys?

   a. caudal fold test
   b. intravenous test
   c. ophthalmic test
   d. comparative test
   e. subcutaneous test

104. Brucella abortus *and* Francisella tularensis
differ in their:

   a. usual mode of transmission
   b. intracellular location in the host
   c. host response
   d. Gram reaction
   e. morphology

105. *Concerning Johne's disease, which*
*statement is **least** accurate?*

   a. Culture is the most reliable means of
      diagnosis.
   b. There are a considerable number of
      asymptomatic carriers.
   c. Sheep and goats are highly resistant.
   d. It can be manifested as genital infections.
   e. Examination of rectal smears is unreliable
      for definitive diagnosis.

106. *From an economic standpoint, which of the*
following is the greatest deficiency in use of
strain 19 vaccine for prevention of brucellosis
in cattle?

   a. Male calves may become sterile.
   b. Live organisms may infect people.
   c. The resulting low-grade infections may be
      transmissible.

   d. A small percentage of animals have
      persistent agglutination titers.
   e. Calves become hypersensitive to *Brucella*
      protein.

107. *Which* Mycobacterium *species grows most*
slowly and least luxuriantly?

   a. *Mycobacterium avium*
   b. *Mycobacterium tuberculosis*
   c. *Mycobacterium fortuitum*
   d. *Mycobacterium bovis*
   e. *Mycobacterium intracellulare*

108. *Microscopic examination of a sectioned*
"sulfur granule" from a suppurating lesion on
a cow's jaw is most likely to reveal a:

   a. colony of filamentous organisms
   b. colony of short rods
   c. collection of spiral organisms
   d. colony of spore-forming organisms
   e. colony of Gram-negative bacteria

109. *Severe infectious atrophic rhinitis in swine*
is caused by:

   a. *Bordetella bronchiseptica* and *Pasteurella*
      multocida
   b. toxigenic *Pasteurella multocida* alone
   c. toxigenic *Bordetella bronchiseptica* alone
   d. *Bordetella bronchiseptica* and
      Pseudomonas aeruginosa
   e. *Bordetella parapertussis*

110. Anaplasma marginale *infects:*

   a. monocytes
   b. neutrophils (polymorphonuclear leukocytes)
   c. eosinophils
   d. red blood cells
   e. hepatocytes

111. *Swine dysentery is most conveniently and*
rapidly diagnosed in the laboratory by:

   a. stained smear from intestinal mucosa
   b. immunodiffusion test

c. growth inhibition test

d. culture

e. complement-fixation test

112. *Concerning Potomac horse fever (monocytic ehrlichiosis), which statement is* **least** *accurate?*

a. It is caused by *Ehrlichia equi.*

b. It tends to occur during the winter.

c. It induces diarrhea.

d. It has been observed in a number of states.

e. The indirect fluorescent antibody test on serum is useful for detecting specific antibodies.

113. *Concerning use of* Leptospira *bacterins in dogs, which statement is* **least** *accurate?*

a. They consist of killed organisms.

b. A monovalent bacterin gives adequate protection.

c. Dogs should be vaccinated at least annually.

d. Vaccines elicit relatively low levels of agglutinating antibodies.

e. Bacterins may not prevent shedding of leptospires in the urine.

114. *Concerning chlamydiae, which statement is* **least** *accurate?*

a. They occur widely in domestic animals.

b. Only one species infects domestic animals.

c. When present, they do not always cause clinical signs.

d. They are intracellular parasites.

e. The principal mode of transmission is by the bite of arthropods.

115. *Leptospirosis in cattle is usually diagnosed by:*

a. demonstration of leptospires in urine

b. demonstration of leptospires in aborted fetuses

c. demonstration of leptospires on culture

d. the agar-gel precipitin test

e. the microscopic agglutination test

116. *Concerning ehrlichiosis in dogs, which statement is* **least** *accurate?*

a. The causal agent multiplies in mononuclear cells.

b. It may be characterized by epistaxis.

c. The causal agent is transmitted by mites.

d. Human infections have been reported.

e. The indirect fluorescent antibody procedure is a useful serologic test.

117. *Mercaptoethanol is used in the* Brucella *agglutination test to remove:*

a. IgE

b. IgG

c. IgM

d. serum lipid

e. IgA

118. *Concerning* Chlamydia psittaci, *which statement is* **least** *accurate?*

a. It contains a number of serologically different strains.

b. It has a predilection for epithelial cells.

c. Toxins have been isolated from *Chlamydia psittaci* organisms.

d. Infections can be diagnosed by complement-fixation test.

e. It is unaffected by sulfonamides.

119. Actinomyces viscosus *is best differentiated from* Nocardia asteroides *by:*

a. acid-fast stain

b. Giemsa stain

c. demonstration of spores

d. Gram stain

e. motility test

120. *Concerning* Actinomyces viscosus, *which statement is* **least** *accurate?*

a. It is usually transmitted by ticks.

b. It is Gram-positive.

c. It is aerobic.

d. It is commensal in the mouth.

e. It causes disease in dogs.

Correct answers are on pages 127-130.

121. *Concerning* Neorickettsia helminthoeca *infection, which statement is **least** accurate?*

    a. It has a relatively narrow geographic distribution.

    b. It is best diagnosed (presumptively) by demonstration of trematode eggs in feces.

    c. It is best treated with anthelmintics.

    d. It depends on dogs, snails and fish for its perpetuation.

    e. The intestine and lymphoid tissues are mainly involved.

122. *The easiest and quickest way to confirm a diagnosis of dermatophilosis is to:*

    a. use an extract in an immunodiffusion test

    b. demonstrate characteristic organisms in smears made from skin crusts or scabs

    c. isolate and identify the organism

    d. examine biopsies of skin for the characteristic organisms

    e. perform an enzyme-linked immunosorbent assay on serum

123. *Concerning* Nocardia asteroides *and* Actinomyces viscosus, *which statement is **least** accurate?*

    a. They are both Gram positive.

    b. Their infections can be effectively treated with penicillin and streptomycin.

    c. They both produce granulomatous lesions.

    d. They both infect animals via wounds.

    e. They both cause infections in dogs.

124. *Concerning cat scratch disease or cat scratch fever, which statement is **least** accurate?*

    a. It affects mainly kittens.

    b. It affects mainly children.

    c. It is noncontagious.

    d. A skin test is used in diagnosis.

    e. A small bacterium is considered to be the cause.

125. *Which tissue is most appropriate to submit for examination if you suspected that an animal has Tyzzer's disease?*

    a. liver

    b. brain

    c. lung

    d. blood

    e. duodenum

126. *In addition to elimination of infectious material (crusts, scabs, dander), what is the recommended treatment for dermatophilosis?*

    a. extended treatment with iodide given orally

    b. penicillin and streptomycin by injection

    c. griseofulvin given orally for several weeks

    d. amphotericin B by injection

    e. flucytosine by injection

127. *Erythritol in certain tissues stimulates growth of all of the following **except**:*

    a. *Brucella abortus* strain 19

    b. *Brucella melitensis*

    c. *Brucella suis*

    d. *Brucella canis*

    e. *Brucella abortus*

128. *Concerning collection and culture of urine samples from animals with suspected urinary tract infection, which statement is **least** accurate?*

    a. Urine should be refrigerated as soon as possible after collection.

    b. Aseptic collection is important to minimize contamination with normal flora associated with the urinary tract.

    c. Isolation and identification of bacteria are not sufficient to confirm a causal role.

    d. Urine does not support the growth of bacteria.

    e. A bacterial count is necessary for reliable diagnosis of urinary tract infection.

For Questions 129 through 132, select the correct answer from the 4 choices below.

    a. *Pseudomonas aeruginosa*

    b. *Bordetella bronchiseptica*

    c. *Yersinia pestis*

    d. *Pseudomonas mallei*

129. *Produces pyocyanin.*

130. *Transmitted by fleas.*

131. *Infection diagnosed by delayed hypersensitivity reaction.*

132. *Secondary invader, causing pneumonia in dogs with distemper.*

For Questions 133 through 136, select the phrase most closely associated with the organism.

   a. rabbits are a major source of infection
   b. simulates appendicitis of people
   c. causes respiratory infections in rats and mice
   d. causes "wooden tongue"

133. *Francisella tularensis*

134. *Actinobacillus lignieresii*

135. *Yersinia pseudotuberculosis*

136. *Pasteurella pneumotropica*

137. *Which type of vaccine is used to immunize horses against equine influenza?*

   a. fully virulent
   b. heterotypic live
   c. inactivated
   d. modified live
   e. toxoid

138. *Papillomaviruses:*

   a. usually cause systemic infections, with viremia and widely disseminated replication
   b. cause high mortality
   c. cause pathognomonic lesions

   d. are single-stranded DNA viruses
   e. are readily transmitted via the respiratory route

139. *The Coggins' test is diagnostic for equine infectious anemia by virtue of the high antibody titer found in infected horses. This test is based on:*

   a. enzyme-linked immunosorbent assay
   b. indirect immunofluorescence
   c. immunodiffusion
   d. immunoelectron microscopy
   e. virus neutralization

140. *The seasonal occurrence of bluetongue in sheep in best explained by:*

   a. the lability of the virus during winter
   b. the seasonal occurrence of bird migration
   c. confinement of sheep during winter
   d. the seasonal prevalence of arthropod vectors
   e. antigenic shift

141. *Concerning rabies virus, which statement is **least** accurate?*

   a. It replicates in the cytoplasm.
   b. It travels to the salivary gland by way of the brain.
   c. Wild mammals are the most important reservoir.
   d. It can be transmitted by inhalation of an aerosol.
   e. It is one of the most contagious viruses known.

142. *Equine infectious anemia, caused by a retrovirus, is normally transmitted:*

   a. vertically by milk
   b. vertically by the germ cell
   c. horizontally by contact
   d. by an arthropod vector
   e. as a venereal infection

Correct answers are on pages 127-130.

143. *The feline oncornavirus cell membrane antigen (FOCMA):*

   a. is synonymous with group-specific antigen
   b. is a universal cancer antigen that allows identification of any cancer
   c. stimulates a humoral immune response that seems to protect cats against lymphosarcoma
   d. is never useful in enzyme-linked immunosorbent assay for detection of anti-FOCMA antibody
   e. is of no clinical significance

144. *Viruses that reproduce by "budding" from the host cell nuclear membrane are:*

   a. herpesviruses
   b. togaviruses
   c. retroviruses
   d. orthomyxoviruses
   e. coronaviruses

145. *The most distinctively unusual feature of retroviruses and hepadnaviruses is:*

   a. a single-stranded nucleic acid genome
   b. cell entry by endocytosis
   c. the requirement for reverse transcriptase for replication
   d. oncogenicity
   e. a polyprotein precursor for structural protein synthesis

146. *Concerning the nucleic acid content of viruses, which statement is most accurate?*

   a. Parvoviruses contain double-stranded DNA.
   b. Herpesviruses contain single-stranded RNA.
   c. Reoviruses contain single-stranded RNA.
   d. Adenoviruses contain double-stranded DNA.
   e. Papovaviruses contain double-stranded RNA.

147. *The mechanism that best explains attenuation of a virus by serial passage in vivo or in vitro (eg, passage of rabies virus in duck embryo cells) is:*

   a. viral stimulation of humoral immune response

   b. viral stimulation of a cell-mediated immune response
   c. viral stimulation of complement production
   d. selection of a mutant virus
   e. selection of resistant host cells

148. *The mechanism that best explains the phenomenon of antigenic drift in a virus family is:*

   a. migration of mRNA
   b. deactivation of single DNA strands
   c. point mutations
   d. reassortment of genomic segments
   e. interference of virus growth by interferon

149. *Rabies and vesicular stomatitis viruses are classified in the family:*

   a. Reoviridae
   b. Rhabdoviridae
   c. Coronaviridae
   d. Caliciviridae
   e. Paramyxoviridae

150. *Viruses are constructed in a regular arrangement of identical units, such as helices, cubes or complex symmetry. Which viruses have complex symmetry?*

   a. herpesviruses
   b. poxviruses
   c. paramyxoviruses
   d. picornaviruses
   e. coronaviruses

151. *Concerning interferon, which statement is **least** accurate?*

   a. It is heat stable at 56 C.
   b. It protects primarily cells from the host species in which it was produced.
   c. It inhibits replication of a wide variety of viruses.
   d. Agents other than viruses can induce interferon production.
   e. There is more than one type of interferon.

152. *Which method can be used to quantitate both infectious and noninfectious virus particles?*

a. plaque formation using an agar-medium overlay
b. hemagglutination
c. tissue culture infective dose
d. pock production
e. plaque assay using a carboxymethyl-cellulose overlay

153. *It will take 48 hours for your specimens to arrive at the laboratory for virus isolation. What is the best way to package the specimens?*

a. frozen with dry ice or refrigerated with wet ice
b. in 10% formalin
c. in glycerol
d. in charcoal transport medium
e. in sealed containers (feces separate), not refrigerated

154. *Concerning bluetongue, which statement is least accurate?*

a. The disease in cattle is often inapparent.
b. Only one serotype occurs in the US.
c. The immunodiffusion test is useful in diagnosis.
d. The disease can be confused with contagious ecthyma.
e. The disease in white-tailed deer may be particularly severe.

155. *Concerning rotavirus of cattle, which statement is least accurate?*

a. It usually causes enteritis and diarrhea in calves 1-3 days of age.
b. It is classified in the family Reoviridae.
c. A low concentration of trypsin aids isolation.
d. It causes villus atrophy.
e. It usually causes keratoconjunctivitis in adult cattle.

156. *Of the bovine diseases listed below, which one can be manifested by genital infections in both males and females?*

a. infectious bovine rhinotracheitis
b. bovine virus diarrhea
c. malignant catarrhal fever
d. vesicular stomatitis
e. bovine mammillitis

157. *Which procedure consistently detects bovine leukemia virus infection without a significant number of false positives?*

a. immunodiffusion test (precipitation in agar)
b. immunofluorescence test
c. complement-fixation test
d. lymphocytosis test
e. intradermal test

158. *The principal reason why single serum samples are of questionable value in diagnosis of infectious bovine rhinotracheitis and bovine virus diarrhea is that:*

a. the viruses lack immunogenicity
b. antibody titers to these diseases are found widely in normal cattle
c. the serologic test used is not reliable
d. the antibody to these viruses is highly labile
e. there are anti-complementary factors in bovine serum

159. *Which disease of cattle is usually characterized by a sporadic occurrence?*

a. malignant catarrhal fever
b. rinderpest
c. infectious bovine rhinotracheitis
d. bovine virus diarrhea
e. parainfluenza-3 viral infection

160. *Which species is resistant to infection (inoculation) with the foot and mouth disease virus?*

a. pigs
b. sheep
c. water buffalo
d. horses
e. guinea pigs

Correct answers are on pages 127-130.

161. Concerning malignant catarrhal fever in the United States, which statement is **least** accurate?

   a. It is associated with sheep.

   b. Wild mammals are a reservoir of infection.

   c. The causal agent, presumed to be a virus, has not yet been isolated.

   d. It occurs in acute, subacute and chronic forms.

   e. Definitive diagnosis is based upon histopathologic changes.

162. An acute respiratory infection in a dairy herd is characterized by fever and nasal and ocular discharge. The visible mucous membranes are hyperemic. Several affected cows have pustular vaginitis. The most likely cause of these signs is:

   a. malignant catarrhal fever virus

   b. respiratory syncytial virus

   c. rhinovirus

   d. infectious bovine rhinotracheitis virus

   e. parainfluenza-3 virus

163. The viral agent causing scours or diarrhea of newborn calves is most effectively and rapidly identified by:

   a. electron microscopy

   b. serum neutralization on paired serum samples

   c. fluorescent antibody staining of fecal smears and intestinal sections

   d. histopathologic examination of sections of affected intestine

   e. hemagglutination by virus antigen in feces

164. Cowpox and pseudocowpox both can cause pox lesions on the udder and teats of cows, and are clinically indistinguishable. Concerning these diseases, which statement is **least** accurate?

   a. Cowpox virus can infect people.

   b. Pseudocowpox virus can infect people.

   c. Both viruses can be propagated on the chorioallantoic membrane of chicken embryos.

   d. Both viruses produce intracytoplasmic inclusions.

   e. Cowpox is rare in the United States.

165. Several 8-month-old steers at pasture have reddish, raised, wart-like lesions on the epithelium of the mouth and muzzle. Cytologic examination of an epithelial scraping reveals large intracytoplasmic inclusions. The most likely cause of these findings is:

   a. ulcerative dermatosis

   b. vesicular stomatitis

   c. foot-and-mouth disease

   d. bovine papular stomatitis

   e. infectious bovine rhinotracheitis

166. Which disease is **not** caused by a poxvirus?

   a. ectromelia

   b. bovine ulcerative mammillitis

   c. myxomatosis

   d. lumpy skin disease

   e. bovine papular stomatitis

167. Approximately 10% of a sheep flock at pasture has an infection characterized by ocular and nasal discharge, and excessive salivation. In the later stages of infection, the tongue and lips are cyanotic and ulcerated. The farmer said he found 2 dead deer in the adjacent woods and thought they may have died from the same infection. The most likely cause of these findings is:

   a. ulcerative dermatosis

   b. bluetongue

   c. contagious ecthyma

   d. foot and mouth disease

   e. vesicular stomatitis

168. Which disease has **not** yet been observed in the United States?

   a. swine infertility and respiratory syndrome

   b. scrapie

   c. progressive pneumonia of sheep

   d. bluetongue

   e. pulmonary adenomatosis

169. Which disease is readily transmissible to people?

    a. caprine arthritis and encephalitis
    b. swine pox
    c. ectromelia
    d. contagious ecthyma
    e. ulcerative dermatosis

For Questions 170 through 174, select the correct answer from the 5 choices below.

    a. bluetongue
    b. foot-and-mouth disease
    c. contagious ecthyma
    d. ulcerative dermatosis
    e. sheep pox

170. Mainly transmitted by vectors.

171. Readily transmitted to people.

172. Has not been observed in the United States and is not a threat to cattle.

173. Sometimes called lip and leg ulceration.

174. Natural hosts include cattle, sheep, goats and swine.

175. Concerning scrapie, which statement is **least** accurate?

    a. It can be diagnosed by a delayed hypersensitivity reaction.
    b. It occurs in the United States.
    c. Vaccination does not protect against scrapie.
    d. Bovine spongiform encephalopathy resembles scrapie.
    e. If allowed to run its natural course, scrapie is fatal.

176. Concerning progressive pneumonia in sheep, which statement is **least** accurate?

    a. Signs are most common in sheep more than 4 years of age.
    b. It is also called maedi-visna.
    c. It is seen in sheep and goats.
    d. It is synonymous with pulmonary adenomatosis.
    e. It is caused by a retrovirus.

177. Concerning porcine parvovirus, which statement is **least** accurate?

    a. It causes abortions in late pregnancy.
    b. It may cause stillbirths and mummified fetuses.
    c. Transplacental infection occurs.
    d. Boars may have subclinical genital infection.
    e. The virus can persist in the environment for a long period.

178. Examination of the carcass of a pig that died reveals petechial hemorrhages in the kidneys, enlarged and hemorrhagic lymph nodes, intestinal ulcers, and perivascular cuffing in the brain. The most likely cause of these findings is:

    a. pseudorabies
    b. hemagglutinating encephalomyelitis virus infection
    c. encephalomyocarditis
    d. hog cholera
    e. rabies

179. Concerning vesicular exanthema, which statement is **least** accurate?

    a. It has not been observed in swine in the United States in recent years.
    b. It is caused by a calicivirus.
    c. Of the domestic animals, it affects only swine.
    d. It has not been reported outside of the United States.
    e. It is enzootic in swine in California.

Correct answers are on pages 127-130.

180. *Concerning Teschen-Talfan disease, which statement is **least** accurate?*

    a. It is caused by a neurotropic strain of enteroviruses.
    b. Mild forms of the disease (Talfan) are seen occasionally in the United States.
    c. Swine of all ages may be susceptible.
    d. Gross lesions are particularly characteristic in the acute Teschen form of the disease.
    e. Definitive diagnosis depends upon isolation and identification of the causal virus.

181. *Concerning swine vesicular disease, which statement is **least** accurate?*

    a. It may be confused clinically with foot-and-mouth disease.
    b. It can be differentiated from foot-and-mouth disease by horse inoculation.
    c. It can be spread by garbage feeding.
    d. It does not occur in the United States.
    e. It is caused by an enterovirus.

182. *Concerning swine influenza, which statement is **least** accurate?*

    a. It is not as economically significant as enzootic pneumonia of swine.
    b. Vaccination is widely practiced.
    c. It is a disease of high morbidity but low mortality.
    d. It is common in the United States.
    e. The virus belongs to the influenza-A group.

183. *Concerning inclusion-body rhinitis in swine, which statement is **least** accurate?*

    a. It is caused by a cytomegalovirus.
    b. It is characterized by large intranuclear inclusions.
    c. It is caused by a herpesvirus.
    d. Lesions are produced by dermonecrotoxin.
    e. The causal virus is ubiquitous in the United States.

184. *The principal reservoir for pseudorabies virus is thought to be:*

    a. pigs
    b. sheep
    c. rats
    d. raccoons
    e. insects

For Questions 185 through 188, select the correct answer from the 4 choices below.

    a. swine pox
    b. vomiting and wasting disease
    c. African swine fever
    d. encephalomyocarditis

185. *Caused by a picornavirus.*

186. *Lesions may resemble those of hog cholera.*

187. *More appropriately called hemagglutinating encephalomyelitis.*

188. *Can be transmitted by* Haematopinus suis.

189. *Concerning eastern, western and Venezuelan equine encephalomyelitis, which statement is **least** accurate?*

    a. Circling and paralysis are common signs.
    b. EEE and VEE have higher mortality than WEE.
    c. VEE is particularly severe in people.
    d. EEE can be confused with rabies.
    e. VEE is usually confined to South and Central America.

190. *Of 15 horses pastured in a wooded area, 1 becomes hyperexcitable and aggressive. The horse rolls on the ground as though it had colic. The most likely cause of these signs is:*

    a. eastern equine encephalomyelitis
    b. western equine encephalomyelitis
    c. rabies
    d. equine monocytic ehrlichiosis
    e. African horse sickness

191. *The primary reservoir of eastern equine encephalomyelitis virus is:*

a. forest rodents
b. wild birds
c. mosquitoes
d. reptiles
e. horses

192. *Concerning equine infectious anemia, which statement is **least** accurate?*

a. The virus is transmitted by blood-sucking insects.
b. Preventive measures include vaccination.
c. An agar-gel immunodiffusion test is used for labroatory diagnosis.
d. The virus may cross the placenta and infect the fetus.
e. Animals that survive infection serve as carriers throughout their lives.

193. *Concerning equine influenza, which statement is **least** accurate?*

a. Low hemagglutination inhibition titers are common.
b. Serious complications are common.
c. It is caused by 1 of 2 antigenic or serologic types of virus.
d. The infections are often enzootic.
e. Paired serum samples are useful in serologic diagnosis.

194. *Which virus has been associated with abortion "storms" in foaling establishments?*

a. virus of equine viral arteritis
b. virus of equine serum hepatitis
c. virus of St. Louis encephalomyelitis
d. equine herpesvirus-3
e. equine papilloma virus

195. *Concerning swine blue eye disease, which statement is **least** accurate?*

a. It is caused by a paramyxovirus.
b. It occurs occasionally in the United States.
c. It has only been observed in Mexico.

d. Among its manifestations are central nervous system disorders.
e. The virus can be identified by a direct fluorescent antibody procedure.

196. *Rotaviral and enteric coronaviral infections in neonates both can cause diarrhea, followed by dehydration and often death. Concerning rotaviral and enteric coronaviral infections, which statement is most accurate?*

a. Clinical disease is mild unless there is secondary infection with enteropathogenic *E coli*.
b. Malabsorption arising from virus-IgA immune complexes causes the clinical signs.
c. Death is caused ultimately by endothelial destruction.
d. Secretory epithelium of the gut is destroyed.
e. Absorptive epithelium of the gut is destroyed.

197. *When paired serum samples (acute and convalescent) from a pig showing clinical signs of swine influenza are tested by hemagglutination inhibition, the titers are 1:4 and 1:32 for acute and convalescent samples, respectively. From these findings, the most appropriate conclusion is that:*

a. hemagglutination inhibition is not a useful test to diagnose swine influenza
b. the results of the test do not provide a definitive diagnosis
c. this animal does not have swine influenza
d. this animal has swine influenza
e. swine influenza virus does not agglutinate red blood cells

198. *Concerning equine herpesvirus-1, which statement is **least** accurate?*

a. It usually causes rhinopneumonitis in young horses.
b. Abortions in infected mares occur in late pregnancy.
c. Fetal tissues have characteristic inclusions.
d. Horses may be reinfected.
e. Ataxia and caudal paresis may be seen in foals.

Correct answers are on pages 127-130.

199. *Which of the following has a major role in fatal adenoviral infections in Arabian foals?*

    a. migration of lungworms
    b. insufficient colostrum consumption
    c. joint ill
    d. B- and T-cell deficiencies
    e. secondary invasion by *Rhodococcus equi*

200. *Concerning infectious tracheobronchitis in dogs, which statement is **least** accurate?*

    a. Parainfluenza virus type 2 may be involved.
    b. It is also known as kennel cough.
    c. Canine adenovirus type 2 is usually involved.
    d. Canine adenovirus type 1 may be involved.
    e. *Bordetella bronchiseptica* may be involved.

201. *Concerning parvoviral infection in dogs, which statement is **least** accurate?*

    a. The causal virus has little resistance to environmental factors.
    b. *Campylobacter jejuni* may cause similar signs.
    c. The virus's capacity to hemagglutinate can be used in laboratory diagnosis.
    d. The virus has been implicated in myocarditis of puppies.
    e. Type-2 parvovirus infects dogs.

202. *Concerning rabies, which statement is **least** accurate?*

    a. It is caused by a rhabdovirus.
    b. Live rabies vaccine for use in dogs may produce rabies if given to cattle.
    c. Demonstration of rabies antigen by immunofluorescence is the most widely used diagnostic test.
    d. The incubation period is never longer than 3 months.
    e. Aerosol infection has been reported.

203. *Concerning herpesviral infection in dogs, which statement is **least** accurate?*

    a. It may be involved in the kennel cough syndrome.

    b. Infection is mild in older dogs.
    c. It can be diagnosed by virus isolation and identification.
    d. Infection is often lethal in puppies.
    e. Bilateral opacification of the lens is a pathognomonic sign.

For Questions 204 through 208, select the correct answer from the 5 choices below.

    a. rabies
    b. canine distemper
    c. infectious canine hepatitis
    d. canine herpesviral infection
    e. canine oral papillomatosis

204. *Transient postvaccinal "blue eye" syndrome may be seen.*

205. *Most likely to be fatal in puppies less than 2 weeks of age.*

206. *Almost invariably fatal, regardless of age.*

207. *A possible sequela in old dogs is encephalitis.*

208. *Caused by papovavirus.*

209. *Concerning distemper in dogs, which statement is **least** accurate?*

    a. The diagnosis is often based on clinical signs.
    b. The virus is readily isolated from cell cultures.
    c. It is sometimes diagnosed by fluorescent antibody staining of the buffy coat.
    d. It is caused by a paramyxovirus.
    e. Old dogs with postinfection encephalitis cannot transmit the virus.

For Questions 210 through 213, select the correct answer from the 4 choices below.

    a. feline viral rhinotracheitis
    b. feline caliciviral infection
    c. feline pneumonitis
    d. feline reoviral infection

210. *Caused by a chlamydia.*

211. *Causes palatine and glossal ulcerations.*

212. *Occasionally causes abortion.*

213. *Caused by a double-stranded RNA virus.*

214. *Feline panleukopenia virus (a parvovirus) does not stimulate DNA synthesis in the infected host cell, as do papovaviruses. Which of the following is **not** explained by this fact?*

   a. Feline panleukopenia virus requires dividing cells for its replication.
   b. Feline panleukopenia virus replication in tissue culture ceases when cells reach confluency and stop dividing.
   c. Feline panleukopenia virus infects granulocytic and erythrocytic precursor cells in the bone marrow.
   d. Feline panleukopenia virus attacks the immature cells lining the crypts of the small intestine.
   e. Feline panleukopenia is highly contagious.

215. *Concerning feline leukemia virus infection, which statement is **least** accurate?*

   a. Appreciable feline oncornavirus cell membrane antigen (FOCMA) titers are thought to indicate immunity.
   b. Enzyme-linked immunosorbent assay of serum for p27 antigen is not as sensitive as indirect fluorescent antibody testing.
   c. Cats with appreciable levels of virus-neutralizing antibodies do not usually develop clinical signs.
   d. The indirect fluorescent antibody test is an assay for p27 antigen in blood smears.
   e. The agar-gel precipitin test is not used in diagnosis.

216. *Concerning feline immunodeficiency virus (FIV) infection, which statement is **least** accurate?*

   a. FIV-infected cats may be concurrently infected with feline sarcoma virus.

   b. It is caused by a lentivirus.
   c. Cats may carry viable FIV for long periods.
   d. The principal mode of infection is probably by aerosol.
   e. A test kit is available to detect antibody to FIV.

217. *Concerning feline infectious peritonitis (FIP), which statement is **least** accurate?*

   a. In-utero infections may result in stillbirths.
   b. A modified-live-virus vaccine is available.
   c. A high titer on indirect fluorescent antibody testing and clinical signs support a diagnosis of FIP.
   d. Feline enteric coronaviruses do not cross-react with FIP virus.
   e. Effusive and noneffusive forms of FIP are seen.

For Questions 218 through 221, select the correct answer from the 4 choices below.

   a. coronavirus
   b. lentivirus
   c. parvovirus
   d. oncovirus

218. *Causes feline leukemia.*

219. *Causes feline immunodeficiency virus infection.*

220. *Causes feline infectious peritonitis.*

221. *Causes feline panleukopenia.*

For Questions 222 through 225, select the correct answer from the 4 choices below.

   a. Newcastle disease
   b. infectious laryngotracheitis
   c. infectious bronchitis
   d. avian encephalomyelitis

Correct answers are on pages 127-130.

222. *Caused by an enterovirus.*

223. *Produces pocks on the chorioallantoic membrane.*

224. *Caused by a coronavirus.*

225. *Caused by a paramyxovirus.*

226. *Viscerotropic Newcastle disease is a very severe, highly contagious infection of poultry. Concerning this disease, which statement is **least** accurate?*

   a. It is also known as the velogenic form of Newcastle disease.
   b. The mesogenic form is enzootic in the United States.
   c. The lentogenic form is enzootic in the United States.
   d. The causal virus is lethal for chicken embryos.
   e. The causal virus results in dwarfing of chicken embryos.

227. *Concerning viroids or prions, which statement is **least** accurate?*

   a. They are the cause of bovine spongiform encephalopathy.
   b. They are impervious to the chemicals and radiation that destroy conventional viruses.
   c. They may be rod-shaped and crystalline.
   d. They are products of viral genes.
   e. They are the cause of "kuru."

Questions 228 through 231

A yearling bull suddenly dies at pasture. The hindquarters are extensively swollen and, on palpation, you note a crackling sound.

228. *Culture of tissue samples is most likely to reveal:*

   a. Gram-positive, nonmotile, anaerobic rods
   b. Gram-negative, nonmotile rods with square ends

   c. Gram-positive, motile, spore-forming rods with rounded ends
   d. Gram-positive, motile, spore-forming rods with square ends
   e. Gram-positive rods with terminal spores giving the appearance of a tennis racquet

229. *The most likely cause of this bull's death is:*

   a. salmonellosis
   b. malignant edema
   c. tetanus
   d. black head
   e. blackleg

230. *The causative agent of this disease is:*

   a. *Clostridium chauvoei*
   b. *Clostridium septicum*
   c. *Clostridium novyi*
   d. *Clostridium tetani*
   e. *Clostridium hemolyticum*

231. *A rapid and reliable test that is commonly used to diagnose this disease is:*

   a. direct smear of affected muscle tissue
   b. fluorescent antibody test
   c. mouse inoculation
   d. complement fixation
   e. hemagglutination inhibition

232. *The organism that produces a characteristic fruity odor when grown on blood agar is:*

   a. *Pseudomonas*
   b. *Pasteurella*
   c. *Proteus*
   d. *Salmonella*
   e. *Corynebacterium*

233. *After the iodine step of Gram staining, Gram-positive organisms are:*

   a. colorless
   b. pink
   c. purple
   d. red

e. black

234. Anaerobic, endospore-forming, nonencapsulated bacteria are found in the genus:

a. *Bacillus*
b. *Hemophilus*
c. *Actinomyces*
d. *Clostridium*
e. *Corynebacterium*

235. Bacteria that grow best between 20 and 40 C are referred to as:

a. psychophiles
b. mesophiles
c. thermodurics
d. capnophiles
e. anaerobes

236. Beta hemolysis on blood agar cultures refers to:

a. partial hemolysis of red blood cells in the medium
b. complete hemolysis of red blood cells in the medium
c. a double zone of hemolysis of red blood cells in the medium
d. no hemolysis of red blood cells in the medium
e. selective hemolysis of undersized red blood cells in the medium

237. Which of the following is not a characteristic of an exotoxin?

a. soluble in water
b. protein in nature
c. heat stable
d. antigenic
e. excreted from the bacteria into the surrounding medium

238. All of the following are characteristics of mycobacteria except:

a. thin, straight rods
b. aerobic
c. acid fast
d. Gram negative
e. nonmotile

239. Concerning Listeria and Erysipelothrix, which statement is most accurate?

a. Both organisms are catalase positive and nonmotile.
b. *Listeria* is catalase positive and *Erysipelothrix* is catalase negative, and both organisms are motile.
c. Both organisms are catalase positive and motile.
d. Both organisms are catalase negative and nonmotile.
e. *Listeria* is catalase positive and motile, while *Erysipelothrix* is catalase negative and nonmotile.

240. Which of the following is not a characteristic of Bacillus anthracis?

a. Gram-positive rod
b. nonmotile
c. anaerobic
d. catalase positive
e. has a central spore

241. Which of the following is an anaerobe?

a. *Bacillus*
b. *Clostridium*
c. *Listeria*
d. *Pseudomonas*
e. *Erysipelothrix*

242. The term ectothrix refers to:

a. dermatophyte spores located on the outside of infected hair shafts
b. bacterial spores located on the inside of infected hair shafts
c. bacterial spores located on the outside and inside of infected hair shafts
d. dermatophyte spores located in the dermis
e. dermatophyte spores located in the germinal bed of claws

Correct answers are on pages 127-130.

243. *How do molds differ from bacteria and yeasts?*

    a. growth curve
    b. plant-like
    c. saprophytes
    d. Gram reaction
    e. multinucleated

244. *The correct sequence of virus replication in animals is:*

    a. attachment, uncoating, penetration, latent period, replication, assembly and release
    b. attachment, penetration, latent period, uncoating, replication, assembly and release
    c. attachment, penetration, uncoating, assembly, replication and release
    d. attachment, penetration, uncoating, latent period, replication, assembly and release
    e. attachment, penetration, uncoating, replication, latent period, assembly and release

245. *On a culture plate inoculated with material from an abscess in a dog, you grow a large number of* Staphylococcus aureus *colonies and several colonies of large Gram-positive rods with Chinese letter arrangement. The colonies of Gram-positive rods are most likely those of:*

    a. *Actinomyces (Corynebacterium) pyogenes*
    b. *Bacillus pisiformis*
    c. *Pasteurella multocida*
    d. *Clostridium novyi*
    e. *Pseudomonas aeruginosa*

246. *The microscopic structures most useful in identification of dermatophytes are:*

    a. septate, branching hyphae
    b. microconidia and nonseptate, nonbranching hyphae
    c. chlamydospores and microconidia
    d. macroconidia and microconidia
    e. macroconidia and colony morphology

247. *The CAMP-esculin test is used to differentiate:*

    a. staphylococci from streptococci
    b. *Streptococus agalactiae* from other streptococci causing mastitis
    c. *Staphylococcus aureus* from *Staphylococcus epidermidis*
    d. *Micrococcus* from staphylococci causing pyoderma
    e. *Streptococcus equi* from *Streptococcus zooepidemicus*

248. *A microorganism that is unique for its bipolar staining is:*

    a. *Pasteurella*
    b. *Listeria*
    c. *Clostridium*
    d. *Bacillus*
    e. *Klebsiella*

249. *Bacteria are most resistant to destruction during the:*

    a. lag phase
    b. logarithmic phase
    c. stationary phase
    d. dormant phase
    e. death phase

250. *The steps involved in bacteriophage replication are similar to those of virus replication. Concerning bacteriophages, which statement is most accurate?*

    a. The entire bacteriophage enters the bacterium.
    b. Bacteriophage uncoating occurs soon after it enters a bacterium.
    c. Only the head of the bacteriophage enters the bacterium.
    d. Bacteriophages enter bacteria with the tail part inserted first.
    e. There is a latent period or eclipse in bacteriophage replication.

251. *Concerning viruses, which statement is least accurate?*

    a. Viruses do not grow on artificial media and require living cells to grow.

b. Viruses do not have cellular organelles for metabolism.
c. Viruses contain both DNA and RNA.
d. Viruses do not contain ribosomes.
e. Viruses are not destroyed by antibiotics.

252. *In the California mastitis test, gel forms when the test reagent reacts with:*

a. proteins in the milk sample
b. cellular DNA in the milk sample
c. fat and protein in the milk sample
d. organic salts in the milk sample
e. trace elements in the milk sample

Answers

1. **d**
2. **c**
3. **a**
4. **e**
5. **b**
6. **a**
7. **a**
8. **a**
9. **c**
10. **b**
11. **e**
12. **d**
13. **c**
14. **c**
15. **d**
16. **a**
17. **c**
18. **c**
19. **b**
20. **a** *Coccidioides immitis* is a dimorphic fungus, but the yeast form is not produced on culture media.
21. **c** *Rhinosporidium seeberi* has not been grown on artificial media.
22. **a**
23. **d**
24. **c**
25. **d**
26. **a**
27. **c**
28. **c**
29. **a** Immunity in fungal infections is primarily cell mediated.

30. **d**
31. **c**
32. **c**
33. **a**
34. **c** Ammonia is released, resulting in an alkaline pH.
35. **d** O-antigens are associated with the cell walls of Gram-negative bacteria.
36. **c**
37. **c**
38. **d**
39. **d**
40. **d**
41. **c**
42. **d** Heterotrophs do not have a need for high carbon dioxide levels.
43. **d**
44. **d**
45. **d** Less denaturation takes place with filtration.
46. **a**
47. **b**
48. **d**
49. **a**
50. **e**
51. **b**
52. **a**
53. **a**
54. **a** *Rhodococcus equi* is not apt to be isolated from blood. Cultures from sources other than tracheal wash are likely to be overgrown with other bacteria.
55. **a**
56. **c**

57. **e**

58. **c** Immunity is predominantly humoral.

59. **b** *Listeria monocytogenes* grows in silage when the pH is above 5.5.

60. **a**

61. **c**

62. **a**

63. **c**

64. **d** For this reason, it is not advisable to open the carcasses of animals that have died from anthrax.

65. **a**

66. **c**

67. **a**

68. **a**

69. **e**

70. **d**

71. **b**

72. **d**

73. **b** *Clostridium septicum* infects animals via wounds, and *Clostridium chauvoei* by ingestion.

74. **b**

75. **a** The carrier state of salmonellosis in animals cannot be readily eliminated.

76. **b** The mallein test depends upon a delayed hypersensitivity reaction.

77. **c**

78. **a** The toxin by which laboratory diagnosis is made is labile and present in fresh small intestine.

79. **d**

80. **e**

81. **a**

82. **d** Atrophic rhinitis of swine is now thought to depend upon infection by *Bordetella bronchiseptica* and toxin-producing strains of *Pasteurella multocida*.

83. **c**

84. **a**

85. **e**

86. **a** *Actinobacillus equuli* is commonly found in equine feces.

87. **d**

88. **a** *Campylobacter fetus* subspecies *venerealis* does not cause abortion in sheep.

89. **a**

90. **b**

91. **c** *Campylobacter jejuni* frequently infects people.

92. **a**

93. **a**

94. **a**

95. **c**

96. **b**

97. **a**

98. **c**

99. **b** *Campylobacter* species can be recovered from the semen of bulls, but lesions are not produced.

100. **b** *Brucella ovis* does not possess the A or M antigen.

101. **e**

102. **b**

103. **c**

104. **a** The usual mode of transmission in tularemia is by biting arthropods, in contrast to *Brucella abortus* infection, which is transmitted venereally or via ingestion.

105. **c**

106. **d**

107. **d**

108. **a** The filamentous organism is the Gram-positive bacterium, *Actinomyces bovis*.

109. **a**

110. **d**

111. **a**

112. **a** Potomac horse fever is caused by *Ehrlichia risticii*.

113. **b** A bacterin containing serovars *Leptospira canicola* and *L icterohaemorrhagiae* should be used.

114. **e** The principal modes of infection are by ingestion and inhalation.

115. **e**

116. **c** Transmission is by the dog tick, *Rhipicephalus sanguineus*.

117. **c**

118. **c**

119. **a** Most strains of *Nocardia asteroides* are partially acid fast.

120. **a**

121. **c**

122. **b**

123. **b** Penicillin and streptomycin are not effective in treatment of nocardiosis.

124. **a**

125. **a**

126. **b**

127. **a** The growth of *Brucella abortus* strain 19 is not stimulated by erythritol.

128. **d** Urine does support the growth of some bacteria.

129. **a**

130. **c**

131. **d**

132. **b**

133. **a**

134. **d**

135. **b**

136. **c**

137. **c**

138. **c** The lesions are sufficiently characteristic to be termed pathognomonic.

139. **c**

140. **d**

141. **e** Rabies, which is mainly transmitted by the bite of a rabid animal, is not considered highly contagious.

142. **d**

143. **c**

144. **a**

145. **c**

146. **d**

147. **d**

148. **c**

149. **b**

150. **b**

151. **a**

152. **b** Hemagglutination quantifies both infectious and noninfectious virus particles.

153. **a**

154. **b** At least 5 serotypes have been identified in the United States.

155. **e**

156. **a**

157. **a**

158. **b**

159. **a**

160. **d**

161. **b**

162. **d**

163. **c**

164. **c**

165. **d**

166. **b**

167. **b**

168. **a**

169. **d**

170. **a**

171. **c**

172. **e**

173. **d**

174. **b**

175. **a**

176. **d**

177. **a**

178. **d**

179. **e**

180. **d** Gross lesions are not apparent in acute Teschen disease.

181. **b**

182. **b**

183. **d**

184. **a**

185. **d**

186. **c**

187. **b**

188. **a**

189. **c**

190. **c** Though the clinical signs of rabies and eastern equine encephalomyelitis may be similar, these signs are more consistent with rabies.

191. **b**

192. **b**

193. **b** Serous complications are infrequent.

194. **a**

195. **b**

196. **e**

197. **d**

198. **a** Rhinopneumonitis in young horses is generally considered to be due to EHV-1, subtype 2.

199. **d**

200. **d**

201. **a**

202. **d**

203. **e**

204. **c**

205. **d**

206. **a**

207. **b**

208. **e**

209. **b** The virus of canine distemper is not readily cultivated in cell cultures.

210. **c**

211. **b**

212. **a**

213. **d**

214. **e** The highly contagious nature of feline panleukopenia is considered to be due to dissemination of the highly resistant virus.

215. **b**

216. **d**

217. **d**

218. **d**

219. **b**

220. **a**

221. **c**

222. **d**

223. **b**

224. **c**

225. **a**

226. **e**

227. **d**

228. **c**

229. **e** Swelling over the hindquarters and gas in the tissues causing crackling sounds on palpation suggest blackleg (malignant edema, gas gangrene).

230. **a**

231. **b**

232. **b** This is a characteristic of *Pasteurella*.

233. **c** The iodine fixes the crystal violet in the bacterial cell wall, producing a purple color. Iodine does not impart its own color to the cell.

234. **d** *Clostridium* is a large, anaerobic, nonencapsulated, endospore-forming rod.

235. **b** Mesophilic bacteria grow at 20-40 C, which is the temperature range preferred by most pathogenic bacteria.

236. **b** Beta hemolysis refers to complete hemolysis of red blood cells in the medium, producing a clear zone around the bacterial colonies.

237. **c** Exotoxins are very heat sensitive.

238. **d** *Mycobacterium* is Gram positive.

239. **e** *Listeria* is catalase positive with tumbling motility, whereas *Erysipelothrix* is catalase negative and nonmotile.

240. **c** *Bacillus anthracis* is aerobic.

241. **b** *Clostridium* is strictly anaerobic.

242. **a**

243. **e**

244. **d**

245. **a** This species was named *pyogenes* (pus producer) because it is commonly associated with pus production. This Gram-positive bacillus is often "clubbed" at one end and occurs in palisades or "Chinese letter" arrangement.

246. **e**

247. **b** *Streptococcus agalactiae* produces an arrow-shaped zone, while *Streptococcus uberis* produces brown colonies. *Streptococcus dysgalactiae* produces no special effects.

248. **a**

249. **c**

250. **e** The cycle of virus replication, including replication of bacteriophages, is characterized by a latent period or eclipse.

251. **c** Viruses may contain DNA or RNA, but never both.

252. **b**

Microscopic Anatomy

S.J. Morgan

Recommended Reading

Banks WJ: *Applied Veterinary Histology.* 2nd ed. Williams & Wilkins, Baltimore, 1986.

Dellman HD: *Textbook of Veterinary Histology.* 4th ed. Lea & Febiger, Philadelphia, 1993.

Meyer DJ *et al: Veterinary Laboratory Medicine: Interpretation and Diagnosis.* Saunders, Philadelphia, 1992.

Willard MD *et al: Small Animal Clinical Diagnosis by Laboratory Methods.* Saunders, Philadelphia, 1989.

Practice answer sheet is on page 261.

Questions

1. *Transitional epithelium is a characteristic feature of the:*

   a. upper respiratory system
   b. urinary bladder
   c. seminiferous tubules
   d. gallbladder
   e. oviduct

2. *There are 3 basic methods of cell secretion. Which type of secretion is **not** characterized by the cell cytoplasm itself contributing to the secretory product?*

   a. holocrine
   b. apocrine
   c. merocrine
   d. anacrine
   e. endocrine

3. *Collagen can be produced by all of the following **except**:*

   a. osteoblasts
   b. fibroblasts
   c. smooth muscle cells
   d. chondroblasts
   e. squamous epithelial cells

Correct answers are on pages 144-146.

4. *Elastin makes up a significant proportion of the:*

    a. cornea

    b. nuchal ligament

    c. myocardium

    d. footpad of dogs

    e. pinna

5. *Which tissue is normally vascular?*

    a. cornea

    b. lens

    c. hyaline cartilage

    d. elastic cartilage

    e. bone

6. *From most immature to most mature, what is the correct order of development in osteoid-forming cells?*

    a. osteoprogenitor cell, osteoblast, osteocyte

    b. osteocyte, osteoblast, osteoprogenitor cell

    c. osteoprogenitor cell, osteocyte, osteoblast

    d. osteoblast, osteoprogenitor cell, osteocyte

    e. osteoblast, osteocyte, osteoprogenitor cell

7. *In red blood cells, a Howell-Jolly body is:*

    a. a remnant of rough endoplasmic reticulum

    b. a nuclear remnant

    c. a form of hemoglobin that has been oxidized

    d. a phagocytized parasite

    e. an accumulation of excessive cell membrane

8. *In which species are red blood cells normally of oval shape?*

    a. cattle

    b. horses

    c. camels

    d. pigs

    e. goats

9. *In mammals, which stage of red blood cell development is the most mature cell containing a nucleus?*

    a. rubricyte

    b. metarubricyte

    c. reticulocyte

    d. rubriblast

    e. prorubricyte

10. *Concerning cardiac and skeletal muscle, which statement is most accurate?*

    a. Cardiac muscle fibers are not striated, whereas skeletal muscle fibers are striated.

    b. Cardiac myofiber nuclei are peripherally oriented, whereas skeletal myofiber nuclei are centrally oriented.

    c. Skeletal muscle myofibers exhibit more prominent branching than cardiac muscle myofibers.

    d. Cardiac muscle contains structures known as intercalated disks.

    e. Skeletal muscle contains structures known as intercalated disks.

11. *Concerning veins and arteries, which statement is most accurate?*

    a. Luminal diameter is greater than mural (wall) thickness in veins, whereas luminal diameter is smaller than mural (wall) thickness in arteries.

    b. Venules, but not arterioles, contain an internal elastic membrane.

    c. Because of the increased amount of smooth muscle in veins, as compared with that in arteries, veins are more frequently contracted and contain less blood.

    d. Elastic fibers are more numerous in large veins than in large arteries.

    e. Valves may be seen in medium-sized arteries, but never in medium-sized veins.

12. *The period of the hair growth cycle in which the hair grows is known as:*

    a. telogen

    b. catagen

    c. anagen

    d. halogen

    e. neogen

13. *In dogs, which structure contains cells referred to as hepatoid or hepatocyte-like?*

    a. circumanal glands
    b. anal glands
    c. ceruminous glands
    d. vomeronasal organ
    e. sebaceous glands surrounding the oral cavity

14. *Corpora amylacea may be found in the:*

    a. ceruminous glands
    b. mammary glands
    c. sebaceous glands
    d. circumanal glands
    e. pineal gland

15. *Concerning the equine hoof, which statement is most accurate?*

    a. Epidermal laminae are classified as insensitive, whereas dermal laminae are classified as sensitive and the primary epidermal laminae are keratinized.
    b. Epidermal laminae are classified as insensitive, whereas dermal laminae are classified as sensitive and the secondary epidermal laminae are keratinized.
    c. Dermal laminae are classified as insensitive, whereas epidermal laminae are classified as sensitive and the primary dermal laminae are keratinized.
    d. Dermal laminae are classified as insensitive, whereas epidermal laminae are classified as sensitive and the secondary dermal laminae are keratinized.
    e. Merocrine sweat glands are present in the digital cushion.

16. *Enamel is formed by:*

    a. odontoblasts
    b. ameloblasts
    c. periodontal membrane lining cells
    d. enamoblasts
    e. alveoloblasts

17. *Concerning gastric cell function, which statement is most accurate?*

    a. Hydrochloric acid is secreted by parietal cells.
    b. Hydrochloric acid is secreted by chief cells.
    c. Argentaffin cells secrete their products directly into the gastric lumen.
    d. Argentaffin cells are present in the nonglandular mucosa.
    e. Chief cells secrete mucus to help protect the mucosa from erosion.

18. *Concerning the mesangial cells of the glomerulus, which statement is most accurate?*

    a. They are of ectodermal origin.
    b. They most likely have a phagocytic and supportive function.
    c. They most likely form a portion of the glomerular filtration barrier.
    d. They are of endodermal origin.
    e. They are not present in avian kidneys.

19. *In the mammalian lung, the airways of smallest diameter in which cilia are **absent** are the:*

    a. primary bronchioles
    b. tertiary bronchioles
    c. secondary bronchioles
    d. alveolar ducts
    e. alveolar saccules

20. *Concerning type-I (membranous) and type-II (granular) pneumocytes, which statement is most accurate?*

    a. Tyep-I pneumocytes are squamous, whereas type-II pneumocytes are cuboidal or round.
    b. Type-II pneumocytes are the primary cell lining of the alveoli in the normal adult lung.
    c. Type-I pneumocytes produce surfactant and other products.
    d. Type-I pneumocytes are cuboidal or round, whereas type-II pneumocytes are squamous.
    e. Type-I and -II pneumocytes cannot be differentiated with a light microscope.

Correct answers are on pages 144-146.

21. *Concerning the air sacs of birds, which statement is most accurate?*

    a. In addition to facilitating movement of air through the lung, they function in exchange of gases.

    b. Most birds have only one air sac.

    c. Air sac diverticula are present in bones.

    d. There is really no functional difference between the air sac and the lung.

    e. Air sacs are limited to the thoracic region.

22. *Concerning the adrenal cortex, which statement is most accurate?*

    a. The zona glomerulosa produces glucocorticoids, the zona fasciculata produces sex hormones, and the zona reticularis produces mineralocorticoids.

    b. The zona glomerulosa produces mineralocorticoids, the zona fasciculata produces glucocorticoids, and the zona reticularis produces sex hormones.

    c. The zona glomerulosa produces mineralocorticoids, the zona fasciculata produces sex hormones, and the zona reticularis produces glucocorticoids.

    d. The zona glomerulosa produces glucocorticoids, the zona fasciculata produces mineralocorticoids, and the zona reticularis produces sex hormones.

    e. The zona glomerulosa produces sex hormones, the zona fasciculata produces mineralocorticoids, and the zona reticularis produces glucocorticoids.

23. *Sertoli cells function in all of the following ways* **except***:*

    a. provide support and probably nutrition to developing gametes

    b. secrete estrogens

    c. facilitate release of gametes

    d. phagocytize damaged gametes

    e. secrete testosterone

24. *What is the correct order of spermatogenesis?*

    a. A spermatogonium, B spermatogonium, I (intermediate) spermatogonium, primary spermatocyte, secondary spermatocyte, spermatid

    b. A spermatogonium, I (intermediate) spermatogonium, B spermatogonium, primary spermatocyte, secondary spermatocyte, spermatid

    c. A spermatogonium, I (intermediate) spermatogonium, B spermatogonium, spermatid, primary spermatocyte, secondary spermatocyte

    d. B spermatogonium, I (intermediate) spermatogonium, A spermatogonium, spermatid, primary spermatocyte, secondary spermatocyte

    e. B spermatogonium, A spermatogonium, I (intermediate) spermatogonium, primary spermatocyte, secondary spermatocyte, spermatid

25. *During spermatogenesis, which cell is the first to become haploid?*

    a. spermatid

    b. primary spermatocyte

    c. secondary spermatocyte

    d. B spermatogonium

    e. A spermatogonium

26. *Concerning the normal uterus, which statement is most accurate?*

    a. The caruncle is a region of the lamina propria-submucosa that is highly vascularized and contains many glands.

    b. The cotyledon is a region of the lamina propria-submucosa that is highly vascularized and contains many glands.

    c. Changes that occur during the estrous cycle include glandular activity, vascularization and leukocyte infiltration.

    d. Changes that occur during the estrous cycle include epithelial keratinization and leukocyte infiltration.

    e. The cotyledon is a region of the lamina propria-submucosa that is highly vascularized but nonglandular.

27. *Diffuse placentation is present in:*

    a. horses and pigs

b. horses and cattle

c. dogs and cats

d. dogs and ferrets

e. horses and dogs

28. *Concerning the trophoblast, which statement is **least** accurate?*

 a. Trophoblast cells form the outer layer of the blastocyst.

 b. During nidation in mares (early attachment to the uterus), trophoblasts invade the uterine mucosa, providing a point of attachment.

 c. Trophoblasts are involved in formation of endometrial cups.

 d. Trophoblasts transport oxygen to the newly fertilized ovum.

 e. Trophoblasts arise from the chorioallantoic placenta.

29. *Concerning reproduction in birds, which statement is **least** accurate?*

 a. Only one functional ovary and oviduct are retained in adults.

 b. A corpus luteum does not form after ovulation.

 c. Both infundibular glands and sperm host glands may store spermatozoa.

 d. The vagina is also known as the "shell gland."

 e. The uterus is responsible for formation of the egg shell.

30. *Concerning the normal cornea, which statement is **least** accurate?*

 a. The rostral epithelium consists of cornified stratified squamous epithelium.

 b. It contains numerous nerve endings.

 c. It is avascular, and diffusion of nutrients is the mechanism for nutritive supply.

 d. In major domestic species, the equine cornea is the most sensitive to injury.

 e. Edema results in separation of tissue within the substantia propria.

31. *Which layer is especially well developed in the footpad of dogs?*

 a. stratum granulosum

 b. stratum basale

 c. stratum lucidum

 d. stratum spinosum

 e. stratum germinativum

32. *The uveal tract consists of the:*

 a. choroid, ciliary body and retina

 b. choroid, iris and retina

 c. choroid, ciliary body and iris

 d. choroid, ciliary body and lens

 e. retina, choroid and lens

33. *Which species does **not** have a tapetum lucidum?*

 a. horses

 b. dogs

 c. cats

 d. cattle

 e. pigs

34. *Another name for interstitial cells of the testis is:*

 a. seminiferous cells

 b. Sertoli cells

 c. accessory cells

 d. Leydig cells

 e. supporting cells

35. *The predominant type of connective tissue in tendons and ligaments is:*

 a. areolar connective tissue

 b. irregular dense white fibrous connective tissue

 c. regular dense white fibrous connective tissue

 d. elastic connective tissue

 e. fibrocartilage

Correct answers are on pages 144-146.

36. *Concerning brown adipose tissue, which statement is **least** accurate?*

   a. It contains numerous mitochondria.
   b. It is histologically distinct from white adipose tissue.
   c. It is less well supplied with blood vessels and nerves than is white adipose tissue.
   d. Thermoregulation is an important feature.
   e. In most species, it is more abundant in neonates than in mature animals.

37. *The multinucleated giant cell responsible for remodeling of osteoid is the:*

   a. osteocyte
   b. osteoblast
   c. osteoclast
   d. chondroclast
   e. foreign-body giant cell

38. *Abnormal transformation of a specific, adult, fully differentiated tissue into another differentiated type is called:*

   a. dysplasia
   b. anaplasia
   c. hyperplasia
   d. metaplasia
   e. neoplasia

39. *Woven bone is also known as:*

   a. lamellar bone
   b. fibrous bone
   c. chondrous bone
   d. mature bone
   e. osseous bone

40. *Osteoclasts are derived from:*

   a. macrophages
   b. osteocytes
   c. osteoblasts
   d. osteoprogenitor cells
   e. chondroclasts

41. *Heinz bodies, also known as erythrocyte refractile bodies, consist of:*

   a. nuclear fragments
   b. mitochondrial remnants
   c. oxidized hemoglobin
   d. phagocytized pigments
   e. accumulations of smooth endoplasmic reticulum

42. *Poikilocytes include all of the following forms of red blood cells **except**:*

   a. acanthocytes
   b. leptocytes
   c. schistocytes
   d. stomatocytes
   e. globulocytes

43. *Rouleaux formation (stacking of red blood cells) is most commonly encountered in normal:*

   a. dogs
   b. cats
   c. cattle
   d. horses
   e. goats

44. *The first site of hematopoiesis during embryonic development is the:*

   a. yolk sac
   b. liver
   c. spleen
   d. thymus
   e. bone marrow

45. *Concerning muscle fibers, which statement is most accurate?*

   a. Red muscle fibers consist primarily of type-I fibers, which contain abundant mitochondria and myoglobin.
   b. White muscle fibers consist primarily of type-I fibers, which contain minimal myoglobin and mitochondria.
   c. Type-I fibers are also known as fast-twitch fibers.

d. Type-II fibers are also known as slow-twitch fibers.

e. There is no difference in myofiber type in the breast muscle of a duck as compared with the breast muscle of a chicken.

46. *In which vessels are valves present?*

a. vena cava and lymph vessels
b. small and medium-sized veins and lymph vessels
c. small and medium-sized arteries and lymph vessels
d. small and medium-sized arteries
e. vena cava and small veins

47. *What species has lymph nodes in which lymphatic nodules are located in the central or medullary regions, and structures described as "medullary cords" are located in the peripheral or cortical region?*

a. pigs
b. horses
c. cattle
d. dogs
e. cats

48. *Hemal nodes are found in:*

a. dogs and cats
b. ruminants
c. horses and cattle
d. horses and sheep
e. dogs and horses

49. *Hassall's corpuscles may be found in the:*

a. spleen
b. thymus
c. thyroid
d. retropharyngeal lymph node
e. mammary gland

50. *Abundant adipose tissue is found in the:*

a. scrotum and eyelid
b. frog of horses and pinna of dogs
c. digital cushion of horses and footpad of dogs
d. point of attachment of the dew claw
e. pharyngeal mucosa

51. *Integumentary melanin pigment is most abundant in the:*

a. stratum basale and stratum spinosum
b. stratum lucidum and stratum folliculosum
c. stratum granulosum and stratum superficialis
d. stratum corneum and stratum dermosum
e. stratum disjunctum and stratum epidermosum

52. *Keratohyaline granules are present in the:*

a. stratum basale
b. stratum lucidum
c. stratum granulosum
d. stratum corneum
e. stratum disjunctum

53. *When mineralized, predentin becomes dentin. Predentin is secreted by:*

a. ameloblasts
b. osteoblasts and osteocytes
c. odontoblasts
d. fibroblasts and fibrocytes
e. amelocytes

54. *Which cells of the gastric mucosa secrete materials into the lamina propria (subsequently taken up by vasculature) rather than into the gastric lumen?*

a. parietal cells
b. zymogen cells
c. argentaffin (enterochromaffin) cells
d. mucous neck cells
e. chief cells

Correct answers are on pages 144-146.

55. Zymogen cells of the gastric mucosa are also known as:

 a. transitional cells
 b. oxyntic cells
 c. extrinsic cells
 d. chief cells
 e. parietal cells

56. Paneth cells are present in the:

 a. small intestine of ruminants and horses
 b. stomach of dogs
 c. pancreas of most domestic species
 d. large intestine of cats
 e. small intestine of cats

57. Brunner's glands are found in the:

 a. duodenal mucosa
 b. ileal mucosa
 c. duodenal submucosa
 d. ileal submucosa
 e. duodenal muscularis

58. Concerning juxtaglomerular cells, which statement is most accurate?

 a. They are modified smooth muscle cells of the glomerular afferent arteriole and they secrete renin.
 b. They are modified smooth muscle cells of the glomerular afferent arteriole and they secrete angiotensin.
 c. They are modified smooth muscle cells of the glomerular afferent arteriole and they secrete aldosterone.
 d. They are modified epithelial cells of the proximal convoluted tubule and they secrete renin.
 e. They are modified epithelial cells of the proximal convoluted tubule and they secrete angiotensin.

59. Cartilaginous rings/plaques are associated with the:

 a. primary bronchi
 b. alveolar saccules
 c. secondary bronchioles
 d. primary bronchioles
 e. tertiary bronchioles

60. Which species has the most well-developed bronchioles?

 a. cattle
 b. pigs
 c. horses
 d. mice
 e. dogs

61. Concerning the lungs of birds, which statement is most accurate?

 a. They are quite similar, histologically, to the lungs of mammals.
 b. Relative to the size of the thoracic cavity, they are extremely small.
 c. Their volume changes with the respiratory cycle.
 d. They are not continuous with the air sacs.
 e. They serve the same function as the air sacs.

62. Insulin is secreted by which type of pancreatic islet cells?

 a. alpha cells
 b. beta cells
 c. C cells
 d. delta cells
 e. gamma cells

63. Amine precursor uptake and decarboxylase cells include all of the following except:

 a. cells that secrete gastrointestinal hormones
 b. C (parafollicular) cells of the thyroid
 c. pancreatic islet cells
 d. cells within the parathyroid gland
 e. adrenal medullary cells

64. Cells that comprise the corona radiata surrounding the primary oocyte are:

 a. granulosa cells of the cumulus oophorus
 b. granulosa cells of the zona pellucida

c. thecal cells of the cumulus oophorus

d. thecal cells of the zona pellucida

e. trophoblasts

65. *Concerning the lens in adult animals, which statement is most accurate?*

a. Epithelium is present on the rostral surface only.

b. Epithelium is present on the caudal surface only.

c. Both the rostral and caudal surfaces have epithelium.

d. Neither the rostral nor the caudal surface has epithelium.

e. The epithelium is stratified squamous.

66. *Concerning the retina, which statement is **least** accurate?*

a. The fundus of birds and some mammals (chinchilla, armadillo, bat) is avascular.

b. Rods are generally distributed throughout the retina, whereas cones are the predominant type of photoreceptor in the area centralis retinae.

c. Astrocytes, oligodendroglia and microglia may be present in the retina.

d. It forms the innermost layer of the eye.

e. It forms a portion of the uveal tract.

67. *The most abundant type of collagen in cartilage is:*

a. type I

b. type II

c. type III

d. type IV

e. type V

68. *Fibroblasts can be differentiated from fibrocytes by their:*

a. larger, more oval nucleus

b. less abundant cytoplasm

c. more eosinophilic cytoplasm

d. less prominent nucleolus

e. more spindle-shaped nucleus

69. *Abundant fibrocartilage can be found in the:*

a. nose

b. larynx

c. trachea and bronchi

d. external ear

e. intervertebral disks

70. *Which type of cartilage **lacks** a distinct perichondrium?*

a. hyaline cartilage

b. elastic cartilage

c. fibrocartilage

d. cartilage of the appendicular skeleton

e. cartilage of the flat bones of the skull

71. *Intramembranous ossification occurs in bones of the:*

a. calvaria

b. extremities

c. pelvis

d. thoracic vertebrae

e. lumbar vertebrae

72. *As one progresses distally toward the diaphysis, the correct order of cartilage zones within the growth plate is:*

a. proliferation, maturation, mineralization and ossification, resting

b. proliferation, maturation, resting, mineralization and ossification

c. resting, proliferation, mineralization and ossification, maturation

d. resting, proliferation, maturation, mineralization and ossification

e. resting, maturation, proliferation, mineralization and ossification

Correct answers are on pages 144-146.

73. *Concerning red blood cells in normal goats, which statement is most accurate?*

    a. They are slightly larger than the red blood cells in normal dogs.
    b. Rouleaux formation is common.
    c. Anisocytosis and even poikilocytosis are common.
    d. Nucleated forms are common.
    e. The percentage of reticulated red blood cells in normal goats is 10-15%.

74. *Concerning the morphology of eosinophils, which statement is most accurate?*

    a. Canine eosinophilic granules stain intensely orange.
    b. Feline eosinophilic granules are nearly perfectly round.
    c. Porcine eosinophilic granules are rod shaped.
    d. Equine eosinophilic granules are round, large and so numerous that they frequently obscure the nucleus.
    e. Equine eosinophils are large and rod shaped, and so numerous that they frequently obscure the nucleus.

75. *In which species do circulating lymphocytes normally outnumber neutrophils?*

    a. horses
    b. dogs
    c. cats
    d. cattle
    e. ferrets

76. *The external elastic lamina of an artery defines the outer limit of the:*

    a. intima
    b. media
    c. adventitia
    d. endothelium
    e. vasa vasorum

77. *A sinusoidal spleen has abundant venous sinuses and can store large amounts of blood for quick release if needed. Which animals do **not** have a sinusoidal spleen?*

    a. horses
    b. dogs
    c. cats
    d. ruminants
    e. zebras

78. *What is the major hematopoietic activity of the spleen in adult animals?*

    a. erythropoiesis
    b. lymphopoiesis
    c. granulopoiesis
    d. erythropoiesis and lymphopoiesis
    e. lymphopoiesis and granulopoiesis

79. *Which animals have the most prominent peribronchiolar mucous glands?*

    a. horses
    b. dogs
    c. pigs
    d. ruminants
    e. cats

80. *Which species has a nonkeratinized esophageal tunica mucosa?*

    a. dogs
    b. horses
    c. rats
    d. cattle
    e. goats

81. *Which species has submucosal glands along the entire length of the esophagus?*

    a. horses
    b. cattle
    c. cats
    d. dogs
    e. goats

82. *Which species does **not** have a nonglandular portion of the stomach?*

    a. cattle
    b. horses

c. pigs

d. rats

e. dogs

83. *The mucosal lining of the omasum, reticulum and rumen consists of:*

    a. stratified squamous epithelium
    b. stratified columnar epithelium
    c. transitional epithelium
    d. cuboidal epithelium
    e. pseudostratified columnar epithelium

84. *Which segment of bowel contains the highest proportion of goblet cells?*

    a. duodenum
    b. cecum
    c. colon
    d. rectum
    e. ileum

85. *Fibrous connective tissue separates each hepatic lobule in:*

    a. pigs
    b. horses
    c. ruminants
    d. dogs
    e. cats

86. *Melanophore-rich caruncular regions are present in:*

    a. cattle
    b. goats
    c. sheep
    d. horses
    e. dogs

87. *Cytologic examination of a vaginal smear from a female dog in heat is most likely to reveal:*

    a. occasional red blood cells and many cornified squamous epithelial cells
    b. occasional red blood cells and scattered cornified squamous epithelial cells
    c. numerous red blood cells and many cornified squamous epithelial cells
    d. occasional red blood cells and many noncornified squamous epithelial cells
    e. numerous red blood cells and many noncornified squamous epithelial cells

88. *Tarsal glands of the eyelid are classified as:*

    a. sebaceous glands
    b. sweat glands
    c. lymphoid tissue
    d. mucous glands
    e. endocrine glands

89. *Which species has a relatively thick pleura?*

    a. horses
    b. dogs
    c. cats
    d. rats
    e. pigs

90. *Concerning the intestinal tract, which statement is **least** accurate?*

    a. The tunica mucosa is thicker in the colon than in the small intestine.
    b. Villi are present in the colon but not in the small intestine.
    c. Goblet cells are more abundant in the colon than in the small intestine.
    d. Aggregates of lymphoid cells (Peyer's patches) are more common in the distal small intestine than in the proximal small intestine.
    e. In the small intestine, cell division occurs at the villus tip.

91. *Which species does **not** have a gallbladder?*

    a. dogs
    b. horses
    c. ferrets
    d. cattle
    e. cats

Correct answers are on pages 144-146.

92. *On histologic examination, the thymic cortex appears darker than the medulla because of:*

    a. melanin pigment in the medulla
    b. lipofuscin pigment in the medulla
    c. the high density of epithelial cells in the medulla
    d. the high density of lymphocytes in the medulla
    e. hemosiderin in the medulla

93. *Myoepithelial cells are most prominent in the:*

    a. apocrine glands of the anal sac
    b. harderian glands
    c. mammary glands
    d. tarsal glands
    e. meibomian glands

94. *Hyaluronic acid is abundant in the:*

    a. skin
    b. synovial fluid
    c. cornea
    d. cartilage
    e. myocardium

95. *Concerning the spleen, which statement is least accurate?*

    a. The red pulp predominates over the white pulp.
    b. Of domestic species, the horse has the thickest capsule.
    c. Periarterial lymphatic sheaths are composed of T-lymphocytes.
    d. The spleen of a ruminant can be classified as sinusoidal.
    e. It is one of the possible sites of extramedullary hematopoiesis.

96. *Which structure is lined with simple squamous epithelium?*

    a. blood vessels
    b. urinary bladder
    c. ventricles of the brain
    d. bronchi
    e. gallbladder

97. *Concerning epithelium, which statement is least accurate?*

    a. With pseudostratified epithelium, not all cells contact the basement membrane, but all reach the surface.
    b. Ciliated cuboidal epithelium is present in the ventricles of the brain (ependymal cells) and in the terminal bronchioles of the lung.
    c. Ciliated columnar epithelium is present in the tertiary bronchi, uterus and oviducts.
    d. The epidermal laminae of horses are composed of squamous epithelial cells.
    e. The peritoneal and pleural cavities are lined by simple squamous epithelium.

98. *What does the term "argyrophilic" mean?*

    a. stains positively with gold impregnation techniques
    b. stains positively with silver impregnation techniques
    c. stains positively with argon-based stains
    d. the ability of a single stain to impart a different color to different granules
    e. abundant arginine in the matrix

99. *Purkinje cells that are histologically distinct are found in the:*

    a. cerebrum and myocardium
    b. cerebellum and myocardium
    c. brainstem and myocardium
    d. testis and ovary
    e. adrenal gland and testis

100. *Which tissue normally involutes with the onset of puberty?*

    a. thyroid
    b. adrenal gland
    c. meibomian gland
    d. thymus
    e. pineal gland

101. *Herring bodies are found in the:*

    a. thymus
    b. neurohypophysis

c. proximal renal tubular epithelium

d. mammary gland

e. cerebrum

102. *Kupffer cells are found in the:*

a. spleen

b. large intestinal mucosa

c. gastric mucosa

d. liver

e. cerebellum

103. *Which cells are **not** found in the retina?*

a. sustentacular cells

b. inner plexiform cells

c. rods

d. cones

e. ganglion cells

104. *Concerning the intestinal tract, which statement is **least** accurate?*

a. Villi serve to increase the surface area for absorption.

b. In the normal maturation process, epithelial cells migrate distally along the contour of the villi.

c. Peyer's patches are found only in the ileum.

d. On sections stained with hemotoxylin and eosin, mucus within the epithelial-cell cytoplasm appears as large, round, clear vacuoles.

e. Brunner's glands are present in the duodenum.

105. *Which cell has an eccentric nucleus?*

a. lymphoblast

b. plasma cell

c. mast cell

d. basophil

e. fibroblast

106. *Concerning megakaryocytes, which statement is **least** accurate?*

a. They contain a relatively large volume of cytoplasm.

b. They are multinucleated.

c. Thrombocytes, or platelets, arise from megakaryocytes.

d. They are most abundant in the bone marrow.

e. They can be found in the spleen of normal animals.

107. *One of the major functions of Kupffer cells is:*

a. production of collagen

b. production of glucagon

c. phagocytosis

d. accumulation of excess vitamin A

e. production of C-reactive protein

108. *Concerning the histologic appearance of smooth muscle, which statement is most accurate?*

a. The nucleus is classically described as "cigar shaped" because of its rounded ends.

b. The nucleus has sharp, angular ends.

c. Smooth muscle cells are arranged in tight whorls.

d. Smooth muscle cells are arranged singly in a loose mucinous background.

e. Smooth muscle cells are typically observed against a collagenous background.

109. *From which embryonic cell layer is the lens derived?*

a. ectoderm

b. phthisoderm

c. mesoderm

d. ophthoderm

e. endoderm

110. *Discontinuous endothelium is found in the:*

a. thymus

b. brain

c. liver

d. nasal cavity

e. testis

Correct answers are on pages 144-146.

Answers

1. **b**

2. **c** Merocrine secretion does not involve incorporation of the cell cytoplasm into the secretory product.

3. **e** Squamous epithelial cells do not secrete collagen. Many cells of mesodermal origin can produce collagen.

4. **b** Though elastin can be found in the other tissues listed, the nuchal ligament contains the greatest proportion.

5. **e** Bone is normally vascular. The other tissues listed are vascular only under pathologic conditions.

6. **a**

7. **b**

8. **c**

9. **b**

10. **d** Cardiac muscle contains structures known as intercalated disks. Both cardiac and skeletal muscle are striated. Cardiac nuclei are centrally oriented, whereas skeletal nuclei are peripherally oriented. Cardiac myofibers are more highly branched.

11. **a** Luminal diameter is greater than mural thickness in veins, whereas luminal diameter is smaller than mural thickness in arteries.

12. **c**

13. **a** The circumanal glands have cells that are histologically similar to hepatocytes.

14. **b**

15. **a** The epidermal laminae are classified as insensitive, whereas the dermal laminae are classified as sensitive and the primary epidermal laminae are keratinized.

16. **b**

17. **a** Hydrochloric acid is secreted by parietal cells. Argentaffin cells secrete their product into the interstitium; it is subsequently taken up by the blood. Chief cells secrete pepsinogen, not mucus.

18. **b** Mesangial cells most likely have a phagocytic and supportive function. They are of mesodermal origin.

19. **b**

20. **a**

21. **c** Air sac diverticula are present in bones. Air sacs are present in the abdominal and thoracic region, are multiple, and do not function in exchange of gases.

22. **b**

23. **e**

24. **b**

25. **c**

26. **c** Changes during the estrous cycle include glandular activity, vascularization and leukocyte infiltration. The caruncle and cotyledon are uterine and placental structures, respectively, that contain few glands. Uterine epithelial keratinization does not occur during the estrous cycle.

27. **a**

28. **d**

29. **d**

30. **a**

31. **c**

32. **c**

33. **e**

34. **d**

35. **c**

36. **b**

37. **c**

38. **d** Metaplasia is the transformation of a specific, adult, fully differentiated tissue into another differentiated tissue. Loss of differentiation is common to dysplasia, anaplasia and neoplasia, whereas hyperplasia refers to increased proliferation.

39. **a**

40. **a**

41. **c**

42. **e** The other cells listed are poikilocytes, or abnormally shaped red blood cells.

43. **d** Equine red blood cells show prominent rouleaux formation. Under abnormal

conditions (inflammation), it may be
encountered in other species.

44. **a**

45. **a** Red muscle fibers consist primarily of
type-I fibers, with abundant mitochondria and
myoglobin. Type-I fibers are slow-twitch fibers
and type-II fibers are fast-twitch fibers. The
breast muscle of a duck contains more red
muscle fibers than does the breast muscle of a
chicken.

46. **a**

47. **a** As compared with other species, pigs have
a reversal of medullary and cortical
components in their lymph nodes.

48. **b**

49. **b**

50. **c**

51. **a**

52. **c**

53. **c**

54. **c**

55. **d**

56. **a**

57. **c**

58. **a**

59. **a**

60. **e**

61. **b** Relative to the size of the thoracic cavity,
the avian lung is extremely small. The lungs do
not actually change in volume. The air sacs
function in actual movement of air.

62. **b**

63. **d**

64. **a**

65. **a**

66. **e**

67. **b**

68. **a**

69. **e**

70. **c**

71. **a**

72. **d**

73. **c** Anisocytosis and even poikilocytosis are
common in normal goat blood. The red blood
cells of goats are smaller than the red blood
cells of dogs.

74. **d**

75. **d**

76. **b**

77. **d**

78. **b**

79. **e**

80. **a**

81. **d**

82. **e**

83. **a**

84. **d**

85. **a**

86. **c**

87. **a**

88. **a**

89. **a**

90. **b** Villi are present in the small intestine, not
in the colon. In the small intestine, cell division
occurs in the crypt.

91. **b**

92. **d** The dark color of the thymic cortex is due
to the high density of lymphocytes.

93. **c** Myoepithelial cells are abundant in the
mammary gland. They are associated with
expulsion of secretory material.

94. **b**

95. **d**

96. **a** The urinary bladder is lined by transitional
epithelium, the gallbladder and bronchi by
columnar epithelium, and the ventricles by
cuboidal epithelium.

97. **a** With pseudostratified epithelium, all cells
contact the basement membrane, but not all
reach the surface.

98. **b** Argyrophilic refers to staining positively
with silver impregnation techniques.
Metachromatic refers to the ability of a single
stain to impart a different color to different
granules.

99. **b**

100. **d**

101. **b**

102. **d**

103. **a**

104. **c** Peyer's patches, though most prominent
     in the ileum, are found in other portions of the
     small intestine, particularly the jejunum.

105. **b**

106. **b**

107. **c**

108. **a**

109. **a**

110. **c**

Notes

Section 6

Neuroanatomy

A. de Lahunta

Recommended Reading

de Lahunta A: *Veterinary Neuroanatomy and Clinical Neurology.* 2nd ed. Saunders, Philadelphia, 1983.

> ***Practice answer sheet is on page 263.***

Questions

1. Which of the following is **not** derived from neural crest?

   a. myenteric ganglia
   b. sympathetic trunk ganglia
   c. spinal ganglia
   d. general somatic efferent neurons
   e. general somatic afferent neurons

2. Communication between the ventricular system and subarachnoid space occurs at the level of the:

   a. telencephalon
   b. diencephalon
   c. mesencephalon
   d. metencephalon
   e. myelencephalon

3. The membranous labyrinth of the inner ear is derived from the:

   a. rhombencephalon
   b. otic placode

   c. diencephalon
   d. paraxial mesoderm
   e. neural crest

4. Which of the following is associated with cyclopian malformation?

   a. cerebellar hypoplasia
   b. myelodysplasia
   c. holoprosencephaly
   d. exencephaly
   e. meningoencephalocele

5. Which of the following is **not** considered to be developed from the neural tube neuroepithelium?

   a. microglia
   b. astroglia
   c. oligodendroglia
   d. ependyma
   e. neurons

Correct answers are on pages 153-155.

6. Which of the following is **not** a feature of radial nerve paralysis?

   a. inability to support weight on the forelimb
   b. walking on the dorsal surface of the forepaw
   c. analgesia of the middorsal surface of the forepaw
   d. atrophy of the cranial forearm muscles
   e. inability to extend the shoulder to advance the limb

7. Which of the following is most likely to occur with sciatic nerve injury?

   a. walking on the dorsal surface of the hind paw
   b. inability to support weight on the pelvic limb
   c. inability to flex the hip to advance the pelvic limb
   d. analgesia on the medial side of the crus
   e. analgesia on the proximocaudal aspect of the thigh

8. Which of the following is **not** a feature of traumatic unilateral avulsion of the spinal roots that provide branches to the brachial plexus?

   a. ipsilateral pupillary constriction
   b. loss of the cutaneous trunci reflex
   c. inability to support weight on the limb
   d. inability to advance the limb
   e. cutaneous analgesia over the pectoral muscles

9. The spinal tract of the trigeminal nerve in the medulla contains:

   a. general visceral efferent neurons
   b. general visceral afferent neurons
   c. general somatic afferent neurons
   d. special somatic afferent neurons
   e. general somatic efferent neurons

10. Which of the following does **not** occur with otitis media and otitis interna in small animals?

    a. facial paralysis
    b. facial analgesia
    c. head tilt
    d. deafness
    e. Horner's syndrome

11. In the medulla, the intramedullary course (genu) of axons of the facial neurons passes over the:

    a. abducent nucleus
    b. trigeminal motor nucleus
    c. vestibular nucleus
    d. hypoglossal nucleus
    e. cochlear nucleus

12. A transverse section of the brain at which level shows the trigeminal motor nucleus?

    a. rostral colliculi
    b. obex
    c. lateral and medial geniculate nuclei
    d. rostral and middle cerebellar peduncles
    e. acoustic stria and caudal cerebellar peduncles

13. Which axons are **not** present in the caudal cerebellar peduncles?

    a. olivocerebellar axons
    b. spinocerebellar axons
    c. pontocerebellar axons
    d. vestibulocerebellar axons
    e. cuneocerebellar axons

14. Concerning cerebellar Purkinje neurons, which statement is **least** accurate?

    a. The cell bodies form a single row superficial to the granule-cell layer.
    b. The dendritic zone projects into the molecular layer, transverse to the longitudinal axis of the folium.
    c. Most Purkinje neurons terminate on neurons in the cerebellar nuclei, which they facilitate through release of glutamic acid.
    d. Olivary neurons project directly to the dendritic zone of Purkinje neurons via climbing fibers.
    e. Longitudinally oriented axons of cerebellar granule cells synapse on the Purkinje dendritic zone.

15. Concerning the cerebellar external germinal layer, which statement is **least** accurate?

    a. It is the source of granule-cell neurons.
    b. In calves, it reaches peak mitotic activity before birth.
    c. In cats, it is especially susceptible to infection by panleukopenia virus around the time of birth.
    d. It forms the ependyma of the fourth ventricle beneath the cerebellum.
    e. It covers the external surface of all the cerebellar folia beneath the pia.

16. The palpebral reflex involves which pairs of cranial nerves (afferent – efferent)?

    a. II and V
    b. II and VII
    c. III and V
    d. V and VII
    e. VII and V

17. Examination of a 3-year-old dog reveals a dilated left pupil. The menace response is normal bilaterally. Light directed into the left eye only elicits constriction of the right pupil. Light directed into the right eye also only elicits constriction of the right pupil. The lesion responsible for these signs involves which structure on the left side?

    a. optic nerve
    b. oculomotor nerve
    c. cranial cervical ganglion
    d. ophthalmic nerve
    e. geniculate ganglion

18. Which of the following is **not** a feature of Horner's syndrome?

    a. miosis
    b. strabismus
    c. ptosis
    d. third eyelid protrusion
    e. enophthalmos

19. Neuronal processes that cross from the neopallium of one cerebral hemisphere to the neopallium of the opposite cerebral hemisphere pass through the:

    a. internal capsule
    b. rostral commissure
    c. caudal commissure
    d. corpus callosum
    e. pyramidal decussation

20. Which of the following is **not** part of the auditory perception pathway?

    a. medial geniculate nucleus
    b. brachium of the caudal colliculus
    c. cochlear nucleus
    d. pretectal nucleus
    e. sylvian gyrus

21. In cats, the left optic tract contains:

    a. 75% of the left optic nerve axons from the medial aspect of the retina
    b. 25% of the right optic nerve axons from the lateral aspect of the retina
    c. 80% of the right optic nerve axons from the lateral aspect of the retina
    d. 65% of the right optic nerve axons from the medial aspect of the retina
    e. all of the axons from the left lateral geniculate nucleus

22. Which of the following is **not** considered part of the limbic system?

    a. amygdala
    b. red nucleus
    c. hippocampus
    d. cingulate gyrus
    e. mamillary body

23. Which of the following is **not** directly related to the lateral ventricle?

    a. falx cerebri
    b. corpus callosum
    c. internal capsule
    d. caudate nucleus
    e. hippocampal fornix

Correct answers are on pages 153-155.

24. Compromise of the middle cerebral artery would cause infarction of the:

    a. cingulate gyrus
    b. hippocampus
    c. epithalamus
    d. ectosylvian gyrus
    e. septal nuclei

25. Which of the following is **not** a feature of the internal carotid artery?

    a. supplies the middle meningeal artery
    b. is rudimentary in cats
    c. courses through the cavernous sinus
    d. anastomoses with the basilar artery
    e. passes into the tympano-occipital fissure

26. Which of the following is **least** likely to be associated with Horner's syndrome?

    a. otitis media
    b. embolic infarction of the lateral funiculus of spinal cord segments C6 and C7
    c. avulsion of the ventral spinal roots from C6 through T2
    d. trigeminal neuritis
    e. retrobulbar optic neuritis

27. Which of the following is **least** likely to be observed after fibrocartilaginous embolic infarction of the entire spinal cord from L6 caudally, through the end of the conus medullaris?

    a. analgesia of the skin of the caudal thigh
    b. anal atonia, areflexia and analgesia
    c. normal perception of the skin of the cranial thigh
    d. normal patellar reflexes
    e. analgesia of the skin of the medial side of the crus

28. Which of the following is **not** involved with general proprioception?

    a. spinocerebellar tract
    b. cuneocerebellar tract

    c. fasciculus gracilis
    d. fasciculus cuneatus
    e. spinothalamic tract

29. A 6-year-old male mixed-breed dog has a sudden onset of inability to use the left pelvic limb. The limb is held in extension and is dragged along on the dorsum of the paw as the dog walks. The limb is not protracted during walking. Examination reveals hypertonia, hyperreflexia and normal nociception. Where is the lesion most likely located?

    a. left sciatic nerve
    b. spinal cord segments T3-L3, on the left
    c. right prosencephalon
    d. spinal cord segments L4-S1, on the left
    e. left femoral nerve

30. A 10-year-old male Beagle occasionally stumbles when negotiating stairs or when getting in and out of the car. The dog's gait, muscle tone and size, and reflexes are normal, but the hopping, hemiwalking and placing responses are slow in the right limbs. What is the **least** likely site of the lesion causing these signs?

    a. left postcruciate gyrus
    b. right internal capsule
    c. left crus cerebri
    d. right lateral medulla
    e. lateral funiculus of spinal cord segments C1-C6, on the right

31. Concerning myelination in the peripheral nervous system, which statement is **least** accurate?

    a. Myelin is a product of Schwann cells.
    b. Each myelinating cell forms one internode of myelin.
    c. Myelinating cells are derived from limb bud mesoderm.
    d. Myelin thickness is related to the size of the axon.
    e. Myelin consists of spirals of the mesaxon of the myelinating cell.

32. *Concerning nociceptive somatic afferent neurons in peripheral nerves, which statement is **least** accurate?*

   a. They are derived from neural crest ectoderm.
   b. They release substance P at their terminations in the dorsal gray column.
   c. Most of them are thinly myelinated or unmyelinated.
   d. Their cell bodies are located in the spinal cord dorsal gray column.
   e. Their axons course through a spinal nerve and its associated dorsal root.

33. *If intramuscular injection of a drug into the caudal thigh completely destroys the sciatic nerve, Wallerian degeneration occurs. Which of the following is **not** a feature of this phenomenon?*

   a. primary segmental demyelination of axons distal to the lesion
   b. preservation of Schwann cells and endoneurium distal to the lesion
   c. degeneration of all axons distal to the lesion and a few internodes proximal to it
   d. secondary demyelination of degenerating axons
   e. central chromatolysis and enlargement of cell bodies in the spinal cord ventral gray column at L7 and S1

34. *Concerning histologic features of normal adult cerebral cortex, which statement is **least** accurate?*

   a. Neuronal cell bodies contain Nissl substance in their cytoplasm and have a prominent nucleolus.
   b. Of the glial cells, astrocyte nuclei are the largest and have the least dense chromatin.
   c. Oligodendrocyte nuclei are typically elongated, with the most dense chromatin.
   d. Microglial nuclei resemble capillary endothelial-cell nuclei.
   e. Immunocytochemical staining for glial acidic fibrillary protein stains astrocyte processes.

35. *Which of the following would **not** be found on a transverse section of the brain at the level of the optic chiasm?*

   a. caudate nucleus
   b. internal capsule
   c. corpus callosum
   d. hippocampal cortex
   e. lateral ventricle

36. *Which of the following would **not** be found on a transverse section of the brain at the level of the rostral colliculi?*

   a. septal nuclei
   b. medial geniculate nucleus
   c. hippocampal cortex
   d. crus cerebri
   e. mesencephalic aqueduct

37. *Which of the following would **not** be found on a transverse section of the brain at the level of the confluence of the peduncles with the cerebellum?*

   a. trapezoid body
   b. vestibular nuclei
   c. facial nerve fibers
   d. pyramids
   e. caudal colliculi

38. *Examination of an 8-year-old male German Shepherd with a sudden onset of a right head tilt and falling to the right reveals resting horizontal nystagmus with the quick phase to the left, a slight tendency to drag the right limbs, and a mild hopping deficit in the right limbs. Where is the lesion most likely located?*

   a. right middle and inner ear
   b. right vestibulocochlear nerve
   c. right third cervical spinal cord segment
   d. right medulla
   e. left crus cerebri

39. *Which of the following is **not** a component of the inner ear concerned with auditory function?*

   a. basilar membrane
   b. spiral ganglion
   c. crista ampullaris
   d. scala vestibuli
   e. tectorial membrane

Correct answers are on pages 153-155.

40. Which of the following is involved in transmission of impulses that are responsible for the normal nystagmus generated when the head is moved side to side?

a. medial longitudinal fasciculus
b. medial lemniscus
c. brachium of the rostral colliculi
d. acoustic stria
e. lateral lemniscus

41. Examination of a dog reveals complete atrophy of the right masseter and temporal muscles, no palpebral reflex on the right but a normal menace response bilaterally, and analgesia of the right side of the face. Where is the lesion most likely located?

a. cranial nerve VII
b. cranial nerve V
c. cranial nerves V and VII
d. mandibular nerve
e. ophthalmic nerve

42. Which group of structures does **not** have a common function or pathway?

a. cochlear nuclei, lateral lemniscus, brachium of the caudal colliculus, medial geniculate nucleus
b. retina, optic nerve, optic tract, lateral geniculate nucleus, internal capsule
c. postcruciate gyrus, internal capsule, crus cerebri, longitudinal fibers of pons, pyramids
d. amygdala, hippocampus, fornix, caudate nucleus, lentiform nucleus
e. fasciculus gracilis, nucleus gracilis, medial lemniscus, ventrocaudomedial nucleus of thalamus, internal capsule

43. Which of the following is **not** a component of the vestibular system?

a. olivary nucleus
b. crista ampullaris
c. fastigial nucleus
d. medial longitudinal fasciculus
e. cranial nerve VIII

44. Examination of a 6-year-old cat with generalized seizures shows lack of a menace response in the right eye but a normal palpebral reflex in both eyes. The pupils are of normal size in ambient light and both respond directly and indirectly to bright light. Findings for the rest of the examination are normal. A lesion at which site would **not** explain these signs?

a. right optic nerve
b. left optic tract
c. left lateral geniculate nucleus
d. left internal capsule
e. left occipital lobe

45. The pigment epithelium of the retina is critical to normal development and function of the:

a. ganglion cells of the retina
b. vitreous body
c. retinal bipolar neurons
d. tapetum lucidum
e. photoreceptor layer of the retina

46. The cell bodies of the axons in the optic nerve that transmit light-induced stimuli are located in the:

a. lateral geniculate nucleus
b. photoreceptor layer of the retina
c. retinal ganglion-cell layer
d. retinal bipolar-cell layer
e. pretectal nuclei of the thalamus

47. Which of the following is **not** involved in normal bladder evacuation and urination?

a. parasympathetic stimulation of detrusor smooth muscle
b. inhibition of adrenergic alpha receptors at the bladder neck and urethral junction
c. inhibition of adrenergic beta receptors in the detrusor muscle
d. stimulation of cholinergic pudendal innervation of the urethralis muscle
e. stimulation of cholinergic peripheral innervation of striated abdominal muscles

48. Which of the following clinical signs would **not** be related to a disturbance of the hypothalamic nuclei?

    a. hemianopsia
    b. hyperthermia
    c. bradycardia
    d. obtundation
    e. diabetes insipidus

49. Which of the following is **not** composed of motor neurons?

    a. trochlear nucleus
    b. spinal cord ventral gray column

    c. hypoglossal nucleus
    d. cuneate nuclei
    e. nucleus ambiguus

50. Congenital laryngeal paralysis is inherited in Bouvier dogs and has been associated with loss of cell bodies in what nucleus in the medulla?

    a. facial nucleus
    b. nucleus ambiguus
    c. solitary nucleus
    d. lateral cuneate nucleus
    e. parasympathetic nucleus of vagus

Answers

1. **d** General somatic efferent neurons are derived from the germinal layer of the neural tube.

2. **e** This occurs through the lateral apertures in the caudal medullary velum, just caudal to the cerebellar peduncles.

3. **b** This ectodermal thickening develops in relation to the rhombencephalon and invaginates to form an otocyst beneath the surface ectoderm.

4. **c** Failure to induce division of the single optic field of neuroectoderm into 2 optic vesicles is associated with failure of 2 telencephalons to develop. Only 1 telencephalon develops; this condition is called holoprosencephaly.

5. **a** Microglia are considered to be mesodermal in origin and reside as potential macrophages in the central nervous system.

6. **e** Extending the shoulder and advancing the limb are functions of the supraspinatus and brachiocephalicus muscles, which are not innervated by the radial nerve.

7. **a** Walking on the dorsal surface of the hind paw results from damage to the peroneal branch of the sciatic nerve to the extensors of the digits.

8. **e** The skin over the pectoral muscles is innervated by cutaneous branches that arise from nerves cranial and caudal to the avulsion.

9. **c** General somatic afferent neurons comprise the spinal tract of V with their cell bodies in the trigeminal ganglion.

10. **b** Facial analgesia involves a trigeminal nerve deficit. This nerve is not related to the middle and inner ear, whereas the facial and sympathetic nerves course through or adjacent to the middle ear.

11. **a**

12. **d** The rostral and middle cerebellar peduncles are located at the caudal aspect of the pons.

13. **c** The pontocerebellar axons reach the cerebellum through the middle cerebellar peduncles.

14. **c** Most Purkinje neurons terminate on neurons in the cerebellar nuclei, which they facilitate through release of glutamic acid. Purkinje neurons are inhibitory to these neurons via the neurotransmitter gamma aminobutyric acid.

15. **d** The cerebellar external germinal layer forms the ependyma of the fourth ventricle beneath the cerebellum. This is derived from the germinal cells that did *not* migrate to the surface of the developing cerebellum to form the external germinal layer.

16. **d** The palpebral reflex involves stimulation of the cutaneous endings of the trigeminal

nerve (afferent V). Eyelid closure is mediated through the palpebral branch of the facial nerve (efferent VII).

17. **b** The general visceral efferent parasympathetic neurons to the left constrictor of the iris are not functioning in this animal. These are present only in the oculomotor nerve.

18. **b** Horner's syndrome is a sympathetic paralysis of ocular smooth muscle. Sympathetic neurons do not innervate extraocular striated muscle.

19. **d**

20. **d** The pretectal nucleus is part of the pupillary light reflex pathway.

21. **d** The remaining 35% of right optic nerve axons course from the lateral retina through the ipsilateral right optic tract.

22. **b** The red nucleus is in the upper motor neuron system and is the origin of the rubrospinal tract.

23. **a** The falx cerebri is an extention of dura in the longitudinal cerebral fissure between the cerebral hemispheres.

24. **a** The ectosylvian gyrus is the only structure listed that is located on the lateral side of the cerebrum, where the middle cerebral artery supplies the neocortex.

25. **a** The middle meningeal artery is a branch of the maxillary artery at the level of the oval formen.

26. **e** Retrobulbar optic neuritis is an inflammation of brain tissue in the optic nerve, where there are no components of the sympathetic pathway to the eye.

27. **e** The skin of the medial side of the crus is innervated by the saphenous branch of the femoral nerve from spinal cord segments L4, L5 and L6. Segments L4 and L5 are normal here.

28. **e** The spinothalamic tract serves in nociception.

29. **b** These are signs of spastic monoplegia, which involves a complete upper motor neuron deficit to the left pelvic limb. With a normal forelimb, the upper motor neuron must be affected by the lesion somewhere between T3 and L3 and on the same side because these tracts cross in the caudal brainstem or are ipsilateral to the site of their cell bodies.

30. **b** Prosencephalic lesions only affect the postural reactions of the contralateral limbs. From the pons caudally, the clinical signs of locomotor abnormality are ipsilateral to the lesion.

31. **c** The myelinating cell is derived from limb bud mesoderm. It is derived from neural crest ectoderm, the Schwann cell.

32. **d** They are located in the spinal ganglia.

33. **a** Primary segmental demyelination is a primary Schwann cell abnormality. In Wallerian degeneration, myelin degenerates secondary to degeneration of the axon.

34. **c** Microglial-cell nuclei are typically elongated, with the densest chromatin. Oligodendrocyte nuclei are medium sized and round, with denser chromatin than that of astrocytes but less dense than that of microglia.

35. **d** The hippocampal cortex is located considerably caudal to this level.

36. **a** The septal nuclei are located rostrally, adjacent to the bending of the body of the fornix to form the columns of the fornix.

37. **e** The caudal colliculi are rostral to the cerebellum, on the caudal aspect of the mesencephalon.

38. **d** A gait deficit and postural reaction deficits do not occur with peripheral vestibular lesions. The vestibular nuclei and upper motor neuron and general proprioceptive pathways can be affected by a lesion on the side of the medulla, ipsilateral to the deficit.

39. **c** The crista ampullaris is a vestibular system end organ.

40. **a** This brainstem tract connects the vestibular nuclei with the nuclei of cranial nerves III and VI that cause the eyes to adduct and abduct.

41. **b** All 3 branches of cranial nerve V (trigeminal) account for normal nociception in the face. The mandibular nerve innervates the masseter and temporal muscles.

42. **d** The first 3 structures in this group are part of the limbic system. The last 2 nuclei are in the extrapyramidal upper motor neuron system.

43. **a** The olivary nucleus is in the upper motor neuron pathway, from cerebrum to cerebellum.

44. **a** If a lesion of the optic nerve causes a menace deficit, there is usually decreased response of the pupil to direct stimulation by light. A lesion here would also not cause seizures.

45. **e** The photoreceptor layer and the pigment epithelium of the retina are intimately related anatomically and functionally.

46. **c**

47. **d** The urethralis muscle is striated muscle that is normally inhibited to relax the urethra, allowing urine to flow.

48. **a** Hemianopsia is a visual deficit. The pathway is mediated through a thalamic nucleus, not the hypothalamus.

49. **d** Cuneate nuclei cell bodies are in the sensory general proprioceptive pathway.

50. **b** Nucleus ambiguus cell bodies innervate the striated muscle of the larynx, pharynx and esophagus.

Notes

Notes

Section 7

Parasitology

D.D. Bowman

Recommended Reading

Georgi JR and Georgi ME: *Canine Clinical Parasitology.* Lea & Febiger, Philadelphia, 1992.

Georgi JR and Georgi ME: *Parasitology for Veterinarians.* 5th ed. Saunders, Philadelphia, 1990.

Foreyt WJ: *Veterinary Parasitology Reference Manual.* 2nd ed. Washington State Univ, Pullman, WA, 1990.

Fraser CM: *The Merck Veterinary Manual.* 7th ed. Merck, Rahway, NJ, 1991.

Ivens VR *et al:* Principal parasites of domestic animals in the United States: Biological and Diagnostic Information. 2nd ed. University of Illinois Publication 52, Urbana, 1988.

> **Practice answer sheets are on pages 265-266.**

Questions

1. *Several littermate Labrador Retriever puppies develop signs of caudal paralysis and polyradiculitis. A likely protozoal cause of this infection is:*

   a. *Giardia duodenalis*

   b. *Neospora caninum*

   c. *Hepatozoon canis*

   d. *Isospora canis*

   e. *Leishmania donovani*

2. *A dog from Arkansas develops severe anemia and icterus. Examination of the blood reveals small organisms within 15% of the red blood cells. The protozoan within the blood cells is most likely to be:*

   a. *Giardia canis*

   b. *Trypanosoma cruzi*

   c. *Sarcocystis capracanis*

   d. *Babesia canis*

   e. *Toxoplasma gondii*

3. *A litter of puppies develops bloody, mucoid diarrhea within a few days after they are moved to the house of their new owner. The most likely cause of diarrhea in these puppies is:*

   a. *Trichodectes canis*

   b. *Hepatozoon canis*

   c. *Toxoplasma gondii*

   d. *Babesia gibsoni*

   e. *Isospora canis*

Correct answers are on pages 183-188.

4. Routine fecal examination performed on a dog reveals sporocysts of Sarcocystis cruzi. The dog most likely acquired this infection from:

   a. the bite of a tabanid fly
   b. ingestion of a beetle intermediate host
   c. ingestion of a murine paratenic host
   d. ingestion of raw beef
   e. ingestion of sporulated oocysts

5. Examination of the feces of a dog with diarrhea reveals trophozoites of a flagellate protozoan identified as Giardia duodenalis (synonyms: Giardia lamblia and Giardia canis). The dog most likely acquired this infection from:

   a. ingestion of a cyst of this parasite
   b. ingestion of a trophozoite of this parasite
   c. ingestion of an infected earthworm
   d. ingestion of an infected cockroach
   e. the bite of a mosquito

6. A hunting dog that has been housed in an outside kennel in Louisiana becomes lethargic. Examination reveals cardiac dilatation and insufficiency. A likely protozoal cause of these signs is:

   a. Babesia canis
   b. Leishmania braziliensis
   c. Hepatozoon canis
   d. Toxoplasma gondii
   e. Trypanosoma cruzi

7. A cat that enjoys hunting develops a rapidly progressive disease with signs including anemia and icterus. Death occurs a few days after the onset of clinical signs. Histopathologic examination of the lungs and liver reveals blood vessels filled with very large cells containing parasitic inclusions. The most likely cause of this cat's death is infection with:

   a. Aelurostrongylus abstrusus
   b. Cytauxzoon felis
   c. Leishmania braziliensis
   d. Paragonimus kellicotti
   e. Eucoleus (Capillaria) aerophila

8. You prepare a direct saline smear of a gingival scraping from a cat with periodontal disease that has developed concomitantly with feline immunodeficiency virus infection. Microscopic examination of the smear is most likely to reveal a commensal flagellate of the genus:

   a. Trichomonas
   b. Giardia
   c. Entamoeba
   d. Hammondia
   e. Sarcocystis

9. In a Persian cat with chronic diarrhea, infection with Giardia duodenalis (synonym: Giardia lamblia) is suspected. An appropriate examination of the feces should include a:

   a. zinc sulfate centrifugal flotation
   b. modified sugar centrifugal flotation
   c. direct saline smear
   d. sodium nitrate stationary flotation
   e. modified sugar stationary flotation

10. The pregnant, cat-owning client most at risk for passing toxoplasmosis to her fetus during gestation is one that:

   a. has repeatedly eaten raw or rare beef
   b. does a lot of backyard gardening
   c. already has a high circulating Toxoplasma antibody titer at the time of her baby's conception
   d. does not have a high circulating Toxoplasma antibody titer at the time of her baby's conception
   e. owns a cat with a high circulating Toxoplasma antibody titer at the time of her baby's conception

11. Microscopic examination of a stained impression smear made from a skin lesion on the ear of a cat in Oklahoma reveals macrophages containing large numbers of amastigote stages of an intracellular organism. The cat has probably become infected by the bite of a psychodid fly (sandfly). This lesion is most likely to be caused by:

   a. Babesia

b. *Sarcocystis*

c. *Cryptosporidium*

d. *Leishmania*

e. *Trichomonas*

12. *An Arabian foal with inherited combined immunodeficiency develops diarrhea. Examination of the feces by sugar flotation reveals large numbers of very small oocysts typical of a parasite known to cause diarrhea in immunocompromised hosts. The name of this parasite is:*

a. *Eimeria leuckarti*

b. *Cryptosporidium parvum*

c. *Klossiella equi*

d. *Trypanosoma brucei*

e. *Parascaris equorum*

13. *Babesia caballi, which causes disease in horses in the southeastern United States, is transmitted via a:*

a. tick

b. tabanid fly

c. louse

d. mite

e. muscid fly

14. *A 4-year-old Standardbred mare develops paralysis of the right side of its face. Despite various treatments, the disease progresses to lameness and paresis, and the owner elects euthanasia. Necropsy reveals lesions in the brain and spinal cord containing protozoal organisms. The most likely cause of these findings is:*

a. *Trypanosoma equiperdum*

b. *Babesia caballi*

c. *Klossiella equi*

d. *Sarcocystis neurona*

e. *Besnoitia jellisoni*

15. *Necropsy of a horse reveals infection of the skeletal and cardiac muscle with* Sarcocystis bertrami. *Typical clinical signs of chronic myositic infection (ie, infection with the*

bradyzoite stage) with this parasite, as with other species of Sarcocystis, *are:*

a. muscle pain and loss of function

b. inappetence and wasting

c. diarrhea and dehydration

d. central nervous system signs

e. absent

16. *The most likely cause of diarrhea without intestinal blood loss in a 2-week-old calf is:*

a. *Sarcocystis cruzi*

b. *Bunostomum phlebotomum*

c. *Eimeria bovis*

d. *Toxoplasma gondii*

e. *Cryptosporidium parvum*

17. *Infection in a beef herd with* Tritrichomonas foetus *is characterized by:*

a. anemia

b. infertility

c. wasting

d. diarrhea

e. neurologic disease

18. *Winter coccidiosis in cattle is characterized by:*

a. anemia and icterus

b. wasting and myositis

c. diarrhea and dysentery

d. cardiac failure

e. fever and loss of hair at the base of the tail

19. *In order of occurrence, the typical pattern of events in the life cycle of a coccidian parasite, such as* Eimeria, *are:*

a. schizont, schizont, gametocyte, oocyst, sporocyst, sporozoite

b. oocyst, gametocyte, schizont, schizont, sporozoite, sporocyst

c. oocyst, sporocyst, sporozoite, gametocyte, schizont, schizont

d. gametocyte, schizont, schizont, oocyst, sporocyst, sporozoite

e. schizont, schizont, oocyst, gametocyte, sporocyst, sporozoite

Correct answers are on pages 183-188.

20. *In cattle,* Eimeria zurnii *causes lesions in the distal small intestine and in the large intestine. Clinical disease is mainly seen in animals confined in crowded conditions because:*

    a. the organism is spread in an aerosol of the saliva of infected animals
    b. the stage passed in the feces is infective when passed
    c. multiplication of the organisms within the intestinal mucosa produces huge numbers of organisms that contaminate the environment
    d. the ticks feeding on infected cattle spread the disease from host to host, especially when imported young infected cattle are housed with older susceptible animals
    e. the feline intermediate host sheds infective oocysts over a contained area, such as an enclosed feedlot

21. *A llama with intermittent bouts of diarrhea has cysts in its feces when the feces are formed and trophozoites of the same parasite when the feces are diarrheic. Microscopic examination reveals that the cysts are ovoid, have a thin wall, contain 4 nuclei, and are about 8 μ long. The trophozoites are flagellate, about 15 μ long, have 2 nuclei, appear flattened, and have a ventral attachment disk. The parasite described, which may or may not be the cause of the diarrhea, is a species of:*

    a. trichomonad
    b. *Giardia*
    c. *Eimeria*
    d. trypanosome
    e. *Isospora*

22. *Necropsy of a lamb from a flock that has recently developed severe diarrhea reveals numerous whitish, raised lesions, 3-6 mm in diameter, in the intestinal mucosa. Fecal examinations have not disclosed any parasites present in great numbers; however, saline smears prepared from the lesions reveal hundreds to thousands of small elongate organisms. A likely cause of the diarrhea and the intestinal lesions is:*

    a. *Eimeria ahsata*
    b. *Giardia duodenalis (Giardia lamblia)*
    c. *Isospora canis*
    d. *Sarcocystis arieticanis*
    e. *Trichuris ovis*

23. *A flock of ewes is experiencing abortion due to focal placentitis. The parasite that typically causes this lesion in sheep is:*

    a. *Trypanosoma ovis*
    b. *Isospora felis*
    c. *Eimeria ovinoidalis*
    d. *Sarcocystis tenella*
    e. *Toxoplasma gondii*

24. *Microscopic examination of blood smears from a sheep reveals a trypanosome identified as* Trypanosoma ovis. *The biological vector of this parasite between sheep is:*

    a. the tick *Dermacentor nitens*
    b. a fly of the genus *Tabanus*
    c. a fly of the genus *Stomoxys*
    d. the sheep ked *Melophagus ovinus*
    e. a mosquito of the genus *Anopheles*

25. *In 5- to 10-day-old piglets, the most likely cause of scours that is unresponsive to antibiotic therapy is:*

    a. *Isospora suis*
    b. *Eimeria suis*
    c. *Trichinella spiralis*
    d. *Trichuris suis*
    e. *Toxoplasma gondii*

26. *Three parasites that can infect people via ingestion of uncooked or undercooked pork are:*

    a. *Toxoplasma gondii, Taenia solium* and *Stephanurus dentatus*
    b. *Trichinella spiralis, Taenia solium* and *Hyostrongylus rubidus*
    c. *Toxoplasma gondii, Taenia solium* and *Trichinella spiralis*
    d. *Trichinella spiralis, Taenia solium* and *Oesophagostomum radiatum*

e. *Toxoplasma gondii, Eimeria deblieki* and *Trichinella spiralis*

27. *Examination of the feces of a clinically normal guinea pig reveals large (100 μ long) ciliate trophozoites and large cysts up to 60 μ in diameter. Similar parasites have also been found in domestic pigs and on rare occasions may have caused disease in dogs. The parasite in question is:*

a. *Entamoeba coli*
b. *Balantidium coli*
c. *Entamoeba histolytica*
d. *Eimeria*
e. *Trichomonas*

28. *Pigs can be infected with several species of* Sarcocystis, *including* Sarcocystis miescheriana *and* Sarcocystis suihominis. *In the described life cycles of* Sarcocystis *species, the final host (the host in which gametogony and sporocyst production occurs) is:*

a. an herbivore
b. a carnivore
c. a mammal
d. a bird
e. a feline

29. *Several rhesus monkeys housed in a local zoo develop progressive dysentery that ultimately leads to death of one monkey. Necropsy reveals hemorrhagic lesions in the colonic wall and yellow lesions in the liver. Histopathologic examination reveals a small protozoan parasite with a nucleus containing a central karyosome. Some of the parasites contain red blood cells. The most likely cause of these findings is:*

a. *Isospora belli*
b. *Entamoeba histolytica*
c. *Entamoeba coli*
d. *Balantidium coli*
e. *Toxoplasma gondii*

30. *Examination of a pig's feces reveals numerous, thin-walled protozoan cysts of several sizes, ranging from 12 to 30 μ in diameter. All of the cysts appear similar, but some contain 1 nucleus, some contain 4 nuclei, and some contain 8 nuclei. These cysts are representative of several species of parasite found in pigs and are classified as:*

a. trichomonads
b. amoebas
c. trypanosomes
d. ciliates
e. coccidia

31. *A flock of young turkeys is moved into an earthen-floored pen on a small farm in which chickens had previously been housed for several years. After about a week in the new pen, the turkeys develop diarrhea and several die. Necropsy of birds that have died reveals inflammation and necrosis of the cecal wall and raised circular yellowish lesions on the surface of the liver. Microscopic examination of the liver lesions reveals a protozoan parasite. The parasite most likely involved in this disease is:*

a. *Hexamita meleagridis*
b. *Cryptosporidium baileyi*
c. *Histomonas meleagridis*
d. *Giardia*
e. *Eimeria meleagridis*

32. *Which flagellate protozoan is a possible cause of fatal diarrhea in budgerigars and cockatiels?*

a. *Giardia*
b. *Eimeria*
c. *Trichomonas*
d. *Histomonas*
e. *Entamoeba*

Correct answers are on pages 183-188.

33. A red-tailed hawk housed in a rehabilitation clinic while its broken wing heals is fed pigeons obtained as culls from a nearby pigeon breeder. After about a week in the clinic, the hawk stops eating and begins to lose weight. Examination of the buccal cavity of the hawk reveals yellowish-green plaques in the back of the mouth. Microscopic examination of a direct saline smear of material from one of the plaques reveals numerous flagellate parasites. The probable cause of these plaques is a species of:

a. *Giardia*
b. *Eimeria*
c. *Trichomonas*
d. *Histomonas*
e. *Entamoeba*

34. Goslings of a lesser snow goose begin to die a few weeks after hatching. Examination of the blood of the survivors reveals a species of Leucocytozoon. *The biological vector of this parasite is a:*

a. black fly (family Simulidae)
b. mosquito (family Culicidae)
c. tabanid fly (family Tabanidae)
d. hippoboscid fly (family Hippoboscidae)
e. flea (order Siphonaptera)

35. Repeated examination of the blood of a pigeon over a 2-day period reveals red blood cells containing elongate gametocytes of a protozoan parasite; no other stage is identified. The parasite in question is probably a species of:

a. trypanosome
b. *Hemoproteus*
c. *Leukocytozoon*
d. *Plasmodium*
e. *Babesia*

36. Penguins in a group housed in a zoo with an attached outside pool begin to die with signs of fever and anemia. Hematologic examination reveals that the red blood cells contain trophozoites, schizonts and gametocytes of a protozoan parasite. The parasite causing

disease in these penguins is probably a species of:

a. trypanosome
b. *Hemoproteus*
c. *Leukocytozoon*
d. *Plasmodium*
e. *Babesia*

37. A backyard flock of chickens develops bloody diarrhea that results in death of about 30% of the birds. Examination of some of the birds that die reveals the ceca to be filled with blood and thousands of coccidial oocysts. The species of Eimeria responsible for these deaths is most likely:

a. *Eimeria necatrix*
b. *Eimeria tenella*
c. *Eimeria brunetti*
d. *Eimeria maxima*
e. *Eimeria acervulina*

38. Histologic examination of the kidneys of horses at necropsy reveals apicomplexan parasites within the cells of the tubules and the loops of Henle. Some of the parasites resemble petals of a flower surrounding a central body (merozoites surrounding a central residuum). These parasites are usually considered nonpathogenic, though they have been reported to cause renal disease in an immunocompromised pony. This parasite is:

a. *Trypanosoma equiperdum*
b. *Babesia caballi*
c. *Klossiella equi*
d. *Sarcocystis neurona*
e. *Besnoitia jellisoni*

39. A mechanical vector of a parasite is one that transmits the parasite:

a. directly, without development or multiplication of the parasite
b. after internal multiplication of the parasite
c. after required development has occurred
d. after external multiplication of the parasite
e. and is not alive (*eg*, a syringe or needle)

40. The red blood cells of a giraffe are found to be infected with a species of Theileria. The giraffe was most likely infected from the bite of a:

   a. flea
   b. tse-tse fly
   c. tick
   d. mosquito
   e. louse

41. A Beagle housed in an outdoor doghouse with straw bedding develops ventral papular dermatitis characterized by crusts and scales. Treatment with corticosteroids and antifungal agents does not resolve the lesions. Skin scrapings reveal nematode larvae that are all the same size and have a short esophagus with a bulb at its base. No parasites are detected in repeated fecal examinations. Treatment with an organophosphate dip removes the parasites, and the disease resolves. The skin disease in this dog was most likely caused by:

   a. *Rhabditis strongyloides*
   b. *Strongyloides stercoralis*
   c. *Demodex caninum*
   d. *Ancylostoma caninum*
   e. *Uncinaria stenocephala*

42. Fecal examinations performed on a closed research colony of Labrador Retrievers that have experienced occasional bouts of diarrhea reveal larvae in a zinc sulfate centrifugal flotation. Additional larvae are found using Baermann analysis. Examination of the larvae reveals that the genital primordium is longer than the larva is wide. Charcoal cultures of the feces reveal longer larvae with an esophagus about one-half the total length of the larva and a tip of the tail that appears notched. These dogs are most likely infected with:

   a. *Rhabditis strongyloides*
   b. *Strongyloides stercoralis*
   c. *Crenosoma vulpis*
   d. *Filaroides hirthi*
   e. *Uncinaria stenocephala*

43. You and your spouse own a clinic in a small town, and your 3-year-old daughter

accompanies you to the office every day, where she plays in the reception area. After about 6 months, you note that your daughter is not sleeping well and is complaining that her anal area itches. Your pediatrician diagnoses pinworm infection. Your daughter probably obtained her infection from:

   a. your family dog
   b. a dog visiting your clinic
   c. eggs in feces-contaminated soil in your backyard
   d. another child
   e. your family horse

44. The most likely cause of death in Ancylostoma caninum-infected puppies that die of peracute hookworm disease during the second week of life is:

   a. renal failure
   b. diarrhea
   c. anemia
   d. pneumonia
   e. hepatic failure

45. Puppies with hookworm eggs in their feces 2 weeks after birth have typically become infected with Ancylostoma caninum by:

   a. ingestion of infective larvae from soil
   b. transmammary migration of larvae from the bitch
   c. transplacental migration of larvae from the bitch
   d. penetration of the skin by infective larvae
   e. ingestion of hookworm eggs containing infective larvae

46. The eggs of Uncinaria stenocephala can be differentiated from those of Ancylostoma by their:

   a. different shape
   b. smaller size
   c. larger size
   d. embryonated state when passed
   e. much thicker shell

Correct answers are on pages 183-188.

47. *Examination of feces from a Toy Poodle with Cushing's disease (hyperadrenocorticism) reveals a larva identified as that of* Filaroides hirthi. *In such immunocompromised hosts,* Filaroides hirthi *infection is likely to cause:*

    a. neurologic signs
    b. anemia
    c. a nonproductive cough and harsh lung sounds
    d. renal insufficiency
    e. hepatic dysfunction

48. *You find larvae of* Crenosoma vulpis *in a dog's feces and transtracheal washes. To become infective to another dog after they are passed in the feces, the larvae of* C vulpis *must be ingested by a:*

    a. snail or slug
    b. mouse
    c. beetle
    d. cockroach
    e. flea

49. *Puppies that develop patent* Toxocara canis *infection at the beginning of their fourth week of life have most likely become infected with this parasite by:*

    a. ingestion of infective larvae
    b. transmammary migration of larvae from the bitch
    c. transplacental migration of larvae from the bitch
    d. penetration of the skin by infective larvae
    e. ingestion of roundworm eggs containing infective larvae

50. *A dog obtained originally from a local humane shelter in Illinois develops a weeping, pustular lesion on its right carpus. Microscopic examination of a direct saline smear of material from the lesion reveals nematode larvae that are over 500 μ long, with a long pointed tail. Surgical exploration of the lesion reveals a white worm about 30 cm in length. The dog probably became infected by drinking water containing the infected intermediate host, a copepod. The parasite causing the lesion is:*

    a. *Dipetalonema reconditum*
    b. *Dracunculus insignis*
    c. *Spirocerca lupi*
    d. *Angiostrongylus vasorum*
    e. *Dictophyma renale*

51. *A dog infected with* Spirocerca lupi *is most likely to develop:*

    a. diarrhea
    b. anemia
    c. dysphagia
    d. pulmonary insufficiency
    e. right heart failure

52. *The prepatent period of* Dirofilaria immitis *poses problems in diagnosis of heartworm infection in dogs. By definition, the prepatent period of heartworms is that period between:*

    a. the time the mosquito ingests a microfilaria and the time the infective-stage larva is fully developed
    b. the time the adult worms have died and the time the microfilariae are ultimately cleared from the blood due to old age and natural death
    c. the time a dog has been chemotherapeutically cleared of its microfilariae and the time the microfilariae from the existing adults return to detectable levels in the circulation
    d. the time infective-stage larvae are inoculated by a mosquito and the time adult worms first appear in pulmonary vessels
    e. the time infective-stage larvae are inoculated by a mosquito and the time microfilariae first appear in the bloodstream

53. *In a dog with disease caused by* Dirofilaria immitis, *common clinical findings include:*

    a. hepatic dysfunction
    b. renal dysfunction
    c. coughing, decreased exercise tolerance and weight loss
    d. vomiting
    e. edema of the extremities

54. *The prepatent period of whipworm (*Trichuris vulpis*) infection is:*

a. 1 week
b. 1 month
c. 3 months
d. 5 months
e. 1 year

55. A woodchuck dies after showing signs suggestive of rabies; however, postmortem tests for rabies are negative. Histologic examination of sections of the brain reveals rather large larval nematodes resembling ascarids. The most likely cause of disease in this woodchuck is:

a. *Parascaris equorum*
b. *Toxocara canis*
c. *Toxascaris leonina*
d. *Toxocara cati*
e. *Baylisascaris procyonis*

56. You are performing routine fecal examinations on a group of rainbow trout and find small (45 m) eggs with a thick brown shell that appears pitted and has bipolar plugs. These eggs are most likely those of:

a. *Trichuris*
b. a capillarid nematode
c. an acanthocephalan
d. a tapeworm
e. a trematode

57. In a large cattery in Oregon, some cats begin vomiting intermittently. Repeated fecal examinations fail to identify any parasites other than a few coccidia and Giardia that are not confined only to the vomiting cats. When one of the affected cats dies from other causes, necropsy reveals small nematodes (less than 1 mm long) within a focal lesion about 3 cm in diameter in the stomach. The male worms have a copulatory bursa. The most likely cause of vomiting in these cats is:

a. *Ancylostoma tubaeforme*
b. *Ollulanus tricuspis*
c. *Strongyloides tumefaciens*
d. *Physaloptera praeputialis*
e. *Gnathostoma spinigerum*

58. In the southeastern United States and the Caribbean, cats are probably the major source of eggs from which the larvae develop that cause the zoonotic syndrome called cutaneous larva migrans. The nematode that most commonly causes this zoonotic disease is:

a. *Ancylostoma tubaeforme*
b. *Ancylostoma braziliense*
c. *Uncinaria stenocephala*
d. *Ancylostoma caninum*
e. *Ollulanus tricuspis*

59. In the leopard collection of a zoologic park in the midwestern United States, the animals are continually reinfected with the roundworm Toxascaris leonina. The reason this worm is a chronic problem in this type of housing arrangement is the:

a. transmammary transmission of larvae
b. transplacental transmission of larvae
c. cockroach paratenic host
d. earthworm paratenic host
e. rapid embryonation of eggs

60. In a cat with coughing and dyspnea, nematode larvae in the feces have dorsally spined tails. This cat is most likely infected with:

a. *Aelurostrongylus abstrusus*
b. *Crenosoma vulpis*
c. *Ollulanus tricuspis*
d. *Physaloptera praeputialis*
e. *Eucoleus aerophilus (Capillaria aerophila)*

61. A cat with gastritis, evidenced by vomiting and anorexia, is passing small (45 μ long) thick-shelled larvated eggs in its feces. Gastroscopy reveals pinkish-white worms 3-4 cm long without any marked spines on the head. This cat is most likely infected with:

a. *Ollulanus tricuspis*
b. *Gnathostoma spinigerum*
c. *Toxocara cati*
d. *Strongyloides tumefaciens*
e. *Physaloptera praeputialis*

Correct answers are on pages 183-188.

62. *The most important route by which kittens become infected with* Toxocara cati *is:*

   a. ingestion of a paratenic host
   b. transmammary migration of larvae from the queen
   c. transplacental migration of larvae from the queen
   d. penetration of the skin by infective larvae
   e. ingestion of eggs containing infective larvae

63. *A cat from central Louisiana rapidly develops severe neurologic signs that include seizures. After the cat dies, necropsy reveals a 15-cm-long, thin, white worm in brain tissue. This worm is most likely:*

   a. *Dirofilaria immitis*
   b. *Toxocara cati*
   c. *Gnathostoma spinigerum*
   d. *Baylisascaris procyonis*
   e. *Toxascaris leonina*

64. *The first intermediate host of* Gnathostoma spinigerum, *a spirurid nematode parasite of cats, is:*

   a. an earthworm
   b. a snail
   c. a mammal
   d. an arthropod
   e. a fish

65. *A lesion on the lip of a horse does not respond to topical corticosteroids or systemic antibiotics. Ultimately, the horse develops central nervous system signs and is euthanized. Histologic examination of brain tissue reveals large numbers of eosinophils and numerous minute, adult female nematodes. The features of the nematode that allow its identification are its size, the rhabditoid esophagus, and the recurved uterus containing a single egg. The nematode causing this disease is:*

   a. *Strongyloides stercoralis*
   b. *Strongyloides westeri*
   c. *Halicephalobus deletrix*
   d. *Habronema muscae*

   e. *Draschia megastoma*

66. *Treatment of mares at parturition with large doses of ivermectin can prevent infection of foals with* Strongyloides westeri. *Such anthelmintic intervention is successful probably because:*

   a. it prevents passage of infective larvae in the mare's milk
   b. it prevents shedding of eggs in the mare's feces, eliminating the stages in the environment that could infect the foal
   c. the drug is transferred to the foal in the mare's milk
   d. it prevents acquisition of arrested larvae by the mare
   e. it kills the infective stages in feces ingested by the foal

67. *Horses that share pastures with cattle infected with* Trichostrongylus axei *and become infected with this parasite are likely to develop:*

   a. summer sores
   b. gastritis
   c. pneumonia
   d. spinal cord disease
   e. ulcerative colitis

68. *Donkeys infected with* Dictyocaulus arnfieldi *are considered a threat to horses because they contaminate the environment with larvae. Grazing horses acquire lungworm infections by ingesting:*

   a. free-living infective larvae
   b. infective larvae in a snail intermediate host
   c. infective larvae in an oribatid mite
   d. infective larvae in an ant
   e. infective larvae within a lungworm egg

69. *Infection of a horse with large numbers of* Oxyuris equi *is likely to lead to:*

   a. verminous arteritis
   b. gastritis
   c. acute diarrhea in late winter and spring
   d. bare patches around the tail and perineum

e. chronic bloody diarrhea

70. *After an egg of* Parascaris equorum *is ingested by the host, the larva that hatches:*

a. develops entirely within the intestinal lumen
b. undergoes early development in the intestinal wall before migrating back to the small intestine
c. migrates to the liver and throughout the abdominal cavity before migrating back to the small intestine
d. migrates from the liver to the lungs before returning to the small intestine
e. develops in the colon and then migrates back to the small intestine

71. *Necropsy of a horse reveals a 5-cm hemispherical swelling in the stomach at the level of the margo plicatus. The swelling contains necrotic material and a large number of worms about 1 cm long. The females lay small, thin-shelled, larvated eggs. The worm within this lesion is most likely:*

a. *Draschia megastoma*
b. *Habronema muscae*
c. *Trichostrongylus axei*
d. *Strongyloides westeri*
e. *Probstmayria vivipara*

72. *A skin lesion on the face of a horse contains large numbers of eosinophils and nematode larvae, and improves markedly after ivermectin therapy. The larvae are probably those of:*

a. *Habronema muscae*
b. *Strongylus vulgaris*
c. *Trichostrongylus axei*
d. *Strongyloides westeri*
e. *Probstmayria vivipara*

73. *Horses become infected with* Draschia megastoma *by:*

a. ingesting infective larvae from pasture
b. ingesting a fly, *Musca domestica*, containing the infective larvae
c. ingesting an earthworm containing the infective larvae

d. the bite of a fly, *Stomoxys calcitrans*, harboring the infective larvae
e. the bite of a tick, *Dermacentor nitens*, harboring the infective larvae

74. *In horses, small strongyles (cyathostomes) can cause disease when present in large numbers or apparently when there is mass emergence of arrested larvae. Where are the hypobiotic larvae (arrested larvae) of these worms located in a parasitized horse?*

a. the lungs
b. the cranial mesenteric arteries
c. caseous nodules in the small bowel
d. the wall of the cecum and colon
e. the wall of the stomach

75. *In horses, the larvae of* Strongylus vulgaris *are the pathogenic stage of this parasite. Damage is caused by migration of larvae within the:*

a. liver
b. pancreas
c. intima of the cranial mesenteric arteries
d. caseous nodules in the small intestine wall
e. spinal cord

76. *The prepatent period of* Strongylus vulgaris *is:*

a. 2 weeks
b. 1 month
c. 2 months
d. 4 months
e. 6 months

77. *A gorilla develops chronic intermittent diarrhea and dies. Necropsy reveals the ileocecal region of the intestine to be studded with small nodules containing worms with rather large buccal capsules. An occasional strongyle-type egg is occasionally found in the feces. These worms most likely are:*

a. oesophagostomins
b. hookworms
c. metastrongyles
d. trichostronglyes
e. filarids

Correct answers are on pages 183-188.

78. *Cattle become infected with* Ostertagia ostertagi *by:*

   a. ingestion of infective larvae
   b. ingestion of infected oribatid mites
   c. transmammary migration of infective larvae
   d. transplacental migration of infective larvae
   e. ingestion of infective larvae encysted in water plants

79. *A winter outbreak of acute parasitic bronchitis in stabled dairy replacement stock is best managed by treatment with ivermectin, fenbendazole or levamisole, and by:*

   a. keeping the animals as warm as possible
   b. increasing the plane of nutrition
   c. exercising the cattle
   d. monitoring the output of larvae in the feces
   e. removing manure and providing adequate ventilation

80. *As a parasite control measure, the principal objective in administering anthelmintics to all members of a herd or flock is to:*

   a. increase the level of nutrition and state of health of host animals by removing the physiologic drain imposed by the parasites
   b. decrease the number of parasite eggs distributed in the environment of the host
   c. reduce the population of parasites so that the host can develop active immunity in the absence of frank clinical disease
   d. totally and permanently eradicate the parasites
   e. prevent development of anthelmintic resistance in the parasites

81. *In cattle, larvae of* Ostertagia ostertagi *produce lesions in the:*

   a. rumen wall
   b. abomasal wall
   c. lungs
   d. small intestine
   e. large bowel

82. *In late winter in Ohio, a group of young cattle develop profuse watery diarrhea, anemia and hypoproteinemia, as evidenced clinically as submandibular edema (bottle jaw). Despite their illness, the cattle continue eating. The parasite most likely responsible for this condition is:*

   a. *Fasciola hepatica*
   b. *Trichostrongylus axei*
   c. *Ostertagia ostertagi*
   d. *Nematodirus helvetianus*
   e. *Bunostomum phlebotomum*

83. *In a calf that died from severe diarrhea associated with high serum pepsinogen levels, necropsy reveals the rumen, reticulum and omasum to be full of feed, while the remainder of the alimentary tract is virtually empty. The mucosa of the abomasum is covered with grayish white, 3- to 5-mm nodules, each of which contains a small worm. The parasite responsible for this type of lesion in cattle is:*

   a. *Hemonchus placei*
   b. *Trichostronglyus axei*
   c. *Ostertagia ostertagi*
   d. *Nematodirus helvetianus*
   e. *Bunostomum phlebotomum*

84. *A horse has worms in its eye that are identified as* Thelazia lacrymalis. *Horses become infected with this parasite by:*

   a. ingestion of an infected fly, *Musca domestica*
   b. ingestion of an infected fly, *Musca autumnalis*
   c. ingestion of infective larvae while grazing
   d. deposition of infective larvae into the eye by the fly, *Musca autumnalis*
   e. deposition of infective larvae into bite wounds by the fly, *Hematobia irritans*

85. *Necropsy of a cow reveals an elevated regular serpiginous tract in the esophagus that spans about 6 cm. The tract contains a worm with cuticular protuberances on its cranial end and ovoid, small (30 µ long), thick-shelled, larvated eggs. The worm responsible for this lesion is:*

a. *Gongylonema pulchrum*

b. *Thelazia gullosa*

c. *Dracunculus insignis*

d. *Strongyloides papillosus*

e. *Rhabditis (Pelodera) strongyloides*

86. Young beef cattle in Mississippi develop anemia and anasarca during a wet period of the summer. None of the animals shows any signs of diarrhea and some seem constipated. One animal dies and necropsy reveals numerous red and white worms, 20-30 mm long, within the abomasum. The worm most likely responsible for the disease in these cattle is:

a. *Hemonchus placei*

b. *Trichostrongylus axei*

c. *Ostertagia ostertagi*

d. *Nematodirus helvetianus*

e. *Bunostomum phlebotomum*

87. In a large confined dairy herd, the cattle are infected with few parasites, including Strongyloides papillosus *and* Trichuris discolor. *One egg noted in the feces of a few cows is distinguishable from other nematode eggs by its morphologic characteristics. The egg is relatively clear shelled, football shaped (a prolate spheroid) and large (200 μ long), and contains 8-10 large cells (about 25 μ in diameter) and a good deal of empty space on both ends. This is most likely the egg of:*

a. *Hemonchus placei*

b. *Trichostrongylus axei*

c. *Ostertagia ostertagi*

d. *Nematodirus helvetianus*

e. *Bunostomum phlebotomum*

88. Trichostrongyles parasitizing cattle can be identified by the stages passed in the feces using:

a. careful measurement of the eggs

b. microscopic examination of first-stage larvae grown in culture

c. microscopic examination of infective larvae grown in culture

d. microscopic examination of the ornamentation of the eggshells

e. microscopic examination of the larva within the eggshell

89. A calf develops dark, watery diarrhea and no parasite eggs are noted in the feces. Necropsy reveals small, caseous nodules in the wall of the small intestine. Each nodule contains a worm or a decaying worm. Living worms have a large buccal capsule. The worms causing this disease are most likely:

a. *Oesophagostomum radiatum*

b. *Bunostomum phlebotomum*

c. *Hemonchus placei*

d. *Strongyloides papillosus*

e. *Dictyocaulus viviparus*

90. A smear of blood collected from a newborn foal contains microfilariae identified as those of Setaria equina. *If the microfilariae in the foal are not killed by anthelmintic treatment, they will:*

a. develop to adults within the abdominal cavity

b. develop to infective larvae in the dermis

c. cause "summer sores" in the saddle area

d. die from natural causes without serious consequences

e. migrate to the brain, causing serious neurologic disease

91. A calf develops severe bloody diarrhea that proves fatal. At necropsy, the mucosa of the colon is lined with thousands of worms. These worms are pinkish-white and about 2-3 cm long, with a caudal end that is free within the lumen of the bowel, and a thin, hair-like cranial end that is threaded into the colonic mucosa. These worms, which occasionally kill cattle by cecal hemorrhage, are most likely:

a. *Trichostrongylus axei*

b. *Trichinella spiralis*

c. *Trichuris discolor*

d. *Oesophagostomum radiatum*

e. *Hemonchus placei*

Correct answers are on pages 183-188.

92. *Some people in France eat rare or under-cooked horse meat from the United States and develop diarrhea 1-3 days later. The affected individuals then develop myositis and very high eosinophil numbers. Muscle biopsies 4 weeks after the meat was ingested reveal nematode larvae within the striated muscle fibers. The worm most likely responsible for this outbreak of disease is:*

   a. *Bunostomum phlebotomum*
   b. *Toxocara canis*
   c. *Toxocara vitulorum*
   d. *Triodontophorus tenuicollis*
   e. *Trichinella spiralis*

93. *Heavy infections of* Trichostrongylus *in sheep cause:*

   a. anemia
   b. pneumonia
   c. sneezing
   d. watery, dark-green diarrhea
   e. hepatic dysfunction

94. *The major clinical sign of hemonchosis in sheep is:*

   a. pale mucous membranes
   b. diarrhea
   c. hypoproteinemia
   d. constipation
   e. bloody diarrhea

95. *Three nematodes found in the lungs of sheep are:*

   a. *Dictyocaulus, Crenosoma* and *Parelaphostrongylus*
   b. *Muellerius, Aelurostrongylus* and *Dictyocaulus*
   c. *Muellerius, Metastrongylus* and *Protostrongylus*
   d. *Muellerius, Protostrongylus* and *Dictyocaulus*
   e. *Muellerius, Oesophagostomum* and *Dictyocaulus*

96. *A llama in northwestern Pennsylvania develops caudal paralysis in late summer. The* llama is euthanized. Examination of the spinal cord reveals a 4-cm-long, reddish-brown nematode within the gray matter. The worm most likely responsible for this condition is:*

   a. *Baylisascaris procyonis*
   b. *Hypoderma lineatus*
   c. *Fascioloides magna*
   d. *Dracunculus insignis*
   e. *Parelaphostrongylus tenuis*

97. *A flock of sheep spends the summer on rangeland in the mountains of Colorado that is occasionally frequented by elk. The sheep develop dermatitis on their face, and have circulating microfilariae in their blood. The problem is diagnosed as* Elaeophora schneideri *infection. The adult worms of this species are found in the:*

   a. mesenteric arteries
   b. nuchal ligament
   c. abdominal cavity
   d. carotid artery
   e. lungs

98. *The concept of "spring rise" refers to:*

   a. increased numbers of larvae on pasture in the spring
   b. increased development from egg to larvae under spring conditions
   c. increased egg output by ewes due to continued development of arrested larvae
   d. development of increased *Hemonchus*-specific antibody levels during spring
   e. movement of larvae that have overwintered in the soil up onto freshly growing grass in the spring

99. *A white-tailed deer infected with* Parelaphostrongylus tenuis *is housed in the same cement-floored enclosure with a sheep. The sheep could become infected with this parasite by:*

   a. eating fresh deer feces containing the typical metastrongyle larvae bearing the diagnostic terminal spine on their tail

b. eating hay contaminated with the infective larvae that have developed in the moisture that collected near the water supply

c. eating ants that have crawled in from surrounding pasture

d. eating snails that have been living under the cement bricks in the corner and that have fed on the deer feces and now contain infective larvae

e. drinking water contaminated with feces from the deer that contains the typical metastrongyle larvae bearing the diagnostic subterminal spine on their tail

100. *Larvae that may be found in fresh sheep feces are those of:*

a. *Dictyocaulus, Trichostrongylus* and *Parelaphostrongylus*

b. *Muellerius, Hemonchus* and *Dictyocaulus*

c. *Muellerius, Metastrongylus* and *Protostrongylus*

d. *Muellerius, Protostrongylus* and *Dictyocaulus*

e. *Muellerius, Oesophagostomum* and *Dictyocaulus*

101. *In a large flock of caged chickens, certain rows of pullets have reduced feed consumption. Mortality levels become higher for these rows than the overall average for the facility. In 7-10 days, another area of the cage rows develops similar mortality. Necropsy of the dead birds reveals necrotic enteritis, with eroded, roughened mucosa of the ileum and rectum. The lesion has a superficial appearance similar to the surface of a "turkish towel." Ultimately, you discover that the pathogen is transmitted between rows of cages by a continuous-belt mechanical feed system. The parasite most likely causing this disease is:*

a. *Eimeria brunetti*

b. *Ascaridia galli*

c. *Heterakis gallinarum*

d. *Histomonas meleagridis*

e. *Syngamus trachea*

102. *Species of* Nematodirus *differ from other trichostrongyloid nematodes in that:*

a. their larvae develop to the infective stage within the egg

b. the adult worms live in the lungs

c. the adult worms live in the small intestine

d. developing larvae migrate through the liver and lungs

e. they require an intermediate host

103. *Pastured swine are anemic and off feed, with occasionally darkened feces. Necropsy reveals small (less than 1 cm long), reddish nematodes within the gastric mucosa. These worms are most likely:*

a. *Trichostrongylus axei*

b. *Hyostrongylus rubidus*

c. *Strongyloides stercoralis*

d. *Ascaris suum*

e. *Ollulanus tricuspis*

104. *A group of swine raised on cement has white "milk spots" on their liver at necropsy and has had previous signs of lung disease (thumps). The worm most likely responsible for these signs is:*

a. *Metastrongylus apri*

b. *Ascaris suum*

c. *Stephanurus dentatus*

d. *Bunostomum phlebotomum*

e. *Strongyloides ransomi*

105. *Scours occurs in 2- to 6-month-old pigs about 3 weeks after they have been moved from confinement to pastures, and does not respond to treatment with antibiotics. A possible cause of the diarrhea is:*

a. *Ascaris suum*

b. *Isospora suis*

c. *Trichinella spiralis*

d. *Trichuris suis*

e. *Stephanurus dentatus*

Correct answers are on pages 183-188.

106. A nematode that may cause diarrhea in nursing piglets is:

   a. *Oesophagostomum dentatum*
   b. *Hyostrongylus rubidus*
   c. *Strongylus ransomi*
   d. *Metastrongylus apri*
   e. *Macracanthorhynchus hirudinaceus*

107. Pigs become infected with Ascaris suum by:

   a. ingestion of infective eggs
   b. ingestion of larvae on pasture
   c. transmammary transmission
   d. transplacental transmission
   e. ingestion of a paratenic host

108. Occasionally, horses develop lesions on the ventral midline that are characterized by alopecia and depigmentation, and that may respond to ivermectin therapy. These lesions are most likely due to the microfilariae of adult filarids that live within the nuchal ligament. The likely cause of these lesions in horses is:

   a. *Setaria digitata*
   b. *Elaeophora schneideri*
   c. *Teladorsagia circumcincta*
   d. *Onchocerca cervicalis*
   e. *Habronema muscae*

109. Necropsies of feral swine in Louisiana reveal red worms, about 3 cm long, in nodules in the perirenal fat. The female worms are fertile and contain typical strongyle-like eggs. The worms most likely are:

   a. *Syngamus trachea*
   b. *Metastrongylus apri*
   c. *Strongylus edentatus*
   d. *Stephanurus dentatus*
   e. *Fascioloides magna*

110. A group of game-farm pheasants is found standing with their head back while holding their mouth open and breathing rapidly. Some of the birds die. Necropsy reveals red worms within the trachea, with the male and female worms joined in copula. These worms most likely are:

   a. *Syngamus trachea*
   b. *Ascaridia galli*
   c. *Heterakis isolonche*
   d. *Heterakis spumosa*
   e. *Capillaria*

111. At necropsy of a military macaw, the small intestine is filled with white worms 4-6 cm long. The male worms have a "pseudosucker" cranial to the anus. These worms are most likely a species of:

   a. *Syngamus*
   b. *Ascaridia*
   c. *Heterakis*
   d. *Capillaria*
   e. *Histomonas*

112. Ingestion of infective Toxocara canis eggs by a mature bitch is most likely to lead to:

   a. patent infection
   b. destruction of the eggs by gastric fluids
   c. spurious positive fecal examinations (pseudoparasitism)
   d. accumulation of arrested larvae in tissues
   e. hepatomegaly and eosinophilia

113. A pet python dies of an impacted intestine, and you discover a large mass of white worms in the stomach and small intestine. The worms are about 10-15 cm long and have large lips. Eggs have a thick shell and contain a single cell when passed from the female. The worms in this python are most likely members of:

   a. Strongylida (hookworms, trichostrongyles, strongyles)
   b. Rhabditida (*Stronglyoides* and relatives)
   c. Oxyurida (pinworms)
   d. Ascaridida (ascarids)
   e. Spirurida (*Gnathostoma*, other spirurids, filarids)

114. You are asked to take care of a pet iguana for several weeks, and find that it occasionally

passes worms that are white and 1-1.5 cm long. The worms have a short esophagus, with a large round bulb at its base where it joins the intestine, and thick-shelled eggs. These nematodes are most likely members of:

a. Strongylida (hookworms, trichostrongyles, strongyles)

b. Rhabditida (*Strongyloides* and relatives)

c. Oxyurida (pinworms)

d. Ascaridida (ascarids)

e. Spirurida (*Gnathostoma*, other spirurids, filarids)

115. *"Salmon poisoning" of dogs in Alaska, Oregon and Washington is caused by:*

a. *Nanophyetus salmincola*, a trematode whose metacercariae encyst in salmonid fishes

b. *Salmonella typhimurium*

c. *Neorickettsia helminthoeca*, a rickettsia transmitted by *Salmonella typhimurium*

d. *Neorickettsia helminthoeca*, a rickettsia transmitted by *Nanophyetus salmincola*

e. ingestion of *Diphyllobothrium latum* larvae, which encyst in salmonid fishes

116. *Dogs, cats, foxes and mink become infected with* Paragonimus kellicotti *throughout the region of the Mississippi drainage system by ingestion of metacercariae within the tissues of a:*

a. fish

b. copepod

c. frog

d. tadpole

e. crayfish

117. *Kittens can become infected with* Alaria marcianae *soon after birth. The mode of transmission of this trematode parasite to kittens is unusual in that:*

a. there is transmammary transmission

b. there is transplacental transmission

c. the life cycle of this trematode is direct

d. cercariae penetrate the skin directly

e. it uses a frog as an intermediate host

118. *In Florida, a cat with hepatic insufficiency has biliary obstruction. During corrective surgery, flukes are found within the bile duct. The trematode causing this disease is identified as* Platynosomum fastosum. *Cats become infected with this parasite by eating:*

a. ants

b. snails

c. fish

d. lizards

e. mice

119. *A hunting dog in Louisiana develops hepatic disease but subsequently dies of unrelated causes. Necropsy reveals a fibrotic, firm liver. You observe small flukes (1 cm long) within the veins of the liver and the mesenteric veins of the abdominal cavity. There are male and female worms, and female worms are held within the gynecophoral canal of males. The worms causing the hepatic fibrosis are most likely:*

a. *Clonorchis sinensis*

b. *Dicrocoelium dendriticum*

c. *Heterobilharzia americana*

d. *Cryptocotyle lingua*

e. *Alaria canis*

120. *Cattle with chronic* Fasciola hepatica *infection typically have:*

a. fibrotic bile ducts

b. rumenitis

c. abomasitis

d. pneumonia

e. renal disease

121. *In cattle with paramphistome infection, the adult flukes are found in the:*

a. rumen and reticulum

b. omasum

c. abomasum

d. small intestine

e. colon

Correct answers are on pages 183-188.

122. Cattle become infected with Dicrocoelium dendriticum, *the lanceolate fluke of the bile duct, by:*

    a. ingesting metacercariae on vegetation
    b. ingesting infected snails
    c. ingesting infected ants
    d. cercariae penetrating the skin
    e. the bite of a mosquito

123. *Outbreaks of clinical* Fasciola hepatica *infection may occur during periods of drought because:*

    a. sheep are forced to eat unpalatable aquatic vegetation that may be covered with infected ants
    b. sheep are forced to eat unpalatable aquatic vegetation that may contain encysted metacercariae
    c. sheep are forced to graze close to ant hills
    d. sheep may enter bodies of water and be penetrated by cercariae
    e. *Fasciola hepatica* causes disease only in malnourished sheep

124. *A Sika deer that is housed in a petting zoo in New York develops acute hepatosis and dies. Necropsy reveals that the liver has been severely damaged by migrating flukes that are several centimeters long. This fluke, which usually has the white-tailed deer as its final host, is:*

    a. *Fasciola buskii*
    b. *Fascioloides magna*
    c. *Dicrocoelium dendriticum*
    d. *Clonorchis sinensis*
    e. *Alaria marcianae*

125. *Examination of a dog's feces reveals a large (120 μ long), ovoid, brown-shelled egg with a marked operculum and containing several developing cells. The parasite from which this egg came is most likely:*

    a. *Heterobilharzia americana*
    b. *Paragonimus kellicotti*
    c. *Spirometra mansonoides*
    d. *Diphyllobothrium latum*

    e. *Taenia pisiformis*

126. *Digenetic trematodes, such as* Fasciola, Dicrocoelium, Paragonimus *and* Platynoso-mum, *use various invertebrates and vertebrates as second intermediate hosts if one is required for completion of the life cycle. The first intermediate host of a digenetic trematode is:*

    a. an annelid, such as an earthworm
    b. a mollusk, such as a snail
    c. an arthropod, such as an insect
    d. a mammal
    e. a fish

127. *Radiographs of the lungs of a cat show circular lesions about 2-3 cm in diameter in the distal lobes. Examination of the feces reveals brown, operculate eggs. This cat is probably infected with:*

    a. *Platynosomum fastosum*
    b. *Paragonimus kellicotti*
    c. *Alaria marcianae*
    d. *Clonorchis sinensis*
    e. *Cryptocotyle lingua*

128. *Adult taeniid tapeworms are found in dogs, cats and people. The life cycle of taeniid cestodes is characterized by the requirement of:*

    a. an annelid intermediate host, such as an earthworm
    b. a molluskan intermediate host, such as a snail
    c. an arthropod intermediate host, such as an insect
    d. a mammalian intermediate host
    e. a fish intermediate host

129. *If you had to move a group of foxes from Ontario to North Carolina, the parasite you should be most concerned about introducing to the new locale with the foxes is:*

    a. *Uncinaria stenocephala*
    b. *Ancylostoma caninum*
    c. *Toxascaris leonina*
    d. *Echinococcus multilocularis*

e. *Taenia hydatigena*

d. ants

e. mice

130. *In Iceland, reduction of the prevalence of* Echinococcus granulosus *virtually to nil required over a century of deworming dogs and cooking sheep offal. Control has failed in parts of Australia and New Zealand because of:*

a. anthelmintic resistance of the parasite
b. lack of cooperation on the part of sheep producers
c. existence of sylvatic and pastoral cycles
d. lack of effective anthelmintic treatment for dogs
e. mechanical transmission of *Echinococus granulosus* eggs from dogs to sheep by the woolstrike fly, *Lucilia cuprina*

131. *A dog in Minnesota is passing operculate eggs identified as those of the tapeworm,* Diphyllobothrium latum. *This dog was most likely infected by ingesting:*

a. fish
b. beef
c. pork
d. mutton
e. mice

132. *Acanthocephalans have a spiny proboscis and lack an intestinal tract. The life cycle of an acanthocephalan is characterized by the requirement of:*

a. an annelid intermediate host, such as an earthworm
b. a molluskan intermediate host, such as a snail
c. an arthropod intermediate host, such as an insect
d. a mammalian intermediate host
e. no requirement for an intermediate host

133. *Macracanthorhynchus ingens is a parasite of raccoons and occasionally dogs. Dogs become infected by ingestion of infected:*

a. earthworms
b. millipedes
c. snails

134. *Cats become infected with* Dipylidium caninum *by ingesting fleas containing cysticercoids. The fleas become infected with this cestode by ingesting:*

a. cysticerci in circulating blood
b. tapeworm eggs in larval fleas
c. tapeworm eggs in young adult fleas
d. mesocercariae in circulating blood
e. infected oribatid mites

135. *Cats become infected with* Taenia taeniaeformis *by ingesting infected:*

a. fleas
b. fish
c. earthworms
d. rodents
e. snails

136. *Necropsy of a horse reveals the intestine to contain a very large number of white tapeworms at the ileocecal valve, though no eggs were detected in the feces before necropsy. This parasite is most likely:*

a. *Taenia hydatigena*
b. *Echinococcus granulosus*
c. *Moniezia expansa*
d. *Anoplocephala perfoliata*
e. *Thysanosoma actinoides*

137. *Cysticerci found in the muscles of cattle usually are those that can develop into adult* Taeniarhynchus (Taenia) saginatus *tapeworms in the small intestine of people ingesting the infected beef. Cysticerci in the muscles of people usually are those that can develop into adult* Taenia solium *tapeworms in the small intestine of:*

a. people
b. swine
c. sheep
d. dogs
e. cats

Correct answers are on pages 183-188.

138. *You find a large cyst (8 cm in diameter) in the lung of a cow in Utah. The cyst contains thousands of microscopic tapeworm scolices. This cyst respresents a:*

a. sparganum
b. cysticerus
c. coenurus
d. hydatid
e. cysticeroid

139. *Occasionally, cattle serve as host to a long adult tapeworm,* Moniezia benedeni. *Cattle become infected by ingesting:*

a. infective eggs
b. infective ants
c. larvae on aquatic plants
d. infected snails
e. infected free-living mites

140. *Cerebral coenurosis of sheep results from ingestion of tapeworm eggs shed in the feces of:*

a. people
b. swine
c. cattle
d. dogs
e. cats

Questions 141 and 142

An outbreak of diarrhea in a group of marmosets is caused by infection with large numbers of acanthocephalan parasites.

141. *Without performing a morphologic diagnosis, the parasite causing the disease is most likely:*

a. *Oncicola*
b. *Macracanthorhynchus*
c. *Moniliformis*
d. *Prosthenorchis*
e. *Aonchotheca*

142. *The parasite mentioned in Question 141 is transmitted from primate to primate by ingestion of:*

a. infective eggs
b. larvae in earthworms
c. larvae in cockroaches
d. larvae encysted on fruit
e. food contaminated with feces

143. *A rhesus monkey has dark, hair-like, serpiginous tracts within its buccal cavity. The lesions contain nematode eggs that superficially resemble* Trichuris vulpis *eggs. The parasite typically associated with this type of lesion is a species of:*

a. *Stronglyoides*
b. *Anatrichosoma*
c. *Ancylostoma*
d. *Trichinella*
e. *Oxyuris*

144. *At necropsy of a dog, you find a tapeworm with no hooks on its proboscis. The segments are small and have no lateral genital opening, and gravid segments contain a central and single thick-walled mass of eggs. This tapeworm is a species of:*

a. *Echinococcus*
b. *Taenia*
c. *Dipylidium*
d. *Hymenolepis*
e. *Mesocestoides*

145. *Necropsy of several sheep in Montana reveals large numbers of cestodes within the bile duct. Examination of the tapeworms reveals that the segments appear "fringed." The tapeworms are most likely specimens of:*

a. *Thysanosoma actinoides*
b. *Hymenolepis diminuta*
c. *Hymenolepis nana*
d. *Taenia hydatigena*
e. *Echinococcus granulosus*

146. *A 12-year-old Pomeranian dog is losing mats of hair on its back, near the base of the tail. You examine the lesion and discover 50-100 maggots in and on the skin. The fly causing this lesion is most likely:*

    a. *Musca*
    b. *Stomoxys calcitrans*
    c. a calliphorid
    d. *Hypoderma lineatum*
    e. a cuterebrid

147. *A puppy adopted from a local shelter is infested with lice, which have a head about as wide as the abdomen. These lice are:*

    a. anopluran lice
    b. mallophagan lice
    c. *Linognathus setosus*
    d. human lice
    e. very difficult to treat

148. *The stage of the flea that becomes infected with the dog tapeworm,* Dipylidium caninum, *lives off the host in soil or bedding. Before becoming an adult, the flea goes through a pupal stage, and the adult flea emerges from the pupal case. The life cycle of fleas is said to involve:*

    a. incomplete metamorphosis
    b. simple metamorphosis
    c. partial metamorphosis
    d. complex metamorphosis
    e. continuous metamorphosis

149. *Adult fleas of dogs and cats usually prefer to be:*

    a. in the bedding of the host
    b. on the host
    c. in the soil
    d. in small cracks in the carpet or floor
    e. within the host's ear canal

150. *Ixodes dammini was described as a new species in 1979. This tick is the vector of Lyme disease (borreliosis) in the northeastern United States. The final host of this tick is typically the white-tailed deer* (Odocoileus virginiana). *The larva of this tick typically feeds on:*

    a. cattle
    b. rabbits
    c. lizards
    d. white-footed mice (*Peromyscus leucopus*)
    e. white-tailed deer

151. Rhipicephalus sanguineus *has been transported around the world along with its canine host, and it now has the largest geographic distribution of any known tick. The reason for the success of this typically tropical African tick is the fact that the larvae, nymphs and adults:*

    a. can overwinter in very cold climates
    b. feed quite contentedly on people
    c. do not need to feed, except as adults
    d. are smaller than most mites
    e. feed quite contentedly on dogs

152. *An army-owned German Shepherd that has served in the Middle East develops splenomegaly and skin lesions. Impression smears from a biopsy of skin lesions reveal* Leishmania. *While in the Middle East, this dog was likely bitten by an infected:*

    a. mosquito
    b. black fly
    c. deer fly
    d. *Culicoides* gnat
    e. psychodid (*Phlebotomus*) sand fly

153. *A nymphal* Ixodes *can be differentiated from a nymph of other genera of hard ticks by its:*

    a. elongated third palpal segments
    b. spur at the base of the tarsal segment of the first pair of legs
    c. 3 pair of legs
    d. pre-anal groove on its ventral surface
    e. spur on the caudal aspect of the tarsal segment of the last pair of legs

Correct answers are on pages 183-188.

154. Examination of nasal mucus secreted by a Boxer dog with upper respiratory disease reveals rather large mites. These mites are most likely:

a. Sarcoptes scabiei
b. Otodectes cynotis
c. Trixacarus caviae
d. Raillietia auris
e. Pneumonyssoides caninum

155. Mites in the ear of a dog are typically:

a. Sarcoptes scabiei
b. Notoedres cati
c. Otodectes cynotis
d. Lynxacarus radovskyi
e. Pyemotes tritici

156. Small, dandruff-like flakes in the hair of a dog appear to move. Examination of the apparent dandruff reveals it to be comprised of mites. This "walking dandruff" is associated with infestation by:

a. Sarcoptes scabiei
b. Myocoptes musculinus
c. Cheyletiella yasguri
d. Chirodiscoides caviae
e. Pyemotes tritici

157. Dogs typically acquire Demodex infestations from:

a. association with infested dogs
b. the bitch as pups while nursing
c. wild rodents
d. birds
e. contact with infested people

158. A cat is presented to your clinic in early autumn with a painless lesion on its cheek. The lesion contains a very large maggot (3 cm long) that you surgically remove. The maggot is probably a larva of:

a. Musca
b. Stomoxys calcitrans
c. a calliphorid
d. Gasterophilus intestinalis
e. Cuterebra

159. Examination of a brown tick collected from a cat to determine if the tick is a species of Ixodes reveals that the second palpal segment is laterally flared and the tick has no pre-anal groove. This tick is a member of the genus:

a. Dermacentor
b. Amblyomma
c. Boophilus
d. Haemaphysalis
e. Rhipicephalus

160. A cat develops severe pruritic dermatitis on its ears. Close examination reveals 6-legged mites with plumose setae on their dorsal scutum. These are the larvae of:

a. sarcoptiform mites
b. Demodex
c. Lynxacarus radovskyi
d. trombiculid mites
e. Cheyletiella

161. A cat from Key West, Florida, has a poor haircoat, a generally scruffy appearance, and small slow-moving mites clinging to its hair. These mites are most likely:

a. Sarcoptes scabiei
b. Notoedres cati
c. Otodectes cynotis
d. Lynxacarus radovskyi
e. Pyemotes tritici

162. Microscopic examination of skin scrapings from a cat with localized dermatitis on its face reveals large numbers of small sausage-shaped mites. These mites are most likely:

a. Demodex cati
b. Notoedres cati
c. Lynxacarus radovskyi
d. Cheyletiella blakei
e. Sarcoptes scabiei

163. *A cat from Islamorada Key, Florida, has severely thickened ears and dermatitis that extends onto the back and face. The cause of these lesions is found to be a sarcoptiform mite identified as* Notoedres cati. *These mites can be differentiated from* Sarcoptes scabiei *by the:*

    a. comparative lengths of the pretarsi
    b. location of the anus
    c. number of legs
    d. host they infest
    e. long, jointed pedicles on their pretarsi

164. *Face flies (*Musca autumnalis*) on horses are best controlled by:*

    a. applying insecticides to the horse's face
    b. applying insecticides to the horse's face, in conjunction with use of fly veils
    c. feeding a larvicide (tetrachlorovinphos) to nearby cattle
    d. feeding a larvicide (tetrachlorovinphos) to the horses
    e. feeding a larvicide (tetrachlorovinphos) to the horses and nearby cattle

165. *Horses in a herd develop ventral midline dermatitis that disappears each winter. The shelter where they are fed in the evening is near a stand of rather open forest. After other measures fail, you suggest placing a slowly revolving fan on one end of the shelter. The fan is an overwhelming success during the next spring and summer. Your decision to suggest the fan was based on a guess as to the causative agent from your knowledge of the flight behavior of:*

    a. mosquitos
    b. tabanids
    c. black flies
    d. biting midges (Heleids, Ceratopogonids)
    e. deer flies

166. *The larvae of* Stomoxys calcitrans *develop in:*

    a. fresh cattle manure
    b. damp hay or similar decaying organic matter
    c. soil
    d. quiet bodies of water
    e. rapidly moving streams

167. *Horses with stomach bots can be treated with ivermectin or dichlorvos after the first killing frost. One waits until after this frost because:*

    a. by then larvae have completed their migration through the spinal canal
    b. the cold weather kills the eggs of *Gasterophilus intestinalis* that are attached to hairs
    c. the cold weather kills the egg-laying adult flies
    d. there are no drugs that eliminate the stages developing within the buccal tissues of horses
    e. by then larvae have completed their migration through the liver

168. *In horses, the larvae of* Gasterophilus intestinalis *spend time within the oral mucosa. Ultimately, however, they arrive in the stomach, where they complete their development. The total average stay of* Gasterophilus intestinalis *within a horse is approximately:*

    a. 2 weeks
    b. 2 months
    c. 3 months
    d. 10 months
    e. 23 months

169. Gasterophilus intestinalis *females lay their eggs on the hairs of the:*

    a. neck and intermandibular space of horses; these eggs hatch spontaneously, and the larvae migrate into the animal's mouth
    b. forelimbs of horses; these eggs hatch spontaneously, and the larvae migrate into the animal's mouth
    c. neck and intermandibular space of horses; these eggs hatch in response to a thermal stimulus, and the larvae migrate into the animal's mouth
    d. forelimbs of horses; these eggs hatch in response to a thermal stimulus, and the larvae migrate into the animal's mouth
    e. hind pasterns of horses; these eggs hatch spontaneously, and the larve actively penetrate the animal's skin

Correct answers are on pages 183-188.

170. *A skin lesion in the saddle area of a horse contains a large maggot (bot). This is most likely a species of:*

a. *Gasterophilus*
b. *Hypoderma*
c. *Oestrus*
d. *Stomoxys*
e. *Hematobia*

171. Damalinia equi *is a louse found on horses. The eggs of this louse are most likely to be found:*

a. in the feces
b. glued to the hairs
c. in water containers within the box stall
d. in the bedding of the box stall
e. in soil surrounding the stable

172. *Where are you most likely to find an adult* Hematobia irritans?

a. in the barn
b. resting on flowers
c. resting on a steer's back
d. resting on the inside walls of a cool milking shed
e. resting on outside walls in bright sunshine

173. Hematobia irritans *lays its eggs in:*

a. rapidly running streams
b. straw contaminated with urine or manure, or decaying organic matter on beaches
c. slow-moving or still bodies of water
d. soil
e. fresh cattle manure

174. Hypoderma bovis *females lay their eggs on the hairs of:*

a. neck and intermandibular space of cattle; these eggs hatch spontaneously, and the larvae migrate into the animal's mouth
b. forelimbs of cattle; these eggs hatch spontaneously, and the larvae migrate into the animal's mouth
c. neck and intermandibular space of cattle; these eggs hatch in response to a thermal stimulus, and the larvae migrate into the animal's mouth
d. forelimbs of cattle; these eggs hatch in response to a thermal stimulus, and the larvae migrate into the animal's mouth
e. hind pasterns of cattle; these eggs hatch spontaneously, and the larvae actively penetrate the animal's skin

175. *The larvae of* Hypoderma lineatum *overwinter within the loose connective tissue of the submucosa of the caudal one-third of the esophagus. The larvae of* Hypoderma bovis *overwinter in the:*

a. soil
b. loose connective tissue of the submucosa of the caudal one-third of the esophagus
c. oral cavity
d. rodent intermediate host
e. epidural adipose tissue between the dura mater and periostomum, near the first lumbar vertebra

176. *You look in the ear of a cow and note what appear to be very large mites (about 1 cm in diameter). You subsequently identify the parasites as a stage of the soft tick* Otobius megnini. *The stages present in the ear of this cow are:*

a. larvae, nymphs and adults
b. nymphs and adults
c. nymphs and eggs
d. eggs, larvae and nymphs
e. larvae and nymphs

177. *If you find mites in the ear of a cow, they are most likely:*

a. *Sarcoptes* or *Otodectes*
b. *Chorioptes* or *Psoroptes*
c. *Knemidokoptes* or *Otodectes*
d. *Otodectes* or *Raillietia*
e. *Psoroptes* or *Raillietia*

178. Boophilus annulatus *has been eradicated from the United States by routine dipping of cattle in solutions of arsenicals. Dipping has been successful because* B annulatus *is:*

a. a 1-host tick
b. a 2-host tick
c. a 3-host tick
d. a tick found originally on the American bison that became extinct throughout most of its range, along with its indigenous host
e. only found in the ear canal of cattle

179. Cochliomyia hominivorax *screwworm was first introduced to Africa (Libya) from South America in 1987. It is now causing disease in over 2000 livestock animals a year and has caused disease in companion animals and people. This parasite will cause serious devastation to the wildlife of Africa if it extends its range south of the Sahara. The parasite is deadly because it:*

a. transmits *Trypanosoma rhodesiense* much more successfully than *Stomoxys calcitrans*
b. is a major cause of primary myiasis
c. is a major cause of tertiary myiasis
d. serves as a mechanical vector of anthrax
e. can use almost any mosquito as an intermediate host

180. *The most efficient means of protecting cattle against attack by tabanids is by:*

a. regularly applying repellents
b. stabling animals during peak fly activity
c. placing animals in bright sunlight
d. providing access to water
e. placing animals near the border of a wooded area during peak fly activity

181. *Skin scrapings of a lesion at the base of the tail of a cow reveal mites. You identify the mites as* Chorioptes bovis *by their:*

a. long, jointed pedicles of the pretarsi
b. long, nonjointed pedicles of the pretarsi
c. short pedicels of the pretarsi
d. elongate body

e. lack of caruncles on the pretarsi

182. *Mites of the genus* Demodex *cause mange in various animals. In dogs, the lesions are often generalized and may spread over the entire body surface. In cattle and goats, the lesions are:*

a. large, pustular, subcutaneous masses containing thousands of mites
b. generalized areas of inflammation at the base of the tail
c. found most commonly on the distal legs
d. not unlike the lesions caused by *Sarcoptes*
e. found mainly inside the mouth, along the gingivae

183. *Pupae of the sheep ked,* Melophagus ovinus, *are found:*

a. in pasture soil
b. in the uterus of the female ked
c. stuck to vegetation around rodent and rabbit burrows
d. attached to the host's wool
e. in the sheep's frontal sinuses

184. Oestrus ovis *overwinters as:*

a. third-stage larvae in the frontal sinuses of sheep
b. second-stage larvae in the frontal sinuses of sheep
c. adults in lofts and attics
d. eggs deposited on vegetation in sheep pastures
e. first-stage larvae in the nasal cavity and as pupae in soil

185. *Primary myiasis is defined as myiasis:*

a. requiring a living host
b. caused by the primary maggot present during an outbreak
c. caused by larvae that infest preexisting lesions
d. caused by fly larvae
e. developing in lesions due to an initial bacterial infection

---

Correct answers are on pages 183-188.

186. Oestrus ovis *females deposit:*

    a. eggs that become attached to the wool of the foreleg

    b. larvae onto the back of sheep

    c. larvae directly into the nasal passages of sheep

    d. larvae into the mouth of sheep

    e. eggs that become attached to the lips of sheep

187. *Tick paralysis occurs in a tick-infested animal when the ticks inject a:*

    a. neural toxin

    b. neurotropic virus

    c. rickettsial agent

    d. toxigenic bacterium

    e. substance that induces anaphylaxis

188. *A mite that has long, jointed pedicels and is occasionally found in the ears of llamas is a species of:*

    a. *Sarcoptes*

    b. *Psoroptes*

    c. *Chorioptes*

    d. *Otodectes*

    e. *Knemidokoptes*

189. *An old sow that cannot walk because of severe arthritis has large numbers of very large lice at the base of its ears and on the back of its neck. The lice on this pig are most likely of the genus:*

    a. *Hematopinus*

    b. *Damalinia*

    c. *Linognathus*

    d. *Solenopotes*

    e. *Trichodectes*

190. *In a pig with markedly thickened skin on the inner aspect of the pinnae, skin scrapings of the affected tissue reveal large numbers of mites. The mite most likely causing this lesion is:*

    a. *Sarcoptes*

    b. *Otodectes*

    c. *Psoroptes*

    d. *Chorioptes*

    e. *Cheyletiella*

191. *Ear canker in rabbits is typically caused by:*

    a. *Psoroptes cuniculi*

    b. *Sarcoptes scabiei*

    c. *Chorioptes ovis*

    d. *Cheyletiella blakei*

    e. *Otodectes cynotis*

192. *A budgerigar that develops greatly thickened ceres and feet is found to be infested with skin-dwelling mites. The mites that typically cause this condition are of the genus:*

    a. *Sarcoptes*

    b. *Psoroptes*

    c. *Chorioptes*

    d. *Knemidokoptes*

    e. *Myobia*

193. *Mites of the genus* Ornithonyssus *are infesting people and pets in a household. Control measures should be based on:*

    a. insecticidal treatment of the people and pets

    b. application of insecticides throughout the house

    c. removal of rodent and wild bird nests

    d. vacuum cleaning the house several times each day

    e. use of pesticide strips and flea collars

194. *Hemorrhagic ulcerative stomatitis of the throat pouch of pelicans has been associated with louse infestation. The type of louse most likely involved is:*

    a. an anopluran or a mallophagan

    b. an anopluran

    c. a mallophagan

    d. an ischnoceran

    e. *Pediculus*

195. Mosquito larvae typically develop in:

a. water
b. leaf litter
c. soil
d. feces
e. decaying organic material

196. A nestling red-tailed hawk dies from a suppurative lesion within its aural canals. Examination of the ears reveals large numbers of maggots. The spiracles on the caudal end of the maggots have the inner slit directed ventrolaterally. These maggots, which occasionally cause many deaths among nestling hawks, are a species of:

a. Calliphoridae
b. Gasterophilidae
c. Sarcophagidae
d. Muscidae
e. *Stomoxys*

197. The early larvae of a sarcophagid fly are most likely to be found:

a. in meat
b. attached to a mosquito's leg
c. in sandy soil
d. in fresh cow manure
e. in rotting organic matter

198. An outbreak of Dermanyssus gallinae, *the red mite of poultry, occurs on a modern broiler* breeder farm. To diagnose an infestation with this parasite, it is best to examine:

a. the base of the chicken's leg
b. the base of the chicken's beak
c. cracks and crevices in the cages
d. scrapings of skin just caudal to the oil gland
e. scrapings from skin around the vent

199. A chicken in Alabama has fleas that are attached to the skin around its eyes and on its wattles. The flea that is responsible for this type of infestation is a member of the genus:

a. *Xenopsylla*
b. *Echidnophaga*
c. *Ctenocephalides*
d. *Pulex*
e. *Cediopsylla*

200. Necropsy of a python reveals large (8 cm long) worms within the lungs. The worms appear somewhat segmented and have a mouth bordered on each side by a pair of large hooks. Eggs found in the female worms are the same as eggs found in the snake's feces before death; the eggs appear to contain a mite-like embryo. These worms of the genus Armillifer are representative of which group of parasites?

a. cestodes
b. pentastomids
c. acanthocephalans
d. monogenetic trematodes
e. myxosporidians

Answers

1. **a** Another possible cause is *Toxoplasma gondii.*

2. **d** This organism should be differentiated from *Hemobartonella.*

3. **e** Other species of *Isospora* would also be likely causes of these signs.

4. **d** Bradyzoites (chronic cyst stages) of this parasite are found mainly in striated muscle cells of cattle.

5. **a** *Giardia* has an environmentally resistant cyst that persists well in cool, clear water; hence the concern of water-source contamination.

6. **e** Infection in the United States is transmitted among sylvatic opossums and raccoons by the bite of reduviid bugs; occasionally, dogs are bitten by these vectors.

7. **b** Cats acquire fatal infections with this parasite from tick bites; the sylvatic cycle is tick-bobcat-tick.

8. **a** Trichomonads of a nonpathogenic nature can be found in the mouth of many animals, including people.

9. **c** Another approach would be a fecal ELISA, but these have not yet been verified for use in domestic animals.

10. **d** The fetus of an immune woman or sheep is protected unless the mother is immunosuppressed, such as by corticosteroids or, in people, AIDS.

11. **d** Autochthonous cases of this parasite have been reported in cats in the United States. In impression smears, amastigotes are characterized by a nucleus and a large kinetoplast.

12. **b** Immunosuppressed horses, not unlike dogs, cats and people, can develop severe diarrhea due to cryptosporidiosis.

13. **a**

14. **d** Equine protozoal myeloencephalitis is associated with this species of *Sarcocystis*.

15. **e** Though acute disease may occur, chronic infections only rarely cause significant signs.

16. **e** In certain housing situations, it is not uncommon for 100% of calves to be infected by the third week of life. *Cryptosporidium muris*, another mammalian parasite, also is found in cattle, but usually in older animals. The oocysts of *C parvum* are 5 μ, and those of *C muris* are 7 μ.

17. **b** Reproductive problems may be the first indication that this is a potential problem.

18. **c**

19. **a**

20. **c** Problems arise when animals are confined to small areas, causing accumulation of large infectious doses of oocysts within the soil or cage litter.

21. **b**

22. **a** Disease is likely to occur before oocysts are being shed in the feces. Diagnosis requires examination of the intestinal mucosa of dead animals.

23. **e**

24. **d**

25. **a** *Eimeria* species are seldom pathogenic in pigs. Other parasites that can induce diarrhea in nursing pigs are *Cryptosporidium* and *Strongyloides*.

26. **c**

27. **b** The large size of this parasite typically raises concern, but it often does not cause disease. A similar protozoan parasite of cattle, *Buxtonella sulcata*, is similar in that its discovery often initially raises questions about possible pathogenicity.

28. **b** The carnivore may be a reptile, bird or mammal.

29. **b** *Entamoeba histolytica* is mainly a human pathogen. It occasionally causes disease in housed primates. It also has been reported in dogs and can cause severe disease in experimentally infected kittens. In primate medicine, because the disease produced by *E histolytica* may be so devastating, it is important to distinguish the many species of amoebas that may be found in fecal examinations.

30. **b** Pigs have many nonpathogenic amoebas that may be detected on fecal examination.

31. **c** *Histomonas meleagridis* tends to be less pathogenic in chickens; thus, the parasite is often not detected until turkeys share the same enclosure. It has an unusual life cycle in that the protozoan is often transmitted between birds through infected nematode (*Heterakis*) eggs or *Histomonas*-infected larvae of this nematode that persist within earthworm paratenic hosts in the soil.

32. **a**

33. **c** Hawks sometimes become infected with this parasite from their prey, such as pigeons, and occasionally develop severe diarrhea.

34. **a**

35. **b** *Hemoproteus* differs from *Plasmodium* in that only gametocytes are found in the circulating red blood cells at any time after infection. With *Plasmodium*, several different stages are found in blood smears.

36. **d** *Plasmodium*, probably acquired from local birds, has been responsible for deaths among caged penguins.

37. **b** *Eimeria tenella* causes the classic cecal lesions. Lesions caused by the different species of coccidia parasitizing chickens are

sufficiently distinct to allow recognition of the causative species from the lesions in the intestinal tract. Thus, due to the nature of the industry and the ease with which different species can be identified by lesion appearance, a diagnosis is often made by necropsy of several animals.

38. **c**

39. **a**

40. **c** *Babesia, Theileria* and *Cytauxzoon* (the piroplasms) are all tick transmitted.

41. **a** This is a free-living nematode that occasionally becomes a facultative parasite of the skin.

42. **b** *Strongyloides stercoralis* and *Filaroides* are the 2 most likely possibilities in a closed colony. The larvae of *Filaroides* are sluggish and typically are not recovered by Baermann analysis; also, they would not proliferate in a charcoal culture due to their different life history. *Crenosoma vulpis* also produces larvae, but typically is not transmitted in closed colonies and would not proliferate in charcoal cultures. *Rhabditis strongyloides* is found in skin. *Uncinaria stenocephala* produces eggs that would be found in the feces.

43. **d** People often refuse to accept that their pet is not at fault.

44. **c**

45. **b**

46. **c**

47. **c** Typically disease does not develop in immunologically intact animals. The other species of *Filaroides, F osleri,* causes nodules within the trachea.

48. **a** Paratenic hosts include amphibians and reptiles.

49. **c** Transplacentally acquired *Toxocara canis* larvae can be pathogenic *in utero* or after parturition.

50. **b**

51. **c**

52. **d** The diagnostic dilemma is that there are no detectable microfilariae and antigen tests do not begin to detect infection until several weeks to months after the mosquito bite.

53. **c** The other findings could be present, but they would typically represent more severe or advanced stages of disease.

54. **c**

55. **e** *Baylisascaris procyonis* is a parasite of the raccoon. Other hosts become infected by ingesting the embryonated eggs. Similar lesions have been noted in many other animals and in 2 children.

56. **b** Though the eggs described could be those of *Trichuris, Trichuris* is found in mammals.

57. **b**

58. **b** Geographic distributions are important for certain parasitic diseases. The distribution of cutaneous larva migrans mainly parallels that of *Ancylostoma braziliense;* thus, such lesions would typically not be expected in places where this species of hookworm is not found. This worm is found mainly along the eastern coast of the United States and around the Caribbean. In the dog or cat host, the eggs of the different *Ancylostoma* species are usually indistinguishable.

59. **e**

60. **a**

61. **e**

62. **b**

63. **a** *Dirofilaria immitis* can cause serious disease or death in cats. The disease is usually insidious at the outset, but signs progress rapidly when serious disease does occur.

64. **d** All spirurid nematodes (of which the filarids are a subgroup) undergo development in an arthropod of some type.

65. **c** This rare infection with a free-living nematode is of interest as a curiosity and as a representative case of facultative parasitism, that is, when an organism becomes parasitic only when it has the opportunity.

66. **a**

67. **b**

68. **a**

69. **d** Lesions are related to perianal pruritus caused by the female worms that crawl out to cement their eggs of the perianal region.

70. **d**

71. **a** *Habronema* species live in the same location but do not cause the same type of lesion.

72. **a** Dermal habronemiasis is caused by the larvae of these worms; fortunately, the lesions respond very well to ivermectin therapy.

73. **b**

74. **d**

75. **c**

76. **e**

77. **a**

78. **a** *Ostertagia ostertagi,* like most other trichostrongyles and strongyles, has a direct life cycle.

79. **e** The larvae can develop in the manure pack. Ventilation is good for the cattle.

80. **b**

81. **b**

82. **c**

83. **c**

84. **d**

85. **a** The lesion is pathognomonic.

86. **a** The white reproductive organs of the female can be seen through the red translucent body spiralling about the intestine, giving the worm a "barber pole" appearance.

87. **d** Eggs of the other very large tricho-strongylid, *Marshallagia marshalli,* differ from those of *Nematodirus* in having more parallel sides and being less pointed at the poles; also, this was not offered as a choice.

88. **c** This is the only sure way of identifying the species of parasite involved on the basis of a fecal sample.

89. **a**

90. **d** As with the microfilariae of *Dirofilaria immitis,* microfilariae of *Setaria equina* sometimes pass the placental barrier and enter the developing fetus. These microfilariae may confuse a diagnosis, but they do not cause disease in newborn animals and do not undergo development.

91. **c**

92. **e** It is difficult to imagine how the horse was originally infected, but the scenario is a real one.

93. **d**

94. **a** This is a manifestation of anemia.

95. **d**

96. **e** The adult worms normally can be found in the meninges of the white-tailed deer, where it does not cause disease.

97. **d**

98. **c** It may also be called the periparturient rise.

99. **d**

100. **d**

101. **a** Species of coccidia of chickens, other than *E tenella,* can produce small bowel disease.

102. **a** Most trichostrongyloid nematodes develop on pasture to the infective third-stage larvae from hatched first-stage larvae.

103. **b**

104. **b** The "thumps" is associated with lung migration.

105. **d**

106. **c** Transmammary transmission may lead to signs very early in life.

107. **a**

108. **d**

109. **d**

110. **a**

111. **b** The location in the small intestine and the large size can be used to differentiate *Ascaridia* from *Hemonchus.*

112. **d**

113. **d**

114. **c**

115. **d**

116. **e**

117. **a** This is unusual for a trematode.

118. **d**

119. **c** This is the American schistosome.

120. **a** The lesion in the bile ducts is thought to be due, in part, to secretion of large quantities of proline by the parasite.

121. **a**

122. **c**

123. **b**

124. **b** Sheep and other small ruminants are also affected. In cattle, cysts develop, and the lesions are not as pathogenic.

125. **b** The egg of *Heterobilharzia* has no operculum and contains a developed miracidium when passed in the feces. The eggs of *Spirometra* and *Diphyllobothrium* are very similar and resemble those of *Paragonimus;* however, with experience, they can be distinguished from eggs of *Paragonimus* by

their smaller size, lighter-colored shell, and often less demarcated operculum.

126. **b**

127. **b**

128. **d**

129. **d** *Echinococcus multilocularis* is found only in the northern United States and Canada; hence the concern about moving it to more southern locales.

130. **c**

131. **a**

132. **c**

133. **b** A millipede is an arthropod.

134. **b** Flea larvae that feed on undigested blood passed in the feces of the adult fleas and detritus in the environment are attracted to the egg balls of *Dipylidium caninum* that are passed in the feces of dogs and cats. Tapeworm larvae in the larval, pupal and adult fleas do not become infective until adult fleas have been on the mammalian host for a couple of days.

135. **d** A taeniid tapeworm has a mammalian intermediate host.

136. **d**

137. **a** People are the final host of this parasite; they can also serve as intermediate hosts.

138. **d**

139. **e** One tapeworm of people and rats, *Vampirolepis nana,* has no need of an intermediate host.

140. **d**

141. **d**

142. **c**

143. **b** A capillarid sometimes produces similar lesions in the skin of alligators and crocodiles; these can be problematic under farming conditions.

144. **e**

145. **a** Rapid ligation of the bile duct soon after death limits migration of the worms out of the small intestine. Unless this is done, the worms are usually found in the bile ducts at necropsy.

146. **c**

147. **b**

148. **d**

149. **b** The belief that fleas constantly jump on and off their hosts is a commonly held misconception. Once fleas get on a dog or cat, they tend to stay on the host.

150. **d**

151. **e**

152. **e**

153. **d** The larvae, nymphs and adults of *Ixodes* can all be recognized by the pre-anal groove. This structure is not present in any other ticks. Due to the public awareness of Lyme disease, of which species of *Ixodes* are primary vectors, this characteristic is useful in identifying a tick as a possible vector when it is brought to the clinic for identification.

154. **e**

155. **c**

156. **c**

157. **b**

158. **e** They typically occur at this time of the year because the maggots are leaving the cat to drop onto the soil, where they overwinter.

159. **d** They are often found on rabbits.

160. **d** They are also known as chiggers. Cats sometimes are seriously affected by these mites, which are parasitic on animals only as larvae. Most other vertebrates can also be affected. Lesions are also sometimes reported in horses, turkeys and other animals.

161. **d**

162. **a**

163. **b**

164. **c** The maggots develop in cattle feces.

165. **d** Midges are very weak fliers.

166. **b**

167. **c**

168. **d**

169. **d** Eggs of the other 2 common species hatch spontaneously and crawl into the host's mouth.

170. **b**

171. **b**

172. **c**

173. **e**

174. **e**

175. **e** After a period in deeper tissues, both species of *Hypoderma* migrate to the subcutaneous tissue of the back, where they form a warble. The maggot spends 5-11 weeks completing its development within the warble.

Ophthalmomyiasis interna due to *Hypoderma* has been observed in children. People, like cattle, become infected with larvae that penetrate the skin.

176. **e**

177. **e**

178. **a** All stages prefer to feed on a single host.

179. **b**

180. **b** Repellents may work with repeated application.

181. **c**

182. **a**

183. **d**

184. **e** Larvae gaining access to the nasal sinuses of sheep in late spring or early summer leave the nose in the fall and overwinter in the soil. Any larvae deposited in late summer await spring within the nasal passages.

185. **a**

186. **c**

187. **a** A tick injects a considerable volume of saliva at the feeding site; this saliva contains toxin(s) capable of producing paralysis. One tick is sufficient in the case of small animals and people, whereas several or many may be required in cattle. In Australia, there is a species of ixodid tick capable of causing severe paralysis that requires treatment with a specific antitoxin and supportive therapy.

188. **b** This is how these mites are differentiated.

189. **a** This is the only louse typically found on pigs.

190. **a** This is a pathogen in pigs.

191. **a**

192. **d**

193. **c** These typically become a problem when young birds or rodents have left the nest and the mites are looking for a blood meal.

194. **c** Birds tend to be hosts only to mallophagan lice.

195. **a**

196. **a**

197. **a**

198. **c** The mites tend to infest the birds only to feed, typically at night.

199. **b** This is the stick-tight flea of poultry.

200. **b** These worms are often reported as located in the abdominal cavity, but they are actually found in the air sac-like portion of the snake's lungs.

Notes

Section 8

Pathology

R.D. Hunt

Recommended Reading

Cheville NF: *Cell Pathology.* 2nd ed. Iowa State University Press, Ames, 1983.

Cotran RS *et al: Pathologic Basis of Disease.* 4th ed. Saunders, Philadelphia, 1989.

Jones TC and Hunt RD: *Veterinary Pathology.* 5th ed. Lea & Febiger, Philadelphia, 1983.

Jubb KVF *et al: Pathology of Domestic Animals.* 3rd ed. Academic Press, New York, 1985.

Slauson DO and Cooper BJ: *Mechanisms of Disease – A Textbook of Comparative General Pathology.* Williams & Wilkins, Baltimore, 1982.

Thomson RG: *Special Veterinary Pathology.* Decker, Philadelphia, 1988.

> *Practice answer sheets are on pages 267-268.*

Questions

1. *Tissue specimens mailed to a laboratory for histopathologic examination should be submitted:*

   a. intact in formalin or other fixative
   b. frozen
   c. as thin slices in formalin or other fixative
   d. fresh
   e. in physiologic saline

2. *In which of the following diseases is the tissue reaction granulomatous?*

   a. coccidiosis
   b. strangles
   c. listeriosis
   d. sporotrichosis
   e. leptospirosis

3. *The histopathologic characteristics of toxoplasmosis in dogs are almost identical to those of infection with:*

   a. *Neospora caninum*
   b. *Babesia canis*
   c. *Cryptosporidium*
   d. *Encephalitozoon cuniculi*
   e. *Pneumocystis carinii*

Correct answers are on pages 210-213.

4. *If a necropsy must be delayed for 24 or more hours, it is best to:*

   a. freeze the body
   b. maintain the body at near-normal body temperature
   c. refrigerate the body
   d. not do a necropsy
   e. maintain the body at above-normal body temperature

5. *Feline viral rhinotracheitis is caused by:*

   a. an adenovirus
   b. a herpesvirus
   c. a rhinovirus
   d. a picornavirus
   e. a togavirus

6. *Both intranuclear and intracytoplasmic inclusion bodies are found in:*

   a. African horsesickness
   b. hog cholera
   c. canine distemper
   d. infectious canine hepatitis
   e. cowpox

7. *Which disease is **not** characterized by vesicles?*

   a. pemphigus vulgaris
   b. infectious myxomatosis of rabbits
   c. cowpox
   d. sarcoid in horses
   e. foot and mouth disease

8. *Gout is characterized by tissue deposits of:*

   a. silicon
   b. urates
   c. calcium carbonate
   d. lipofuscin
   e. biliverdin

9. *Carcinomas can originate in the:*

   a. brain
   b. heart
   c. stomach
   d. bone marrow
   e. spinal cord

10. *The single most differentiating feature of malignant neoplasms is their:*

    a. ability to metastasize
    b. large size
    c. anaplastic microscopic appearance
    d. origin from epithelial tissues
    e. tendency to regress

11. *Lipofuscin is also known as:*

    a. hemosiderin
    b. biliverdin
    c. "wear and tear" pigment
    d. apoferritin
    e. bilirubin

12. *Increased vascular permeability due to bradykinin occurs mainly in:*

    a. arteries and veins
    b. capillaries
    c. lymphatics
    d. venules
    e. arterioles

13. *Histamine is produced by:*

    a. mast cells
    b. fibroblasts
    c. T cells
    d. neutrophils
    e. macrophages

14. *Which cellular change is **not** reversible?*

    a. fatty change
    b. glycogenolysis
    c. atrophy
    d. karyorrhexis
    e. potassium loss

15. *Fat necrosis is characterized by formation of:*

   a. calcium soaps
   b. oxalate crystals
   c. amyloid
   d. hyalin
   e. lipofuscin

16. *Atrophy is characterized by:*

   a. increased size of an organ or cells
   b. karyomegaly
   c. decreased size of an organ or cells
   d. karyolysis
   e. postmortem autolysis

17. *Chronic inflammation is:*

   a. characterized by a short course
   b. characterized by a long course
   c. usually restricted to the central nervous system
   d. very rare in animals
   e. characterized by pus

18. *Which cell type most characterizes granulomatous inflammation?*

   a. fibroblasts
   b. neutrophils
   c. mast cells
   d. endothelial cells
   e. epithelioid cells

19. *Macrophages, Langhans' giant cells and epithelioid cells are derived from:*

   a. myeloblasts
   b. monocytes
   c. mast cells
   d. megakaryocytes
   e. melanoblasts

20. *A fatal pulmonary embolus can result from:*

   a. fracture of a long bone
   b. a benign neoplasm
   c. thrombocytopenia
   d. dicumarol poisoning
   e. pneumonia

21. *Caseous necrosis is a feature of:*

   a. toxoplasmosis
   b. tuberculosis
   c. candidiasis
   d. warfarin poisoning
   e. Johne's disease

22. *Red (hemorrhagic) infarcts characteristically occur in the:*

   a. heart
   b. kidney
   c. lung
   d. skin
   e. skeletal muscle

23. *Metaplasia is characterized by replacement of:*

   a. differentiated tissue with another type of undifferentiated tissue
   b. undifferentiated tissue with another type of differentiated tissue
   c. differentiated tissue with another type of differentiated tissue
   d. undifferentiated tissue with another type of undifferentiated tissue
   e. aplastic tissue with neoplastic tissue

24. *Hypertrophy of an organ can result from cellular:*

   a. hyperplasia
   b. dysplasia
   c. metaplasia
   d. aplasia
   e. hypoplasia

25. *Benign neoplasms:*

   a. tend to metastasize
   b. are often encapsulated
   c. are most often caused by viruses
   d. are characterized by marked cellular pleomorphism
   e. of no clinical concern

Correct answers are on pages 210-213.

26. *Carcinomas tend to metastasize via:*

    a. capillaries
    b. veins
    c. arteries
    d. lymphatics
    e. airways

27. *Which type of virus has **not** been associated with neoplastic disease?*

    a. herpesviruses
    b. myxoviruses
    c. oncornaviruses
    d. papovaviruses
    e. adenoviruses

28. *Infarcts are:*

    a. restricted to the heart
    b. caused by interference with blood supply
    c. any well-demarcated area of necrosis
    d. reversible
    e. restricted to the kidney

29. *Necrosis is:*

    a. reversible
    b. a postmortem tissue change
    c. irreversible
    d. synonymous with autolysis
    e. limited to viral infections

30. *In a tissue section of liver from a dog, you observe centrilobular and paracentral necrosis. What is the most likely cause of these findings?*

    a. viral hepatitis
    b. heart failure
    c. distemper
    d. pancreatitis
    e. leptospirosis

31. *Interferons are a class of proteins generally known for their:*

    a. therapeutic effect for fever
    b. antiviral potential

    c. role in iron transport
    d. role in hemostasis
    e. antibacterial potential

32. *Tumor necrosis factor is:*

    a. a factor released from tumor cells undergoing necrosis
    b. a pro-inflammatory factor released from stimulated macrophages
    c. a generic drug used to treat neoplasms
    d. a factor responsible for muscle atrophy in aging
    e. important in initiating metatasis

33. *A chemotactic factor for neutrophils is:*

    a. interleukin 8
    b. interleukin 1
    c. prothrombin
    d. Hageman factor
    e. lysozyme

34. *Endotoxin is:*

    a. a polysaccharide component of the wall of Gram-negative bacteria
    b. a polysaccharide component of the wall of Gram-positive bacteria
    c. a polysaccharide released from endothelial cells
    d. responsible for endometrial necrosis
    e. used to treat ectoparasites

35. *Diapedesis refers to:*

    a. bilateral laminitis
    b. escape of erythrocytes from congested blood vessels
    c. twinning
    d. emigration of leukocytes in inflammation
    e. bilateral footrot

36. *Which feature would allow you to differentiate an area of liquefaction necrosis in a kidney from postmortem autolysis?*

    a. presence of bacteria

b. size of the lesion

c. presence of acute inflammation in surrounding tissue

d. absence of acute inflammation in surrounding tissue

e. presence of karyorrhexis

37. *Under conditions of hypoxia, cells:*

a. shrink, lose water, lose potassium and gain sodium

b. shrink, lose water, lose sodium and gain potassium

c. swell, gain water, lose sodium and gain potassium

d. swell, gain water, lose potassium and gain sodium

e. usually remain normal in size and composition

38. *Fatty change in the liver (fatty liver) is characterized by accumulation of:*

a. cholesterol esters

b. neutral fat

c. lipoproteins

d. glycolipids

e. calcium soaps

39. *Multiple focal accumulations of macrophages and multinucleated giant cells in the lung are most probably a form of:*

a. granulation tissue

b. granulomatous inflammation

c. pulmonary dysplasia

d. pulmonary metaplasia

e. lymphoma

40. *Which cell type is important in intracellular destruction of bacteria?*

a. lymphocytes

b. macrophages

c. plasma cells

d. Langhans' cells

e. melanocytes

41. *Tissue necrosis heals by way of:*

a. emigration of neutrophils

b. regeneration and/or scarring

c. liquefaction

d. bacterial enzymes

e. interferons

42. *In a tissue section of the stomach from a dog that died, you find extensive calcification of the middle one-third of the mucosa. The most likely cause of this finding is:*

a. hypovitaminosis D

b. acute necrotizing pancreatitis

c. chronic renal failure with uremia

d. starvation

e. *Toxocara canis* larval migration

43. *In an aborted bovine fetus, you observe disseminated foci of encephalitis, with small (2-3 µ) basophilic bodies in the cytoplasm of endothelial cells adjacent to the lesions. The most likely cause of these findings is:*

a. brucellosis

b. leptospirosis

c. sarcosporidiosis

d. trichomoniasis

e. lead poisoning

44. *Nigropallidal encephalomalacia is:*

a. a toxicosis caused by consumption of yellow star thistle or Russian knapweed

b. the result of acute central nervous system anoxia

c. caused by equine herpesvirus type 1

d. most common in the eastern United States

e. a form of rabies, with Negri bodies restricted to the globus pallidus

45. *Viral inclusion bodies are:*

a. cytoplasmic or nuclear in location

b. restricted to the nucleus

c. restricted to the cytoplasm

d. seen in all viral diseases

e. composed of lead acetate

Correct answers are on pages 210-213.

46. *In animals with scurvy, copper poisoning or chronic protein malnutrition, bone sections may exhibit:*

    a. osteopetrosis
    b. osteoporosis
    c. osteosarcoma
    d. osteomalacia
    e. osteitis

47. *Extensive hemorrhage is **not** a feature of:*

    a. bracken fern poisoning
    b. halogeton poisoning
    c. septicemia
    d. leptospirosis
    e. infectious canine hepatitis

48. *In dogs, eosinophils are often a prominent feature in:*

    a. transmissible venereal tumors
    b. lymphomas
    c. mast-cell tumors
    d. histiocytomas
    e. papillomas

49. *Male cats with a haircoat comprised of both yellow and black hair have a karyotype with:*

    a. twice the normal diploid number of chromosomes
    b. 2 X chromosomes
    c. 2 Y chromosomes
    d. no chromosome number 17
    e. no chromosome number 12

50. *Anthracosis is:*

    a. characterized by accumulation of silicon dioxide in the lung
    b. synonymous with any form of pneumoconiosis
    c. characterized by accumulation of carbon in the lung
    d. characterized by accumulation of iron pigments in the lung
    e. synonymous with anthrax

51. *Abnormally high serum levels of indirect bilirubin indicate:*

    a. toxic jaundice
    b. hemolytic anemia
    c. obstructive jaundice
    d. primary photosensitization
    e. myelophthisic anemia

52. *A carcinoma that has invaded the basement membrane but not metastasized is referred to as a:*

    a. benign carcinoma
    b. carcinoma *in situ*
    c. squamous-cell carcinoma
    d. carcinoid
    e. basal-cell carcinoma

53. *In a large herd of cattle in the midwestern United States, severe death losses occur over a period of several weeks. Clinical signs include increased lacrimation, depression, anorexia, emaciation and diarrhea. The most striking pathologic findings are extensive epithelial hypertrophy, hyperplasia and metaplasia of multiple organ systems. The most likely cause of these signs is:*

    a. poisoning by fluorides
    b. poisoning by nitrogen trichloride
    c. poisoning by polychlorinated naphthalenes or polychlorinated biphenyls or chlorinated dibenzodioxins
    d. infection with *Absidia corymbifera* or *Sporotrichum schenckii*
    e. hypervitaminosis A

54. *Hypertrophy is characterized by:*

    a. increased size and number of cells
    b. increased number of cells
    c. decreased size of cells
    d. increased size of cells
    e. decreased number of cells

55. *Fat necrosis is often a feature of:*

    a. acute hepatitis
    b. a high-calorie diet

c. acute pancreatitis

d. acute splenitis

e. shipping fever

56. Amyloidosis is most likely to be found in animals with:

a. infectious canine hepatitis

b. canine leptospirosis

c. *Pasteurella multocida* pneumonia

d. tuberculosis

e. vitamin E deficiency

57. Globoid-cell leukodystrophy (Krabbe's disease) results from a deficiency of:

a. hexosaminidase enzymes

b. beta-galactocerebrosidase

c. alpha-glucosidase

d. alpha-mannosidase

e. arylsulfatase B

58. Deficiency of the enzyme uricase is associated with:

a. gout

b. Chediak-Higashi disease

c. Sudanophilic leukodystrophy

d. dystrophic calcification

e. leukopenia

59. Increased circulating levels of phylloerythrin are associated with:

a. congenital porphyria

b. photosensitization

c. buckwheat poisoning

d. anemia

e. pemphigus vulgaris

60. Elevated serum alkaline phosphatase activity is a feature of:

a. any form of jaundice

b. cholestasis

c. hemolytic anemia

d. hepatitis

e. acute renal failure

61. The chronic neurodegenerative diseases in sheep and cattle known as spongiform encephalopathies are caused by:

a. myxoviruses

b. viroids

c. prions

d. disseminated intravascular coagulation

e. picornaviruses

62. Helminth infections may be characterized by any of the following except:

a. lack of an inflammatory response

b. eosinophilia

c. anemia

d. intestinal obstruction

e. myasthenia gravis

63. Trichinella spiralis is the only metazoan parasite that:

a. has an intracellular form

b. can cause myositis

c. has intestinal and tissue stages

d. can affect multiple species

e. can occur in adult and larval forms in the same host

64. The anemia of copper deficiency results from:

a. hemolysis

b. reduced conversion of cyanocobalamin to its active form

c. interference with the availability of iron for synthesis of hemoglobin

d. shortened erythrocyte life span

e. deficiency of tyrosinase

65. The injurious effects of radiation are greatest on:

a. cells of fully differentiated tissues

b. cells with a high rate of replication

c. neurons

d. cells of highly vascularized tissues

e. fibroblasts

Correct answers are on pages 210-213.

66. *The most distinguishing radiographic feature of rickets results from:*

   a. failure of degeneration of the cartilaginous growth plate
   b. premature degeneration of the cartilaginous growth plate
   c. necrosis of osteoblasts
   d. cartilaginous metaplasia of osteoid
   e. decreased thickness of osteoid seams

67. *The single pathologic feature characteristic of most types of viral encephalitis is:*

   a. inclusion bodies
   b. neuronal necrosis
   c. demyelination
   d. hydrocephalus
   e. vasculitis

68. *An acute inflammatory response is dependent upon:*

   a. neutrophils
   b. macrophages
   c. blood vessels
   d. eosinophils
   e. bacteria

69. *Necrosis of small arteries and arterioles without significant inflammation is the outstanding feature of:*

   a. edema disease
   b. salmonellosis
   c. equine viral arteritis
   d. thallium poisoning
   e. listeriosis

70. *Degeneration of skeletal muscle is a feature of all of the following* **except***:*

   a. coyotillo poisoning
   b. coffee senna poisoning
   c. gossypol poisoning
   d. selenium deficiency
   e. milkweed poisoning

71. *Exostoses and ankylosing osteodystrophy of cervical vertebrae in a cat are features of:*

   a. vitamin D toxicity
   b. vitamin A deficiency
   c. vitamin A toxicity
   d. vitamin D deficiency
   e. vitamin E toxicity

72. *The lesions of strangles in horses are best described as:*

   a. granulomatous lymphadenitis
   b. purulent lymphadenitis
   c. necrotizing lymphadenitis
   d. purulent pharyngitis
   e. proliferative tonsillitis

73. *The findings of chronic proliferative synovitis, degenerative arthritis and vegetative valvular endocarditis in a pig are most likely to be caused by:*

   a. salmonellosis
   b. brucellosis
   c. erysipelas
   d. hog cholera
   e. leptospirosis

74. *Myelophthisic anemia results from:*

   a. space-occupying lesions in the bone marrow
   b. iron deficiency
   c. bone marrow aplasia
   d. copper deficiency
   e. osteoporosis

75. *After a dog fractures its tibia, you immobilize the affected limb in a plaster cast for 4 weeks. The fracture heals without complication. However, prolonged immobilization of the limb would also result in:*

   a. adaptive hypertrophy of the leg muscles
   b. adaptive atrophy of the leg muscles
   c. adaptive aplasia of the leg muscles
   d. adaptive necrosis of the leg muscles
   e. adaptive neoplasia of the leg muscles

76. *In acute inflammation, various chemical mediators initiate and sustain the acute inflammatory response. All of the following are important mediators of acute inflammation* **except**:

a. histamine
b. serotonin
c. bradykinin
d. complement
e. collagenase

77. *Loss of hair pigment is seen in copper-deficient animals because:*

a. melanin contains copper
b. tyrosinase contains copper
c. phenylalanine contains copper
d. copper is required for erythrogenesis
e. tyrosine contains copper

78. *A severely ill cat in New Mexico has a history of depression, fever, anorexia, mild leukocytosis and enlarged mandibular and cervical lymph nodes. You euthanize the cat. At necropsy and subsequent histopathologic examination, you identify abscesses in the affected lymph nodes. The most likely cause of these findings is:*

a. feline viral rhinotracheitis
b. togavirus infection
c. bubonic plague
d. feline leukemia virus infection
e. actinobacillosis

79. *You find dorsal root ganglioneuritis, characterized by lymphocytic infiltration, neuronal necrosis and intranuclear inclusion bodies, in spinal cord sections from a cow that died following an acute paralytic illness. The most likely cause of these findings is:*

a. pseudorabies
b. rinderpest
c. malignant catarrhal fever
d. parainfluenza-3 infection
e. rabies

80. *Neutrophils can engulf and kill bacteria through the action of:*

a. myeloperoxidase in their granules
b. RNA-ase in their granules
c. acidic phosphatase in their granules
d. alkaline phosphatase in their granules
e. DNA-ase in their granules

81. *Neutrophils and macrophages ordinarily do not phagocytize invading bacteria until:*

a. the bacteria have died
b. the cells are activated
c. the bacteria have been opsonized
d. fever has developed
e. the cells degranulate

82. *All of the following are important in the pathway leading to neutrophil chemotaxis* **except**:

a. the presence of a specific receptor on the chemotactic agent
b. activation of phospholipase C
c. activation of protein kinase C
d. formation of inositol triphosphate
e. increased intracellular concentrations of calcium

83. *All of the following are platelet agonists* **except**:

a. adenosine diphosphate
b. thrombin
c. collagen
d. prostacyclin
e. thromboxane A$_2$

84. *Any of the following may be associated with hepatic necrosis in mice* **except**:

a. ectromelia virus
b. mouse hepatitis virus
c. murine cytomegalovirus
d. *Corynebacterium kutscheri*
e. murine rotavirus

Correct answers are on pages 210-213.

85. *Venereal spirochetosis of rabbits is mainly a disease of the:*

  a. uterus and oviducts
  b. liver and spleen
  c. skin and mucous membranes
  d. brain
  e. kidney and bladder

86. *Duck plague, Marek's disease and Pacheco's disease are all caused by:*

  a. adenoviruses
  b. herpesviruses
  c. togaviruses
  d. oncornaviruses
  e. morbilliviruses

87. *Which of the following is most likely to cause demyelinating peripheral neuropathy in chickens?*

  a. riboflavin deficiency
  b. vitamin A deficiency
  c. vitamin C deficiency
  d. niacin deficiency
  e. pullorum disease

88. *The most specific lesions of avian encephalomyelitis (epidemic tremor) are found in the:*

  a. cerebrum
  b. spinal cord
  c. midbrain
  d. peripheral nerves
  e. dorsal root ganglia

89. *Viruses, often called immunodeficiency viruses, similar to the cause of AIDS in people have been found in all of the following species except:*

  a. horses
  b. cattle
  c. monkeys
  d. cats
  e. dogs

90. *The most common neoplasm of laboratory rabbits is:*

  a. adenocarcinoma of the mammary gland
  b. lymphoma
  c. adenocarcinoma of the uterus
  d. adenocarcinoma of the stomach
  e. leiomyosarcoma

91. *Hypovitaminosis E may lead to any of the following except:*

  a. encephalomalacia in chicks
  b. necrosis of skeletal muscle in mink
  c. steatitis in cats
  d. hepatic necrosis in pigs
  e. renal tubular necrosis in dogs

92. *Parvovirus-induced myocarditis is most likely to be seen in:*

  a. young dogs
  b. old dogs
  c. Greyhounds
  d. dogs with secondary bacterial infections
  e. pregnant bitches

93. *Fibrosarcomas in dogs have been associated with adult:*

  a. *Toxocara canis*
  b. *Spirocerca lupi*
  c. *Diphyllobothrium latum*
  d. *Ancylostoma caninum*
  e. *Linguatula serrata*

94. *The earliest histopathologic change in endocardial fibroelastosis in Burmese cats is:*

  a. myocardial-cell necrosis
  b. endocardial edema
  c. endocardial calcification
  d. coronary artery occlusion
  e. myocardial-cell calcification

95. *Chediak-Higashi syndrome in Persian cats is characterized by recurrent bacterial infections and:*

  a. dysfunction of neutrophils

b. neutropenia

c. dysfunction of monocytes

d. hypogammaglobulinemia

e. eosinophilia

96. *The breeds predisposed to ventricular septal defects are the:*

a. Boxer and Cocker Spaniel

b. Chihuahua and Pekingese

c. Great Dane and Bull Mastiff

d. English Bulldog and Keeshond

e. Irish Setter and English Foxhound

97. *The most common oral neoplasm of cats is the:*

a. fibrosarcoma

b. malignant melanoma

c. squamous-cell carcinoma

d. chondrosarcoma

e. histiocytoma

98. *In addition to dogs, canine distemper virus is also an important cause of disease in:*

a. raccoons and seals

b. cats and rabbits

c. ferrets and porpoise

d. skunks and coyotes

e. mink and gerbils

99. *The lesions of canine distemper closely resemble those of:*

a. bluetongue

b. feline panleukopenia

c. Aleutian disease

d. bovine virus diarrhea

e. rinderpest

100. *Which lesion is most characteristic of bacillary hemoglobinuria in cattle?*

a. hepatic necrosis

b. pulmonary embolism

c. myocardial necrosis

d. vesicular dermatitis

e. cirrhosis

101. *Atherosclerosis (deposition of cholesterol) is not nearly as common in dogs as in people, but it may by encountered in dogs with:*

a. hypothyroidism

b. hyperthyroidism

c. hyperadrenocorticism

d. hypoadrenocorticism

e. renal failure

102. *Multifocal hepatic necrosis in a horse is most likely to be associated with:*

a. azoturia

b. tetanus

c. Tyzzer's disease

d. locoweed poisoning

e. viral arteritis

103. *In swine, the mycotoxin zearalenone causes:*

a. multifocal hepatic necrosis and cirrhosis

b. encephalomalacia

c. hyperplasia of the uterus, vagina and mammary glands

d. cardiac necrosis

e. agalactia

104. *Multiple keratotic skin lesions that fluoresce on exposure to ultraviolet light are most likely caused by:*

a. ringworm due to *Trichophyton mentagrophytes*

b. pemphigus vulgaris

c. protot[h]ecosis

d. ringworm due to *Microsporum canis*

e. geotrichosis

105. *Ethylene glycol poisoning in cats and* Halogeton gloveratus *poisoning in sheep are both characterized by:*

a. urate nephrosis

b. oxalate nephrosis

c. centrilobular hepatic necrosis

d. peripheral lobular hepatic necrosis

e. disseminated intravascular coagulation

Correct answers are on pages 210-213.

106. Which cutaneous neoplasm of dogs can be transmitted by inoculation with tumor-cell-free filtrates?

   a. histiocytoma
   b. transmissible venereal tumor
   c. mast-cell tumor
   d. hemangiopericytoma
   e. fibrosarcoma

107. Necropsy of a young Landrace piglet that died at 1 week of age reveals elevated, rough, hairless plaques on the distal extremities, and diffuse interstitial pneumonia characterized by numerous multinucleated giant cells. The most likely cause of these findings is:

   a. atypical mycobacterial infection
   b. generalized viral infection
   c. foreign-body reaction
   d. allergic reaction
   e. autosomal recessive trait

108. In hereditary parakeratosis of Shorthorn beef calves, which organ is consistently hypoplastic?

   a. kidneys
   b. cerebellum
   c. eyes
   d. thymus
   e. adrenal glands

109. Increased size of erythrocytes (increased mean corpuscular volume) is seen in:

   a. hemorrhagic anemia
   b. iron-deficiency anemia
   c. myelophthisic anemia
   d. polycythemia vera
   e. copper deficiency

110. A rise in serum alkaline phosphatase activity could indicate disease of the:

   a. skeleton or liver
   b. skeleton or kidneys
   c. liver or kidneys
   d. heart or liver
   e. skeleton or lungs

111. Which neoplasm occurs in both male and female animals?

   a. arrhenoblastoma
   b. dysgerminoma
   c. teratoma
   d. granulosa-cell tumor
   e. luteal-cell tumor

112. Clear vacuoles in the cytoplasm of neurons are an important diagnostic feature of:

   a. viral encephalomyelitis in horses
   b. sporadic encephalomyelitis in cattle
   c. listeriosis
   d. Borna disease
   e. scrapie

113. Spongiform encephalopathy, a relatively newly recognized disease of cattle in England and Europe, is caused by:

   a. an agent comparable to the one that causes scrapie
   b. a poisonous plant
   c. air pollution
   d. a virus of the same family as rabies virus
   e. a species of *Hemophilus*

114. Oral papillomatosis is most common in:

   a. horses and cattle
   b. horses and dogs
   c. dogs and cats
   d. dogs and rabbits
   e. rabbits and cats

115. In contrast to mast-cell tumors in dogs, mast-cell tumors in cats:

   a. are often generalized
   b. do not stain with metachromatic dyes
   c. are caused by a virus
   d. histologically resemble squamous-cell carcinoma
   e. typically involve the spinal cord

116. *Concerning white muscle disease, which statement is **least** accurate?*

   a. It may affect both cardiac and skeletal muscle.
   b. It is caused by vitamin E/selenium deficiency.
   c. It is characterized by hyaline necrosis and calcification of muscle fibers.
   d. It affects calves, lambs and piglets.
   e. It results from arteriolarsclerosis and infarction.

117. *Edema may result from any of the following **except**:*

   a. hyperproteinemia
   b. lymphatic obstruction
   c. increased capillary and venous blood pressure
   d. renal insufficiency
   e. allergic reaction

118. *In response to histamine, fluid leaks from the vascular tree are:*

   a. exclusively from arterioles
   b. exclusively from venules
   c. exclusively from capillaries
   d. from both arterioles and venules
   e. from both arterioles and capillaries

119. *In acute inflammation, adhesion of white blood cells to endothelial cells before their emigration depends upon:*

   a. complement
   b. nonspecific receptor sites on the surface of interstitial cells
   c. specific adhesion molecules on the surface of thrombocytes and interstitial cells
   d. specific adhesion molecules on the surface of endothelial cells and leukocytes
   e. chemotactic agents in the interstitium

120. *All of the following factors are present in granules of neutrophils and are important in the inflammatory process or destruction of bacterial pathogens **except**:*

   a. myeloperoxidase
   b. complement
   c. lysozyme
   d. cationic proteins
   e. proteases

121. *Characteristics of chronic inflammation include all of the following **except**:*

   a. infiltration of macrophages
   b. fibrosis
   c. long duration
   d. marked hyperemia
   e. infiltration of lymphocytes

122. *Multinucleated giant cells are a common component of the cellular inflammatory response in all of the following diseases **except**:*

   a. tuberculosis in cattle
   b. interstitial pneumonia associated with distemper in dogs
   c. coccidioidomycosis in cattle
   d. aspergillosis in dogs
   e. strangles in horses

123. *Dystrophic calcification:*

   a. is seen in areas of tissue necrosis
   b. results from hypercalcemia
   c. is a frequent feature of lead poisoning
   d. results from hypocalcemia
   e. is the chronic form of metastatic calcification

124. *Cells subjected to hypoxic injury may recover if oxygenation is restored. However, if oxygenation is not restored, the cells die. Such damage is termed irreversible injury. Which pathologic feature of damaged cells is most indicative of irreversible injury?*

   a. cell swelling
   b. detachment of ribosomes from endoplasmic reticulum
   c. severe vacuolization of mitochondria
   d. decreased generation of adenosine triphosphate
   e. increased concentration of intracellular sodium

Correct answers are on pages 210-213.

125. *Granulation tissue is:*

    a. pathognomonic of tuberculosis
    b. synonymous with granuloma
    c. important to healing and repair
    d. limited to skin wounds
    e. avascular

126. *Reddening of the skin or other tissue may indicate any of the following **except**:*

    a. hyperemia
    b. congestion
    c. acute inflammation
    d. hemorrhage
    e. arterial thrombosis

127. *The most important event in the pathogenesis of thrombosis is:*

    a. blood stasis
    b. endothelial injury
    c. hypercoagulability
    d. hypercalcemia
    e. hyperviscosity

128. *Red thrombi are most commonly encountered in:*

    a. arteries
    b. veins
    c. lymphatics
    d. neoplastic masses
    e. hypoxic tissues

129. *An embolus may have any of the following features **except**:*

    a. composed of air
    b. composed of fibrin
    c. composed of neoplastic cells
    d. can lead to infarction
    e. attached to the endothelium

130. *Which of the following is **not** a usual feature of a red infarct?*

    a. occurs in loose tissues
    b. occurs in tissues with redundant circulation
    c. usually associated with venous occlusion
    d. usually associated with arterial occlusion
    e. occurs in tissues already congested

131. *Concerning female pseudohermaphrodites, which statement is **least** accurate?*

    a. They have an XX karyotype.
    b. Female pseudohermaphroditism results from the dam's exposure to androgenic steroids early in gestation.
    c. They have normal internal genitalia.
    d. They have external genitalia resembling that of a male.
    e. They have both ovarian and testicular tissue.

132. *Cryptosporidiosis is most commonly associated with:*

    a. cholangiohepatitis
    b. enteritis
    c. pneumonia
    d. pancreatitis
    e. stomatitis

133. *Which neoplasm is **not** of mesenchymal origin?*

    a. meningioma
    b. leiomyosarcoma
    c. osteoma
    d. melanoma
    e. myxoma

134. *All of the following are pathologic features of malignant neoplasms **except**:*

    a. anaplasia
    b. slow growth rate
    c. metastasis
    d. large number of mitoses
    e. cellular pleomorphism

135. *Monoclonal proliferation of cells is typical of:*

    a. a granuloma
    b. a neoplasm

c. a foreign-body reaction

d. a lysosomal storage disease

e. endometrial hyperplasia

c. Glasser's disease

d. streptococcal septicemia

e. leptospirosis

136. *In general, most neoplasms are:*

a. restricted to older animals

b. of monoclonal origin

c. caused by viruses

d. restricted to young animals

e. of polyclonal origin

137. *Serum aspartate aminotransferase, lactic dehydrogenase and creatine kinase activities are most likely to be increased with:*

a. hepatic necrosis

b. renal necrosis

c. myocardial necrosis

d. pulmonary infarction

e. lymphoma

138. *Features of tetralogy of Fallot include all of the following **except**:*

a. ventricular septal defects

b. aorta overriding the venticular defect

c. patent ductus arteriosus

d. obstruction of right ventricular outflow

e. right ventricular hypertrophy

139. *Persistent right aortic arch in a dog is most likely to cause:*

a. dysphagia

b. uremia

c. hypertension

d. cyanosis

e. icterus

140. *A number of pigs die after transport to another farm. At necropsy you find serofibrinous pericarditis, pleuritis, peritonitis and synovitis. The most likely cause of these findings is:*

a. erysipelas

b. hog cholera

141. *Focal myocardial necrosis or myocarditis may be a feature of any of the following **except**:*

a. Chagas' disease

b. foot and mouth disease

c. gossypol poisoning

d. thiamin deficiency

e. vitamin A deficiency

142. *The anemia associated with dietary iron deficiency is characterized as:*

a. macrocytic hyperchromic

b. macrocytic hypochromic

c. normocytic normochromic

d. microcytic hypochromic

e. microcytic hyperchromic

143. *Megaloblastic anemia is characteristic of a deficiency of dietary:*

a. vitamin B_{12} or folic acid

b. vitamin B_{12} or niacin

c. vitamin B_{12} or vitamin B_6

d. vitamin D

e. vitamin E

144. *Multiple myeloma is characterized by neoplastic proliferation of:*

a. myeloid cells

b. erythroid cells

c. plasma cells

d. monocytes

e. thymocytes

145. *Urticaria is characterized by multifocal:*

a. epidermal ulceration and serous effusion

b. dermal hyperemia and edema

c. epidermal vesiculation

d. dermal vesiculation

e. epidermal erosions without serous effusion

Correct answers are on pages 210-213.

146. *Glomerulonephritis associated with persistent and chronic viral diseases results from:*

a. viral invasion of mesangial cells
b. viral invasion of glomerular epithelial cells
c. viral invasion of glomerular endothelial cells
d. deposition of virus-antibody complexes
e. IgE-mediated immediate hypersensitivity

147. *Feminization in a male dog may result from:*

a. Leydig-cell tumor
b. Sertoli-cell tumor
c. seminoma
d. teratoma
e. testicular lymphoma

148. *The ovarian counterpart of a seminoma is the:*

a. choriocarcinoma
b. teratoma
c. granulosa-cell tumor
d. dysgerminoma
e. theca-cell tumor

149. *Hyperparathyroidism may be associated with any of the following* **except**:

a. chronic renal insufficiency
b. vitamin D deficiency
c. prolonged consumption of a high-calcium diet
d. intestinal malabsorption
e. prolonged consumption of a high-phosphorus diet

150. *C-cell or parafollicular-cell tumors are most frequently encountered in:*

a. aged heifers
b. dogs
c. bulls
d. cats
e. mules

151. *The principal pathologic finding in pemphigus vulgaris is:*

a. dermal infiltration with B-lymphocytes
b. dermal infiltration with T-lymphocytes
c. dermal infiltration with eosinophils
d. intradermal vesicles
e. intraepidermal vesicles

152. *Hypertrophic osteoarthropathy is typically associated with:*

a. mycoplasmal infections
b. vitamin D deficiency
c. parathyroid carcinoma
d. pulmonary neoplasms
e. coccidioidomycosis

153. *Concerning macrophages, which statement is* **least** *accurate?*

a. They differentiate into epithelioid cells.
b. They are derived from circulating monocytes.
c. They can phagocytize bacteria.
d. They release factors that stimulate blood vessel growth.
e. They can synthesize collagen.

154. *In which tissue is repair limited by lack of effective replication of parenchymal cells?*

a. epidermis
b. myocardium
c. liver
d. bone marrow
e. pancreas

155. *Which feature can be used to help differentiate a postmortem clot from an antemortem venous thrombus?*

a. A postmortem clot has lines of Zahn.
b. A postmortem clot is infiltrated with leukocytes.
c. A postmortem clot is infiltrated with fibroblasts.
d. A postmortem clot is usually recanalized.
e. A postmortem clot is not attached to the vessel wall.

156. After a prolonged gestation of 11 months, a Holstein cow delivers a large calf that dies immediately after birth. Aside from being large, the dead calf appears grossly normal. What lesion is most likely to be observed at necropsy of the calf?

a. hypoplasia of the thyroid gland
b. hypoplasia of the adrenal glands
c. hypoplasia of the thymus
d. hydrocephalus
e. intranuclear inclusion bodies in hepatocytes

157. A Jersey cow aborts a fetus late in gestation. The principal pathologic finding in the fetus is bronchopneumonia. Which organism is the most likely cause of the abortion?

a. *Brucella abortus*
b. *Campylobacter fetus*
c. *Listeria monocytogenes*
d. *Trichomonas fetus*
e. *Salmonella dublin*

158. Fatty liver is a prominent finding in all of the following disorders **except**:

a. ketosis in cattle
b. diabetes mellitus
c. *Senecio* poisoning
d. phosphorus poisoning
e. carbon tetrachloride poisoning

159. Nephroblastoma is the most common primary renal tumor of:

a. dogs and cats
b. dogs and chickens
c. pigs and chickens
d. pigs and cattle
e. horses and mules

160. Prostatic adenocarcinoma in dogs:

a. only occurs in monorchids
b. only occurs in cryptorchids
c. occurs in both intact and castrated males
d. only occurs in young dogs

e. is caused by a virus

161. Interstitial emphysema is:

a. the principal lesion in horses with heaves
b. most common in cattle
c. most common cats
d. usually allergic in origin
e. a type-II pneumocyte necrosis

162. Following viral pneumonia, the pulmonary alveoli are repaired by:

a. endothelial-cell metaplasia to alveolar cells
b. proliferation of fibroblasts
c. proliferation of Type-I pneumocytes
d. proliferation of Type-II pneumocytes
e. emigration of bronchiolar epithelium

163. Miliary tuberculosis describes:

a. tuberculosis characterized by multiple lesions, each about the size of a millet seed
b. tuberculosis caused by *Mycobacterium miliarium*
c. metastatic tuberculosis
d. tuberculosis caused by *Mycobacterium avium*
e. tuberculosis without calcification

164. In contrast to lesions seen with other fungal diseases, lesions of cryptococcosis are:

a. granulomatous
b. characterized by a profound cellular reaction
c. characterized by a very minimal cellular reaction
d. limited to the central nervous system
e. positive on acid-fast staining

165. Uremia may lead to lesions in body systems other than the kidneys. Which extrarenal lesion is **not** typically associated with uremia?

a. hemorrhagic gastritis
b. calcification of the gastric mucosa
c. endocarditis
d. pericardial effusion
e. glaucoma

Correct answers are on pages 210-213.

166. Hemoglobinuria may be a feature of any of the following disorders in cattle **except**:

a. anaplasmosis
b. leptospirosis
c. babesiosis
d. *Clostridium hemolyticum* infection
e. chronic copper poisoning

167. White heifer disease is characterized by hypoplasia of the:

a. uterine horns, cervix and vagina
b. hair follicles
c. skeletal muscles
d. adenohypophysis
e. parathyroid glands

168. Developmental defects of the central nervous system may be caused by any of the following **except**:

a. bluetongue virus
b. bovine virus diarrhea virus
c. feline parvovirus
d. *Veratrum californicum*
e. *Agave lechuguilla*

169. Alopecia is a pathologic feature of all of the following **except**:

a. jumbay tree poisoning
b. diabetes insipidus
c. thallium poisoning
d. hypothyroidism
e. zinc deficiency

170. Cholesteatomas (cholesteatosis) most commonly occur in the:

a. choroid plexus of old horses
b. choroid plexus of old dogs
c. choroid of the eye of young horses
d. choroid of the eye of young dogs
e. liver of obese cats

171. In a commercial fox colony, a large number of animals die from a disease characterized by ataxia, incoordination and paralysis. On

sections of brain tissue, you observe bilaterally symmetric foci of malacia in the periventricular gray matter. The most likely cause of these findings is:

a. canine distemper
b. canine parvovirus infection
c. thiamin deficiency
d. carbon monoxide poisoning
e. cerebrospinal nematodiasis

172. Secondary amyloidosis differs from primary amyloidosis in that:

a. the protein of secondary amyloidosis contains immunoglobulin light chains
b. the protein of secondary amyloidosis contains immunoglobulin heavy chains
c. the protein of secondary amyloidosis contains glycine
d. secondary amyloidosis is not associated with inflammatory conditions
e. secondary amyloidosis is restricted to the kidney and liver

173. The most useful stain to differentiate amyloid from hyalin is:

a. Von Kossa
b. Gomori's methenamine silver
c. Congo red
d. hematoxylin and eosin
e. Giemsa

174. A hematoma is defined as:

a. a malignant neoplasm of erythroid cells
b. a benign neoplasm of erythroid cells
c. a roughly spherical confined hemorrhage
d. hemorrhage into the peritoneal cavity
e. hemorrhage into the pericardium

175. In chickens, extensive infiltration of the sciatic nerve with lymphoblasts is most characteristic of:

a. avian encephalomyelitis virus infection
b. riboflavin deficiency
c. avian leukosis

d. thiamin deficiency

e. Marek's disease

176. A young dog has generalized disease of the skin, consisting of patches of erythema, alopecia and hyperkeratosis. Biopsy reveals distention of the hair follicles by elongated mites with stubby legs. The most likely cause of these findings is:

a. *Sarcoptes scabiei*

b. *Demodex canis*

c. *Dermacentor variabilis*

d. *Otodius megnini*

e. *Otodectes cynotis*

177. A gray horse has multiple raised, papillary, cornified lesions about the face and neck. Microscopically these lesions are composed of extensively thickened epidermis, with hyperkeratosis and long rete pegs extending into the dermis, but confined by a basement membrane. A rare intranuclear inclusion body is seen in the affected epidermis. The most likely cause of these findings is:

a. squamous-cell carcinoma

b. sarcoid

c. papillomatosis

d. *Dermatophilus congolensis* infection

e. malignant melanoma

178. The mucosa of the nasal passages of a young pig with rhinitis of 2 weeks' duration contains areas of necrosis and lymphocytic infiltration. The epithelial cells and submucosal glands of the nasal mucosa contain large intranuclear inclusion bodies. The most likely cause of these findings is:

a. atrophic rhinitis

b. parvovirus infection

c. rotavirus infection

d. cytomegalovirus infection

e. pseudorabies

179. A 5-month-old Standardbred foal dies from disease characterized by respiratory distress and diarrhea. At necropsy, multiple nodular lesions in the lung consist of abscesses sur-

rounded by macrophages and multinucleated giant cells. Similar lesions are found in the kidney and mesenteric lymph nodes. The most likely cause of these findings is:

a. strangles

b. rhinopneumonitis

c. adenovirus infection

d. *Rhodococcus equi* infection

e. *Pasteurella multocida* infection

180. Which disease of dogs is most likely to cause thrombocytopenia, extensive hemorrhage and lymphadenopathy?

a. ehrlichiosis

b. babesiosis

c. *Ancylostoma caninum* infection

d. distemper

e. parvovirus infection

181. Hydropericardium is often an important feature of all of the following disorders **except**:

a. pulmonary hypertension

b. renal failure

c. hypoproteinemia

d. mulberry heart disease

e. diabetes insipidus

182. Squamous-cell carcinoma occurring in metaplastic urinary bladder epithelium of a cow with hematuria is typically associated with:

a. *Clostridium hemolyticum* infection

b. anthrax

c. bracken fern poisoning

d. trichlorethylene-extracted soybean meal poisoning

e. papillomatosis

183. The primary pathologic change in the syndrome of dwarfism in cattle and dogs is in the:

a. osteoblasts

b. osteoclasts

c. chondrocytes

d. fibroblasts

e. osteoid

Correct answers are on pages 210-213.

184. Inherited deafness in white cats and dogs
     results from:

     a. aplasia of cranial nerve VIII
     b. degeneration of the organ of Corti
     c. degeneration of the vestibular labyrinth
     d. osteopetrosis of the temporal bone
     e. degeneration of the stapes

185. In a cat that developed impaired vision at 3
     years of age, ophthalmoscopic examination
     reveals degeneration in the photoreceptor cells
     of the retina. The most likely cause of these
     findings is:

     a. inherited retinal dystrophy
     b. dietary taurine deficiency
     c. dietary linoleic acid deficiency
     d. parvovirus infection
     e. hypervitaminosis A

186. Hypertrophy, hyperplasia and squamous
     metaplasia of the prostate gland are commonly
     observed in dogs with:

     a. interstitial-cell tumors
     b. seminomas
     c. Sertoli-cell tumors
     d. dysgerminomas
     e. perianal-gland tumors

187. Which of the following is **not** a feature of
     necrotic cells?

     a. karyorrhexis
     b. pyknosis
     c. karyolysis
     d. karyomegaly
     e. absence of a nucleus

188. At necropsy, the wall of a dog's small
     intestine is yellow-brown. On histopathologic
     examination, you find accumulations of
     yellow-brown pigment within the cytoplasm of
     smooth muscle cells. The most likely cause of
     these findings is:

     a. vitamin E deficiency
     b. parvovirus infection

     c. vitamin K deficiency
     d. coccidiosis
     e. pseudomelanosis

189. Microscopic examination of a dog's lungs
     reveals severe congestion and numerous
     hemosiderin-laden macrophages within the
     alveoli. The most likely cause of these findings
     is:

     a. *Pneumocystis carinii* infection
     b. vitamin E deficiency
     c. heart failure
     d. renal failure
     e. infectious canine hepatitis

190. Saddle embolus or thrombus at the iliac
     bifurcation of the aorta is a common finding in
     cats with:

     a. panleukopenia
     b. hypertrophic cardiomyopathy
     c. renal failure
     d. hypertension
     e. feline infectious peritonitis

191. The basic histopathologic defect in Collie eye
     anomaly is:

     a. optic disk coloboma
     b. photoreceptor-cell rosettes
     c. choroidal hypoplasia
     d. scleral ectasia
     e. focal retinal atrophy

192. The histopathologic features of Aleutian
     disease of mink could be confused with those of:

     a. canine distemper
     b. Chediak-Higashi syndrome
     c. malignant lymphoma
     d. multiple myeloma
     e. salmon poisoning

193. Swayback and enzootic ataxia of sheep are
     characterized by:

     a. cavitating lesions in the cerebral white
        matter

b. laminar necrosis of the cerebrum

c. cerebellar hypoplasia

d. spina bifida

e. hydrocephalus

b. a xenograph

c. viral oncogenesis

d. autoimmunity

e. absence of histocompatability antigens

194. *Demyelination or dysmyelination are features of all of the following diseases* **except**:

a. globoid-cell leukodystrophy

b. allergic encephalomyelitis

c. visna

d. canine distemper

e. listeriosis

195. *In dogs, so-called mixed tumors (neoplasms consisting of neoplastic epithelial and mesenchymal elements) are most common in the:*

a. liver and kidney

b. mammary gland and thyroid gland

c. mammary gland and salivary gland

d. mammary gland and lung

e. pituitary gland and adrenal gland

196. *Feline leukemia virus is a primary cause of all of the following pathologic findings* **except**:

a. lymphoma

b. leukopenia

c. anemia

d. enteritis

e. encephalitis

197. *Uroliths in cats are most commonly composed of:*

a. oxalate

b. urate

c. struvite

d. apatite

e. cystine

198. *Transmissible venereal tumor of dogs is an example of:*

a. an allograph

199. *The pulmonary lesion of ovine progressive pneumonia is characterized by:*

a. purulent bronchopneumonia

b. fibrinous pleuritis

c. lymphocytic interstitial pneumonia

d. sequestered zones of necrosis

e. adenomatosis

200. *The most common neoplasm of the equine testicle is the:*

a. interstitial-cell tumor

b. Sertoli-cell tumor

c. seminoma

d. teratoma

e. mesothelioma

201. *Necrotizing vasculitis in a section of a pig's brain is most likely caused by:*

a. edema disease, hog cholera or mercury poisoning

b. edema disease, hog cholera or arsenic poisoning

c. edema disease, erysipelas or mercury poisoning

d. water intoxication, hog cholera or cocklebur poisoning

e. Teschen disease, hog cholera or organophosphate poisoning

202. *In swine, laminar necrosis of the cerebral cortex and extensive infiltration of the meninges and Virchow-Robin spaces are characteristic histopathologic features of:*

a. organomercurial poisoning

b. moldy-feed toxicosis

c. salt poisoning

d. organophosphate poisoning

e. Talfan disease

Correct answers are on pages 210-213.

203. *The most common neoplasm of the appendicular skeleton of dogs is the:*

   a. chondrosarcoma
   b. osteosarcoma
   c. synovioma
   d. giant-cell tumor
   e. fibrosarcoma

204. *The most common neoplasms of the central nervous system of cats are the:*

   a. meningioma and glioma
   b. meningioma and metastatic carcinoma of the mammary gland
   c. meningioma and lymphoma
   d. lymphoma and metastatic carcinoma of the mammary gland
   e. meningioma and ependymoma

205. *In cattle, diffuse and extensive infiltration of histiocytes in the lamina propria of the small intestine and colon is characteristic of:*

   a. salmonellosis
   b. campylobacteriosis
   c. rotavirus infection
   d. calicivirus infection
   e. Johne's disease

206. *In a tissue section of bone from a dog with rickets, you are most likely to find:*

   a. increased activity of osteoblasts and osteoclasts, and wide osteoid seams
   b. decreased activity of osteoblasts, increased activity of osteoclasts, and narrow osteoid seams
   c. increased activity of osteoblasts, decreased activity of osteoclasts, and wide osteoid seams
   d. decreased activity of osteoblasts and osteoclasts, and narrow osteoid seams
   e. decreased activity of osteoblasts, increased activity of osteoclasts, and wide osteoid seams

207. *Benign neoplasms generally remain benign and do not become malignant. An **exception** to this is:*

   a. fibromas that become fibrosarcomas
   b. ostoeomas that become osteosarcomas
   c. papillomas that become squamous-cell carcinomas
   d. lipomas that become liposarcomas
   e. chondromas that become chondrosarcomas

208. *Transmissible venereal tumor of dogs:*

   a. is caused by a virus
   b. contains 58-59 chromosomes, as compared with the normal complement of 78
   c. contains 156 chromosomes, as compared with the normal complement of 78
   d. is highly malignant
   e. is also transmissible to cats

Answers

1. **c**	8. **b**
2. **d**	9. **c**
3. **a**	10. **a**
4. **c**	11. **c**
5. **b**	12. **d**
6. **c**	13. **a**
7. **d**	14. **d**

15. **a**	57. **b**
16. **c**	58. **a**
17. **b**	59. **b**
18. **e**	60. **b**
19. **b**	61. **c**
20. **a**	62. **e**
21. **b**	63. **a**
22. **c**	64. **c**
23. **c**	65. **b**
24. **a**	66. **a**
25. **b**	67. **b**
26. **d**	68. **c**
27. **b**	69. **a**
28. **b**	70. **e**
29. **c**	71. **c**
30. **b**	72. **b**
31. **b**	73. **c**
32. **b**	74. **a**
33. **a**	75. **b**
34. **a**	76. **e**
35. **b**	77. **b**
36. **c**	78. **c**
37. **d**	79. **a**
38. **b**	80. **a**
39. **b**	81. **c**
40. **b**	82. **c**
41. **b**	83. **d**
42. **c**	84. **e**
43. **c**	85. **c**
44. **a**	86. **b**
45. **a**	87. **a**
46. **b**	88. **c**
47. **b**	89. **e**
48. **c**	90. **c**
49. **b**	91. **e**
50. **c**	92. **a**
51. **b**	93. **b**
52. **b**	94. **b**
53. **c**	95. **a**
54. **d**	96. **d**
55. **c**	97. **c**
56. **d**	98. **a**

99. **e**		140. **c**	
100. **a**		141. **e**	
101. **a**		142. **d**	
102. **c**		143. **a**	
103. **c**		144. **c**	
104. **d**		145. **b**	
105. **b**		146. **d**	
106. **c**		147. **b**	
107. **e**		148. **d**	
108. **d**		149. **c**	
109. **a**		150. **c**	
110. **a**		151. **e**	
111. **c**		152. **d**	
112. **e**		153. **e**	
113. **a**		154. **b**	
114. **d**		155. **e**	
115. **a**		156. **b**	
116. **e**		157. **a**	
117. **a**		158. **c**	
118. **b**		159. **c**	
119. **d**		160. **c**	
120. **b**		161. **b**	
121. **d**		162. **d**	
122. **e**		163. **a**	
123. **a**		164. **c**	
124. **c**		165. **e**	
125. **c**		166. **a**	
126. **e**		167. **a**	
127. **b**		168. **e**	
128. **b**		169. **b**	
129. **e**		170. **a**	
130. **d**		171. **c**	
131. **e**		172. **a**	
132. **b**		173. **c**	
133. **d**		174. **c**	
134. **b**		175. **e**	
135. **b**		176. **b**	
136. **b**		177. **c**	
137. **c**		178. **d**	
138. **c**		179. **d**	
139. **a**		180. **a**	

181. **e**
182. **c**
183. **c**
184. **b**
185. **b**
186. **c**
187. **d**
188. **a**
189. **c**
190. **b**
191. **c**
192. **d**
193. **a**
194. **e**

195. **c**
196. **e**
197. **c**
198. **a**
199. **c**
200. **d**
201. **a**
202. **c**
203. **b**
204. **c**
205. **e**
206. **a**
207. **c**
208. **b**

Notes

Notes

Physiology

J.E. Breazile, T.P. Colville

Recommended Reading

Berne RM and Levy MN: *Physiology.* Mosby, St. Louis, 1988.

Cunningham JG: *Textbook of Veterinary Physiology.* Saunders, Philadelphia, 1992.

Patton HD *et al: Textbook of Physiology.* 21st ed. Saunders, Philadelphia, 1989.

Ruckebusch Y *et al: Physiology of Small and Large Domestic Animals.* Decker, Philadelphia, 1991.

Swenson MJ: *Dukes' Physiology of Domestic Animals.* 10th ed. Comstock Publishing, Ithaca, NY, 1984.

West JB: *Best and Taylors' Physiological Basis of Medical Practice.* 12th ed. Williams & Wilkins, Baltimore, 1991.

Practice answer sheets are on pages 269-270.

Questions

1. *The major intracellular storage site for calcium in skeletal muscle is:*

   a. rough endoplasmic reticulum
   b. mitochondria
   c. smooth endoplasmic reticulum
   d. cytoplasm
   e. lysosomes

2. *The major site of energy metabolism in a cell is:*

   a. nucleus
   b. mitochondria
   c. centrioles
   d. microsomes
   e. endoplasmic reticulum

3. *Intrinsic cell membrane proteins that serve as ionic pumps:*

   a. contain an ATPase domain
   b. allow passive diffusion of ions
   c. are fixed in number for a given cell type
   d. maintain a constant rate of ionic transport
   e. are located only in the surface membranes of cells

4. *Sodium pumps of cells:*

   a. are unaffected by hormones
   b. actively transport only sodium ions
   c. transport sodium into the cytoplasm
   d. transport potassium into cells
   e. have a fixed rate of sodium transport

Correct answers are on pages 237-241.

5. Lipid-soluble substrates move across cell membranes through a process known as:

   a. facilitated diffusion
   b. active transport
   c. passive co-transport with water-soluble substrates
   d. simple diffusion
   e. exchange diffusion

6. Facilitated diffusion of substrates across cell membranes:

   a. can move substrates against electrochemical gradients
   b. represents an "aqueous" route for hydrophilic substances
   c. represents a form of active transport
   d. is always a form of co-transport
   e. cannot be saturated

7. Co-transport of organic substrates across mammalian cell membranes:

   a. can occur with potassium diffusion
   b. can involve only 2 organic compounds
   c. requires sodium diffusion
   d. must transport only one substrate at a time
   e. cannot produce a concentration gradient for the organic substrate

8. Blood:

   a. contains cells and plasma
   b. is not important for CO_2 transport
   c. consists of cells and serum
   d. has no excretory function
   e. consists mostly of cells

9. Blood proteins are:

   a. comprised of fewer than 50 individual proteins
   b. produced only in the liver
   c. produced only by bone marrow stem cells
   d. produced only by hepatocytes, leukocytes and vascular endothelia
   e. all of a single type

10. The osmolality of plasma relative to extravascular fluid is provided by:

    a. carbohydrates
    b. albumins
    c. lipids
    d. apoproteins
    e. inorganic ions

11. Plasma albumin:

    a. is produced by hepatocytes and lymphocytes
    b. is entirely limited to intravascular distribution
    c. cannot serve as a transport protein
    d. has a half-life of about 19 days
    e. does not contribute to lipid transport

12. Resting membrane potentials of skeletal muscle and nerve cell membranes are produced primarily by:

    a. concentration gradients of various ions
    b. outward diffusion rate of potassium
    c. inward diffusion of sodium
    d. diffusion of chloride
    e. sodium-potassium pumping

13. The equilibrium potential for potassium ions is a membrane potential produced when there is:

    a. most rapid diffusion of potassium
    b. impermeability to potassium ions
    c. no effect of potassium diffusion on the membrane potential
    d. potassium diffusion more rapid than that of other ions
    e. no net diffusion of potassium

14. Blockage of the sodium-potassium pumps of excitable cells with digitalis derivatives results in:

    a. reduced cell size
    b. increased resting cell membrane potentials
    c. depolarization
    d. blockage of all cellular transport
    e. decreased excitability of cells

15. *Receptor-sensitive ion channels of cell membranes:*

    a. are responsive to cell membrane potentials
    b. always utilize G peptides
    c. always utilize second messengers
    d. may be sensitive to more than one type of receptor
    e. are fixed in number in a given cell type

16. *Increasing excitability of peripheral nerve axons is associated with:*

    a. decreased connective tissue sheaths in the nerve
    b. decreased diameter of nerve axons
    c. lack of myelin in nerve axons
    d. increased connective tissue sheaths in the nerve
    e. increased diameter of nerve axons

17. *In motor neurons, excitability increases with the:*

    a. diameter of axons
    b. diameter of the dendritic tree
    c. diameter of individual dendrites
    d. diameter of the soma
    e. size of the motor unit

18. *A somatic motor unit is defined as:*

    a. all neurons and muscle fibers in a muscle fascicle
    b. a motor nucleus and the muscle fibers innervated
    c. a single motor neuron and all muscle fibers innervated
    d. a single sensory neuron and all motor neurons excited
    e. the least activity in a muscle that will cause movement

19. *Voltage-sensitive calcium channels:*

    a. are N-type channels blocked by cadmium and dihydropyridine class drugs
    b. are L-type channels blocked only by cadmium
    c. are T-type channels blocked by dihydropyridine
    d. of all types are found in a single nerve cell
    e. all exhibit the same threshold Em for activation

20. *Excitatory postsynaptic potentials of neurons:*

    a. are all-or-none responses of the cell membrane
    b. are decreased in amplitude by maintained hyperpolarization
    c. have an equilibrium potential near that for potassium ions
    d. have an equilibrium potential near zero
    e. are produced by decreased permeability to potassium ions

21. *Strychnine poisoning results in:*

    a. blockage of presynaptic inhibition in the central nervous system
    b. hyperactivity of excitatory neurons of the central nervous system
    c. blockage of potassium ion channels of excitatory neurons
    d. blockage of direct synaptic inhibition
    e. blockage of Renshaw cell inhibition

22. *The average number of muscle cells innervated by each motor neuron is called the:*

    a. motor unit
    b. myotatic unit
    c. innervation ratio
    d. size principle for motor neurons
    e. summation ratio

23. *The theory of muscle contraction involving interaction of actin and myosin is called the:*

    a. sliding filament theory
    b. cross bridge theory
    c. continuous filament theory
    d. folding theory
    e. telescoping theory

Correct answers are on pages 237-241.

24. The period during an action potential during which a second action potential cannot be produced by any means is called:

    a. absolute refractory period
    b. subnormal period
    c. relative refractory period
    d. spike potential
    e. supernormal period

25. Temporal summation of muscle contraction is primarily due to:

    a. increased size of the positive afterpotential
    b. increased intracellular sodium concentration
    c. decreased intracellular potassium concentration
    d. increased intracellular calcium concentration
    e. increased amplitude of the action potential

26. To produce prepotentials in nodal cells of the heart, permeability is:

    a. increased to slow calcium channels
    b. increased to fast sodium channels
    c. decreased to slow sodium channels
    d. decreased to slow calcium channels
    e. increased to slow potassium channels

27. The effect of digitalis derivatives on cell membranes is to:

    a. increase sodium-potassium pumping
    b. decrease sodium-potassium pumping
    c. increase permeability to calcium ions
    d. decrease permeability to potassium ions
    e. increase permeability to sodium ions

28. The positive inotropic effect of digitalis derivatives is due to:

    a. decreased intracellular concentration of sodium
    b. increased intracellular concentration of potassium
    c. increased intracellular concentration of sodium
    d. decreased intracellular concentration of calcium
    e. increased intracellular concentration of calcium

29. Epinephrine increases the heart rate by:

    a. increasing permeability of nodal cells to calcium ions
    b. decreasing permeability of nodal cells to calcium ions
    c. increasing permeability of nodal cells to potassium ions
    d. decreasing permeability of nodal cells to sodium ions
    e. increasing permeability of nodal cells to sodium ions

30. Thyroid hormones alter the effect of epinephrine by:

    a. increasing the number of alpha receptors per cell
    b. decreasing the density of enzymes destroying epinephrine
    c. increasing the activity of enzymes destroying epinephrine
    d. increasing the number of beta receptors per cell
    e. decreasing the number of alpha and beta receptors per cell

31. An increase in receptor numbers induced by a deficiency of the hormone specific for those receptors is called:

    a. heterogeneous down regulation
    b. homogeneous up regulation
    c. heterogeneous up regulation
    d. direct up regulation
    e. indirect up regulation

32. Which cells do **not** require insulin for glucose uptake?

    a. skeletal muscle cells
    b. fibroblasts
    c. fat cells
    d. liver cells
    e. neurons

33. *Lusitropy of cardiac muscle cells refers to the:*

    a. rate of action potential production
    b. action potential conduction velocity
    c. force of contraction
    d. rate of relaxation
    e. rate of fiber shortening

34. *Thyroid hormones influence the ionic composition of intracellular fluid by:*

    a. increasing energy availability for pumping ions
    b. up regulating the number of sodium pumps
    c. down regulating the rate of ionic pumping
    d. up regulating the number of ionic channels
    e. down regulating the number of ionic channels

35. *According to the law of circulation, over time, the volume of blood flow:*

    a. is greater in arteries than in veins
    b. is smaller in arteries than in veins
    c. is smaller in the pulmonary circuit than in the systemic
    d. is smaller in the pulmonary circuit than in the systemic
    e. must be equal in all segments of the vascular system

36. *According to Poisuelle's principle, the major determinant of volume of blood flow per unit of time is the:*

    a. cross-sectional radius of the vascular tree
    b. pressure gradient across the vascular tree
    c. viscosity of blood
    d. density of blood
    e. length of the vascular tree

37. *Preload to left ventricular contraction is due to:*

    a. blood pressure in the aorta
    b. peripheral resistance to blood flow
    c. end-diastolic ventricular volume
    d. contractility of cardiac muscle
    e. rate of muscle shortening

38. *Heterometric autoregulation of ventricular contraction describes the relationship between contractility and:*

    a. end-diastolic luminal pressure
    b. end-systolic volume
    c. end-diastolic luminal diameter
    d. end-systolic luminal pressure
    e. end-diastolic wall thickness

39. *Autoregulation of blood flow:*

    a. demonstrates a need for stable blood flow
    b. demonstrates a need for variable blood flow
    c. occurs to the same degree in all organs
    d. is particularly marked in skeletal muscle and skin
    e. represents neural and humoral control

40. *Afterload to left ventricular contraction is defined as the intraventricular pressure:*

    a. at the end of systole
    b. required to open the aortic valve
    c. at the end of diastole
    d. required to close the left atrioventricular valve
    e. required to open the left atrioventricular valve

41. *The chloride shift is necessary for transport of CO_2 in the form of:*

    a. carbamino hemoglobin
    b. soluble gas
    c. plasma $NaHCO_3$
    d. H_2CO_3
    e. carbamino plasma proteins

42. *The major determinant of blood viscosity is the:*

    a. specific gravity of plasma
    b. plasma protein concentration
    c. lipoprotein concentration
    d. hematocrit
    e. number of white blood cells

Correct answers are on pages 237-241.

43. A physical factor in which a decrease in value enhances turbulence of blood flow is the:

a. diameter of blood vessels
b. velocity of blood flow
c. density of blood
d. blood pressure
e. viscosity of blood

44. Reactive hyperemia is due to:

a. decreased adrenergic alpha activity
b. increased adrenergic beta activity
c. increased circulating levels of epinephrine
d. increased circulating levels of acetylcholine
e. increased levels of anaerobic metabolites

45. The mean electrical vector of ventricular depolarization is best measured in the sagittal plane by using electrocardiographic leads:

a. aVF and I
b. aVF and III
c. V10 and I
d. V10 and aVF
e. I and II

46. Concerning normal heart sounds, which statement is most accurate?

a. The first sound corresponds to opening of the atrioventricular valves.
b. The second sound corresponds to closure of the atrioventricular valves.
c. The third sound is produced by ventricular wall tension.
d. The fourth sound is produced by turbulence of blood flow.
e. They can only be heard with amplification.

*47. A factor that does **not** have a major direct influence on ventricular function is:*

a. heart rate
b. preload
c. afterload
d. inotropic state
e. viscosity of blood

48. The major beneficial function of surfactant in the lung is to:

a. slow gas diffusion
b. maintain integrity of the alveoli
c. increase surface tension
d. trap foreign materials
e. provide a medium for movement of macrophages

49. The Bainbridge reflex results from:

a. increased right atrial pressure, which decreases cardiac output
b. decreased right atrial pressure, which increases cardiac output
c. decreased left atrial pressure, which has no effect on cardiac output
d. increased right atrial pressure, which increases cardiac output
e. increased right atrial pressure, which decreases systemic arterial pressure

50. Circulating blood volume is regulated primarily by control of:

a. total body water volume
b. intracellular water volume
c. systemic arterial blood pressure
d. central venous pressure
e. plasma protein concentration

51. Renin is:

a. a pituitary hormone
b. a milk coagulation protein
c. secreted as an active enzyme
d. produced by the adrenal gland
e. a vasoconstrictor

52. The feature that is essential for venous return from dependent body parts is:

a. muscle pumps
b. foot or hoof pumps
c. respiratory pumps
d. venous valves
e. postcapillary blood pressure

53. *The single factor exhibiting dominant control of aldosterone secretion is:*

   a. extracellular potassium ion concentration
   b. neural impulses from the medulla
   c. pituitary secretion of ACTH
   d. atrial natriuretic peptide
   e. angiotensin II

54. *The major effect of myelin is to:*

   a. provide a nutrient source for axons
   b. insulate axons from other axons
   c. limit the frequency of action potentials
   d. enhance the velocity of action potentials
   e. provide physical support of axons

55. *Increased contractility of the heart in response to increased heart rate is called:*

   a. post-tetanic potentiation
   b. Starling's law of the heart
   c. the law of circulation
   d. the ascending staircase
   e. post-extrasystolic potentiation

56. *To increase calcium absorption from the small intestine, parathyroid hormone directly activates or enhances:*

   a. calcium-binding protein synthesis in enterocytes
   b. the effect of vitamin D on enterocytes
   c. liver conversion of previtamin D
   d. enzymes of the skin to produce previtamin D
   e. kidney conversion to active vitamin D

57. *Plasma phosphate concentration influences plasma calcium concentration by:*

   a. binding calcium and making it insoluble
   b. competing for caclium absorption in the intestine
   c. enhancing calcium excretion in the urine
   d. regulating formation of active vitamin D
   e. inhibiting calcium release from bone

58. *The myotatic reflex:*

   a. is activated by muscle contraction
   b. is enhanced by diminished gamma motor activity
   c. results in contraction of heteronomous muscles
   d. results in contraction of homonomous muscles
   e. causes relaxation of synergists to homonomous muscles

59. *The hormone receptor for thyroid hormone (T3) is:*

   a. an intrinsic protein of the cell membrane
   b. located in the cytoplasm of the cell
   c. located in the nuclear membrane
   d. attached to the DNA of the nucleus
   e. associated with RNA molecules

60. *The second messenger associated with the action of antidiuretic hormone (vasopressin) is:*

   a. cAMP
   b. inositol trisphosphate
   c. calcium
   d. cGMP
   e. diacylglyceride

61. *G peptides of the retina are activated by:*

   a. several hormones
   b. inhibitory neurotransmitters
   c. excitatory neurotransmitters
   d. action potentials
   e. light-sensitive pigments

62. *G peptides are so named because they:*

   a. initiate growth
   b. originate from growth hormone
   c. are found in granulocytes
   d. bind guanyl nucleotides
   e. form granules

Correct answers are on pages 237-241.

63. *Intestinal iron absorption:*

    a. is complete, and excess iron is excreted in urine
    b. is complete until plasma transport is saturated
    c. occurs throughout the small intestine
    d. results in storage in absorptive cells
    e. is usually excessive when dietary levels are high

64. *Plasma bilirubin is:*

    a. made soluble by albumin
    b. excreted unconjugated
    c. converted to biliverdin
    d. water soluble
    e. conjugated with amino acids

65. *Plasma bile salts are:*

    a. maintained at a constant level
    b. at highest levels immediately after a meal
    c. a useful indicator of liver function
    d. important in fat metabolism
    e. inhibitors of bile formation

66. *In ruminants, saliva plays an important role in recycling:*

    a. ammonia
    b. urea
    c. sodium
    d. potassium
    e. chloride

67. *Hydrogen ions are secreted from the parietal cells of the stomach by:*

    a. passive diffusion
    b. a hyrogen-potassium exchange pump
    c. a hydrogen-chloride symport
    d. an integral part of the sodium pump
    e. activation of adrenergic receptors

68. *The pancreatic enzyme responsible for auto-activation and activation of other enzymes is:*

    a. phospholipase
    b. carboxypeptidase
    c. elastase
    d. chymotrypsin
    e. trypsin

69. *The second messenger activated by secretin is:*

    a. cAMP
    b. cGMP
    c. calcium
    d. inositol trisphosphate
    e. diacylglyceride

70. *Between meals, pancreatic secretions:*

    a. are controlled by the migrating myoelectric complex
    b. do not contain enzymes
    c. do not contain bicarbonate
    d. contain enzymes only during motility phases of the migrating myoelectric complex
    e. are unrelated to gallbladder contraction

71. *Enterohepatic circulation:*

    a. involves an unusual pattern of arterial and venous blood flow
    b. maintains the pool of bile salts
    c. maintains high levels of bile pigments in plasma
    d. conserves vitamin B_{12}
    e. involves only primary bile salts

72. *Cessation of absorption in the intestines of calves:*

    a. occurs at the same time for all immunoglobulins
    b. involves only immunoglobulins
    c. occurs earlier for IgG than for IgM
    d. involves drugs as well as immunoglobulins
    e. is necessary for passive immunity in all species

73. *Maturation of renal function in calves is complete:*

a. at birth
b. by 1-2 days of age
c. by 1-2 weeks of age
d. by 1 month of age
e. by 2-3 months of age

74. As compared with colostrum produced on the second day of lactation, colostrum produced on the first day of lactation contains:

    a. more lactose
    b. less lipid
    c. less protein
    d. less sodium
    e. more protein

75. Parturition in many species is characterized by a preceding increase in fetal cortisol levels. This increase is associated with:

    a. a decrease in fetal adrenocorticotropic hormone levels
    b. a decrease in fetal corticotropin-releasing factor levels
    c. an increase in maternal progesterone levels
    d. surfactant maturation in the fetus
    e. a decrease in maternal estrogen levels

76. Uteroverdin, a green pigment associated with the fetal membranes of dogs, is:

    a. secreted by the uterine wall
    b. derived from hemoglobin
    c. a degenerative product of the placenta
    d. derived from the placental villi
    e. an indication of fetal resorption

77. Pregnancy testing by radioimmunoassay in farm animals:

    a. is applied only to plasma
    b. tests for estrogens
    c. tests for chorionic gonadotropins
    d. is only effective after the middle of gestation
    e. is effective as early as 3 weeks after insemination

78. During copulation, blood pressure in the corpus cavernosum penis of bulls may be as high as:

    a. 500 mm Hg
    b. 2000 mm Hg
    c. 6000 mm Hg
    d. 10,000 mm Hg
    e. 14,000 mm Hg

79. Pulsatile secretion of pituitary hormones, such as GnRH,:

    a. minimizes up regulation of receptors
    b. maximizes up regulation of recpetors
    c. prevents down regulation of receptors
    d. limits blood levels of hormone
    e. results in pulsatile physiologic effects

80. Cholesterol for synthesis of adrenal steroid hormones is synthesized by adrenal cells and is derived from circulating:

    a. very-low-density lipids
    b. low-density lipids
    c. high-density lipids
    d. chylomicrons
    e. very-high-density lipids

81. Chylomicrons are formed in:

    a. intestinal absorptive cells
    b. liver cells
    c. plasma
    d. lymph
    e. adipocytes

82. In cells, vitamin E:

    a. stimulates growth
    b. enhances protein synthesis
    c. enhances cellular oxidation
    d. limits oxygen utilization
    e. acts as an antioxidant

Correct answers are on pages 237-241.

83. In ruminants, eructation results in passage of rumen gases:

    a. out through the nose
    b. out through the mouth
    c. out through the nose and mouth
    d. into the lung
    e. into the omasum

84. The basic motor activity cycle of the ruminoreticulum begins with:

    a. biphasic contraction of the rumen
    b. biphasic contraction of the rumen and reticulum
    c. rapid biphasic reticular contraction
    d. biphasic contraction of the dorsal sac of the rumen
    e. a single contraction of the ventral sac of the rumen

85. The major source of water in the ruminoreticulum of normal cattle is from:

    a. ingested water
    b. extracellular fluid entering osmotically
    c. fermentation
    d. saliva
    e. backflow from the omasum/abomasum

86. The most powerful control of alveolar ventilation in a resting healthy animal is the:

    a. pH of extracellular fluid
    b. pCO_2 of extracellular fluid
    c. pH of cerebrospinal fluid
    d. pCO_2 of cerebrospinal fluid
    e. pO_2 of extracellular fluid

87. The elastic recoil of lung tissue is primarily attributable to:

    a. connective tissues
    b. pneumocytes
    c. bronchiolar walls
    d. surfactant
    e. blood vessels

88. Atrial natriuretic peptide:

    a. is a pituitary hormone
    b. is produced by cardiac muscle
    c. increases blood volume
    d. controls arterial pressure
    e. decreases urine volume

89. Mucociliary clearance in the respiratory tract refers to:

    a. macrophage action
    b. rate of mucus secretion
    c. volume of mucus secretion
    d. rate of ciliary action
    e. rate of removal of foreign material

90. Lymphokines are:

    a. phospholipids produced by lymphocytes
    b. carbohydrates that act on lymphocytes
    c. lipids that are active in inflammation
    d. peptide hormones produced by lymphocytes
    e. found in high levels in animals with lymphatic neoplasms

91. Interleukins are:

    a. lipids produced by lymphocytes
    b. peptide hormones produced by lymphocytes
    c. carbohydrates that act on lymphocytes
    d. lipids that are active in inflammation
    e. found in high levels in animals with myeloproliferative neoplasms

92. The alveolocapillary membrane characteristically serves:

    a. only as a diffusion barrier for blood gases
    b. to maintain a transcellular electrical potential
    c. to remove amino acids from the plasma
    d. as an endocrine organ
    e. as a detoxifying surface

93. *Pressure within the pleural cavity is negative:*

    a. only during inspiration
    b. during coughing
    c. at all times during eupnea
    d. during vomiting
    e. only during expiration

94. *In domestic animals, the tidal volume per kilogram of body weight is approximately:*

    a. 2-4 ml
    b. 4-6 ml
    c. 6-8 ml
    d. 8-10 ml
    e. 10-12 ml

95. *The major part of airway resistance is attributable to the:*

    a. nasal passages
    b. larynx
    c. trachea
    d. bronchi
    e. bronchioles

96. *By definition, dynamic compliance is measured:*

    a. anytime during inspiration
    b. anytime during expiration
    c. at midpoint during inspiration or expiration
    d. at the end of expiration or inspiration
    e. anytime during the respiratory cycle

97. *In the respiratory tract, physiologic dead space is:*

    a. equal to alveolar dead space
    b. equal to anatomic dead space
    c. less than anatomic dead space
    d. less than alveolar dead space
    e. equal to anatomic dead space plus alveolar dead space

98. *In the "waterfall" region of the lung (region in which downstream pulmonary venous pressure does not influence blood flow rate), pulmonary venous blood pressure:*

    a. is greater than alveolar pressure
    b. is equal to alveolar pressure
    c. equals pulmonary arterial pressure
    d. has no influence on blood flow
    e. controls alveolar blood flow

99. *Theoretically, when 15 grams of pure hemoglobin are saturated with oxygen, the oxygen content is:*

    a. 12.85 ml
    b. 15.55 ml
    c. 17.65 ml
    d. 20.85 ml
    e. 25.25 ml

100. *The effect of increasing CO_2 content of the blood on the affinity of hemoglobin for oxygen is known as the:*

    a. Haldane effect
    b. Bohr effect
    c. Venturi effect
    d. Gibbs effect
    e. Bernoulli effect

101. *As compared with the affinity of hemoglobin for oxygen, the affinity of hemoglobin for carbon monoxide is approximately:*

    a. 50 times greater
    b. 100 times greater
    c. 150 times greater
    d. 200 times greater
    e. 250 times greater

102. *Plasma proteins that inactivate pancreatic enzymes are:*

    a. albumins
    b. globulins
    c. nonspecific proteases
    d. specific proteases
    e. interleukins

Correct answers are on pages 237-241.

103. *Plasma enzymes that inactivate proteins are predominantly:*

    a. serine proteases
    b. tyrosine proteases
    c. arginine proteases
    d. phenylalanine proteases
    e. glycine proteases

104. *Hemopexin is a plasma protein that acts as a carrier for:*

    a. iron
    b. copper
    c. zinc
    d. heme
    e. bilirubin

105. *Haptoglobin is a plasma protein that acts as a carrier for:*

    a. hemoglobin
    b. fatty acids
    c. steroids
    d. bilirubin
    e. iron

106. *Thromboxanes are derived from:*

    a. essential amino acids
    b. glycolipids
    c. any lipid
    d. steroids
    e. essential fatty acids

107. *The integrity of the gastric mucosal barrier to hydrochloric acid is heavily dependent upon:*

    a. bicarbonate in saliva
    b. leukotrienes
    c. prostaglandins
    d. mucus
    e. cell membranes

108. *Production of red blood cells depends upon the hormone, produced in the kidney, called:*

    a. erythropoietin
    b. interleukin-3
    c. granulocyte-macrophage colony-stimulating factor
    d. interleukin-1
    e. prostaglandin F$_2$alpha

109. *The average life span of an erythrocyte in mammalian blood is:*

    a. 80 days
    b. 90 days
    c. 100 days
    d. 110 days
    e. 120 days

110. *The half-life of circulating granulocytes is about:*

    a. 3 days
    b. 2 days
    c. 1 day
    d. 12 hours
    e. 6 hours

111. *Tissue macrophages are derived from:*

    a. neutrophils
    b. fibroblasts
    c. monocytes
    d. lymphocytes
    e. mast cells

112. *Monocytes released from the bone marrow have an intravascular half-life of about:*

    a. 3 days
    b. 2 days
    c. 1 day
    d. 12 hours
    e. 6 hours

113. *Blood cells that are in the blood but not circulating are said to be in the:*

    a. extravasated pool
    b. marginated pool

c. occult pool

d. sequestered pool

e. limited pool

114. *Concerning the smooth muscle of blood vessel walls, which statement is most accurate?*

a. All types have the same properties.

b. Multi-unit muscle is located near the lumen.

c. Single-unit muscle is located near the intima.

d. All types are sensitive to stretch.

e. Only multi-unit muscle is innervated.

115. *Antidiuretic hormone (vasopressin):*

a. is a potent vasopressor

b. is a neurosecretion

c. increases urine production

d. antagonizes aldosterone

e. is a glycoprotein

116. *Reflex activity of the aortic arch and carotid sinus:*

a. may produce only a decrease in arterial pressure

b. may produce only an increase in arterial pressure

c. is phasically active

d. is tonically active

e. responds only to changes in arterial pressure

117. *Measurement of peripheral resistance to blood flow:*

a. requires only arterial pressure and volume of blood flow

b. requires both inflow and outflow pressures

c. requires conversion of volume flow to liters per minute

d. applies only to the systemic circulation

e. pressures are measured in mm Hg

118. *Minute volume:*

a. is tidal volume times respiratory rate

b. is the volume of air entering the alveoli each minute

c. is the volume of air entering the respiratory dead space each minute

d. considers only functional alveoli

e. does not include air volume of the nasal passages

119. *Inspiratory reserve volume is the volume of air that can be inspired with maximal effort after:*

a. normal exhalation

b. maximal exhalation

c. maximal inhalation

d. normal inhalation

e. inhaled dead space volume is subtracted

120. *Anatomic dead space in the respiratory tract:*

a. represents a constant volume in a given animal

b. alone determines alveolar ventilation

c. is variable during the respiratory cycle

d. represents nonfunctional air

e. is easily determined in the live animal

121. *Functional residual capacity of respiration represents:*

a. residual volume

b. minimal volume

c. expiratory reserve volume

d. expiratory reserve plus residual volume

e. expiratory reserve plus minimal volume

122. *At an atmospheric pressure of 760 mm Hg, inhaled dry air that is saturated with water at 37 C:*

a. exerts a pressure of less than 760 mm Hg

b. contains N_2 at a pressure of 608 mm Hg

c. contains O_2 at a pressure of 152 mm Hg

d. exerts a pressure of 713 mm Hg from O_2 and N_2 pressures

e. contains water vapor at 37 mm Hg

Correct answers are on pages 237-241.

123. *Concerning delivery of oxygen to tissues by arterial blood, which statement is most accurate?*

 a. All of the oxygen in arterial blood is delivered.
 b. Most of the oxygen in arterial blood is delivered.
 c. It is enhanced by exercise.
 d. It is inhibited at high altitude.
 e. It is diminished by intracellular 2,3-diphosphoglycerate.

124. *Concerning release of carbon dioxide in the lungs, which statement is most accurate?*

 a. Carbon dioxide release is enhanced by the Haldane effect.
 b. Oxygen diminishes carbon dioxide release.
 c. Plasma becomes more acidic with carbon dioxide release.
 d. Most of the carbon dioxide comes from hemoglobin.
 e. Plasma bicarbonate levels increases with carbon dioxide release.

125. *The basal rate and rhythm of breathing are determined by the:*

 a. pneumotaxic center
 b. apneustic center
 c. chemoreceptor center for respiration
 d. chemoreceptor reflexes
 e. respiratory center of the medulla

126. *The Hering-Breuer reflex:*

 a. is mediated by the glossopharyngeal nerve
 b. is initiated at mid-exhalation
 c. is initiated at the end of exhalation
 d. stimulates inspiration
 e. limits tidal volume

127. *The paradoxic reflex of Head:*

 a. is mediated by thoracic visceral afferents
 b. is initiated by exhalation
 c. is initiated at the end of exhalation
 d. stimulates inspiration
 e. limits tidal volume

128. *The proportion of body weight represented by total body water content in an average adult animal is approximately:*

 a. 40%
 b. 50%
 c. 60%
 d. 70%
 e. 80%

129. *The proportion of body weight represented by total body water content in an extremely obese animal is:*

 a. approximately 60%
 b. greater than 60%
 c. greater than 90%
 d. as much as 75%
 e. as low as 40%

130. *The intracellular fluid volume in a 10-kg animal is approximately:*

 a. 4 liters
 b. 1.5 liters
 c. 2 liters
 d. 5 liters
 e. 1.2 liters

131. *The total intracellular potassium content in a 10-kg animal is approximately:*

 a. 600 mEq
 b. 550 mEq
 c. 500 mEq
 d. 450 mEq
 e. 400 mEq

132. *Because of the Gibbs-Donnan relationship, plasma ionic content differs from that of interstitial fluid in that:*

 a. sodium concentration is lower in interstitial fluid
 b. bicarbonate concentration is higher in plasma
 c. chloride concentration is higher in interstitial fluid
 d. potassium concentration is higher in interstitial fluid

e. calcium concentration is higher in interstitial fluid

133. *Plasma volume is controlled:*

a. independent of interstitial fluid volume
b. by intracellular fluid volume
c. by mechanisms involving the spleen
d. by high-pressure baroreflexes
e. by low-pressure baroreflexes

134. *In regulation of the pH of extracellular fluid, $H_2CO_3/NaHCO_3$ buffering:*

a. has the greatest total buffering capacity of all buffering mechanisms
b. is limited to the extracellular fluid
c. is entirely regulated by alveolar ventilation
d. is entirely regulated by renal mechanisms
e. has relatively low efficiency to buffer at pH 7.4

135. *Concerning calcium balance in the body, which statement is most accurate?*

a. Calcitonin increases the calcium level in extracellular fluid.
b. Vitamin D mobilizes calcium from bone.
c. Parathormone increases the calcium level in extracellular fluid.
d. Parathormone increases deposition of calcium in bone.
e. Calcitonin enhances intestinal absorption of calcium.

136. *Renal clearance of sodium refers to:*

a. the rate at which sodium is excreted in urine
b. the rate at which sodium is removed from plasma
c. the rate at which sodium is resorbed from the renal tubules
d. the volume of plasma required to provide the quantity of sodium excreted per minute
e. the quantity of sodium appearing in the urine each minute

137. *Glomerular filtration rate is best estimated clinically by:*

a. the volume of urine produced per minute
b. free water clearance
c. osmolar clearance
d. creatinine clearance
e. urea clearance

138. *The renal tubular maximum is the:*

a. highest rate at which the tubules can transfer a substance in or out of the interstitial fluid or tubular luminal fluid
b. plasma concentration of substrate
c. mechanism of tubular transport
d. counterport system in the renal tubules
e. secretory mechanism in the renal tubules

139. *Protein in the glomerular filtrate is normally completely resorbed in the:*

a. collecting tubules
b. distal convoluted tubules
c. ascending limb of the loop of Henle
d. descending limb of the loop of Henle
e. proximal convoluted tubule

140. *Protein is resorbed from the glomerular filtrate through a mechanism called:*

a. reverse osmosis
b. pinocytosis
c. passive diffusion
d. facilitated diffusion
e. sodium leaching

141. *"Splay" of renal tubular transport maximum absorptive mechanism is due to variations in:*

a. substrate concentrations in filtrates of different nephrons
b. individual nephron glomerular filtration rate and absorptive capacity
c. renal tubule cell capacity for transport
d. protein binding of the substance
e. concentration of that substance in the renal medulla

Correct answers are on pages 237-241.

142. The osmolality of urine is primarily related to the concentration of:

    a. protein and urea
    b. potassium chloride and calcium chloride
    c. sodium bicarbonate and cystine
    d. cystine and dicalcium phosphate
    e. urea and sodium chloride

143. Production of acidic urine in a state of metabolic alkalosis is referred to as:

    a. paradoxic aciduria
    b. renal tubular alkalosis
    c. renal compensation
    d. renal tubular acidosis
    e. Fanconi syndrome

144. The most common mechanism for acidification of urine is:

    a. resorption of sodium bicarbonate
    b. excretion of titratable acids
    c. excretion of ammonium
    d. excretion of urea
    e. exchange of hydrogen ions for potassium ions

145. To convert ATP to cAMP, adenylate cyclase requires:

    a. calcium
    b. potassium
    c. sodium
    d. magnesium
    e. phosphate

146. Intense exercise in horses results in increased:

    a. numbers of circulating lymphocytes
    b. plasma levels of fatty acids
    c. plasma levels of glucose
    d. plasma levels of protein
    e. numbers of circulating eosinophils

147. Exclusive metabolism of fat results in a respiratory quotient of:

    a. 1
    b. 0.9
    c. 0.8
    d. 0.7
    e. 0.6

148. The primary effect of unilateral excitation of hair cells of the crista ampullaris in the inner ear is:

    a. torticollis
    b. strabismus
    c. anisocoria
    d. opisthotonos
    e. antigravity hypertonicity

149. Dark adaptation of the eye results from:

    a. increased sensitivity of retinal cones
    b. decreased sensitivity of retinal rods
    c. pupillary constriction
    d. destruction of retinal cone pigment
    e. generation of the retinal rod pigment

150. Cocaine affects the sympathetic nervous system by:

    a. blocking secretion of norepinephrine
    b. blocking alpha-adrenergic receptors
    c. stimulating release of norepinephrine
    d. stimulating adrenergic receptors
    e. acting as a beta-adrenergic agent

151. Vitamin B_{12} absorption:

    a. occurs in the duodenum
    b. uses a sodium-linked transport system
    c. requires intrinsic factor
    d. requires bile salts
    e. requires pancreatic enzymes

152. The normal brainstem auditory-evoked response in dogs characteristically:

    a. contains only one deflection
    b. records only ganglionic or nuclear synapses
    c. does not test for the receptor organ
    d. tests the entire neural auditory system
    e. has 3 major deflections

153. *Decerebrate rigidity results from hyperactivity of:*

a. alpha motor neurons
b. the pyramidal tract
c. the rubrospinal tract
d. gamma loops
e. Golgi tendon organs

154. *The area of the brain primarily responsible for circadian rhythm is the:*

a. amygdaloid complex
b. hippocampus
c. paraventricular hypothalamic nucleus
d. suprachiasmatic nucleus
e. mammillary nuclei

155. *The portion of the brainstem that regulates sensory input to the brain is the:*

a. periaqueductal gray matter of the midbrain
b. mesencephalic tectum
c. reticular formation
d. pontine tegmentum
e. medullary tegmentum

156. *Epidermal growth factor:*

a. acts on a nuclear receptor
b. is important only in fetal growth
c. uses cAMP as a second messenger
d. acts through a tyrosine kinase receptor
e. acts only on cells of epidermal origin

157. *Platelet-derived growth factor:*

a. is synthesized only by megakaryocytes
b. stimulates growth of vascular smooth muscle
c. is important only during fetal development
d. uses inositol trisphosphate as a second messenger
e. plays an important role in vasoconstriction

158. *Insulin-like growth factors:*

a. are secreted by the pancreas
b. are secreted by the liver
c. are also called somatostatin
d. have the function and potency of insulin
e. are major metabolic regulators

159. *The major cellular source of plasma creatinine is the:*

a. liver
b. spleen
c. intestine
d. muscle
e. connective tissue

160. *The major source of blood urea is the:*

a. large intestine
b. liver
c. spleen
d. muscle
e. diet

161. *Blood urea is formed by reaction of ammonium with:*

a. nitrogen
b. carbon dioxide
c. oxygen
d. hydrogen
e. bicarbonate

162. *A hormone that inhibits release of prolactin is:*

a. serotonin
b. norepinephrine
c. somatostatin
d. dopamine
e. enkephalins

163. *Action potentials in smooth muscle are primarily produced by changes in permeability to:*

a. calcium
b. chloride
c. sodium
d. potassium
e. organic anions

Correct answers are on pages 237-241.

164. *The pacemaker site for the glandular stomach is located in the:*

    a. cardia
    b. pylorus
    c. fundus
    d. mid-body
    e. lesser curvature

165. *The major determinant of resistance to flow of chyme in the small intestine is:*

    a. diameter of the intestine
    b. viscosity of the bowel contents
    c. specific gravity of the bowel contents
    d. segmentation movements
    e. sphincter activity

166. *The character of plasma that is most important in stimulating the rate of albumin synthesis is:*

    a. globulin concentration
    b. osmolality
    c. viscosity
    d. ionic composition
    e. concentration of fatty acids

167. *Chronic vomiting results in hypochloremia and:*

    a. hyperkalemia
    b. hypernatremia
    c. hyponatremia
    d. hypokalemia
    e. hyperphosphatemia

168. *The migrating myoelectrical complex:*

    a. limits the influence of digestive enzymes on the intestinal mucosa
    b. prevents accumulation of intestinal secretions
    c. limits populations of enteric bacteria
    d. enhances digestion
    e. enhances absorption

169. *In dogs, the stomach contracts:*

    a. once per minute
    b. 5 times per minute
    c. 10 times per minute
    d. 15 times per minute
    e. 20 times per minute

170. *During emesis, small intestinal motility is:*

    a. absent
    b. hyperactive
    c. segmental
    d. peristaltic
    e. antiperistaltic

171. *The major nutrients absorbed from the colon are:*

    a. water-soluble vitamins
    b. glucose and fructose
    c. amino acids
    d. volatile fatty acids
    e. long-chain fatty acids

172. *The basic motor activity cycle of the ruminoreticulum begins in the:*

    a. dorsocaudal ruminal sac
    b. ventrocaudal ruminal sac
    c. cardia
    d. reticulum
    e. ventrocranial ruminal sac

173. *During rumination, the number of ruminoreticular cycles per minute is:*

    a. 5
    b. 4
    c. 3
    d. 2
    e. 1

174. *Secondary ruminal contractions progress:*

    a. cranially from the ventrocaudal sac
    b. cranially from the dorsocaudal sac
    c. caudally from cranioventral sac
    d. dorsally from reticulum

e. caudally from the cardia

175. *The thick segment of the ascending limb of the loop of Henle contains an ion channel that can be blocked by furosemide. This channel is a:*

a. slow sodium channel
b. slow calcium channel
c. sodium and potassium channel
d. sodium, potassium and calcium channel
e. sodium, potassium and chloride channel

176. *What is the most essential agent for stimulation of secretion of hydrochloric acid by parietal cells?*

a. gastrin
b. acetylcholine
c. cholecystokinin
d. histamine
e. prostaglandins

177. *A general name for duodenal secretions that inhibit gastric motility is:*

a. enterokinases
b. enterogastrones
c. enterochalones
d. gastric inhibitory peptide
e. secretin

178. *The increase in plasma bicarbonate levels following a meal is called:*

a. the alkaline tide
b. postprandial alkalosis
c. metabolic alkalosis
d. pancreatic alkalosis
e. gastric alkalinization

179. *Circulatory shock releases a cardiotoxic substance from the pancreas called:*

a. trypsinogen
b. cardiotoxin
c. amylase

d. pancreatic polypeptide
e. lipase

180. *The cephalic phase of pancreatic secretion is mediated by:*

a. cholecystokinin
b. gastrin
c. secretin
d. acetylcholine
e. gastric inhibitory factor

181. *Immunocytes primarily responsible for tissue surveillance are:*

a. plasma cells
b. T-lymphocytes
c. macrophages
d. eosinophils
e. B-lymphocytes

182. *Hepatic bile salts are conjugated with:*

a. sulfate
b. glucuronate
c. amino acids
d. cholesterol
e. lecithin

183. *The proportion of secreted bile salts resorbed from the small intestine is approximately:*

a. 75%
b. 80%
c. 85%
d. 90%
e. 95%

184. *Large quantities of bile salts entering the large intestine produce diarrhea due to:*

a. excessively high osmolality
b. enhanced chloride secretion
c. direct irritation
d. inhibited sodium absorption
e. enhanced potassium secretion

Correct answers are on pages 237-241.

185. *Amino acids are absorbed from glomerular filtrate:*

    a. in the distal convoluted tubule
    b. only partially
    c. by transport maxima mechanisms
    d. by a single transport protein
    e. by simple diffusion

186. *In horses, the intestinal structure in which most water is absorbed is the:*

    a. left ventral colon
    b. left dorsal colon
    c. descending colon
    d. cecum
    e. right dorsal colon

187. *In the small intestine, fatty acids are absorbed in the absence of bile if the fatty acid molecule contains:*

    a. more than 18 carbon atoms
    b. more than 16 carbon atoms
    c. a phosphorus atom
    d. less than 12 carbon atoms
    e. a benzene side chain

188. *Rabbits normally acquire essential amino acids and B vitamins from cecal and colonic fermentation through the process of:*

    a. large intestinal absorption
    b. retropulsion to the small intestine
    c. coprophagy
    d. extensive foraging
    e. enterohepatic circulation

189. *Typically, cardiac ventricular repolarization:*

    a. produces the P wave of the electrocardiogram
    b. progresses from endocardium to epicardium
    c. progresses from base to apex
    d. progresses from epicardium to endocardium
    e. does not produce a deflection on the electrocardiogram

190. *The reference electrode for recording of the aVF lead of the electrocardiogram is attached to the:*

    a. right foreleg
    b. left foreleg
    c. left rear leg
    d. left foreleg and left rear leg
    e. left foreleg and right foreleg

191. *A substance, released by sweat glands, that produces vasodilation is:*

    a. dopamine
    b. prostaglandin
    c. leukotriene
    d. bradykinin
    e. serotonin

192. *Intracellular fluid volume is controlled by:*

    a. Gibbs-Donnan equilibrium
    b. cellular protein concentration
    c. the sodium-potassium pump
    d. aldosterone
    e. extracellular osmolality

193. *The "a" wave of the electroretinogram of the light-adapted eye is produced by:*

    a. depolarization of rods and cones
    b. depolarization of rods alone
    c. depolarization of cones alone
    d. hyperpolarization of cones alone
    e. hyperpolarization of rods alone

194. *The domestic animal that is an induced ovulator is the:*

    a. cow
    b. mare
    c. ewe
    d. sow
    e. queen

195. *Muscle relaxation results from:*

    a. active pumping of calcium from the cytoplasm

b. production of a relaxation factor
c. inhibitory neuromuscular transmission
d. increased levels of cytoplasmic ATP
e. repolarization of the cell membrane

196. *Control of pulmonary vasomotion differs from that of the systemic circulation in that:*

a. increased pCO_2 produces vasodilation
b. decreased pO_2 produces vasodilation
c. increased pH produces vasodilation
d. decreased pCO_2 produces vasoconstriction
e. increased pCO_2 produces vasoconstriction

197. *Pulmonary wedge pressure is a measure of pressure in the:*

a. right atrium
b. pulmonary artery
c. left atrium
d. right ventricle
e. bronchi

198. *Xylose absorption is used to test the integrity of the intestinal mechanism for absorbing:*

a. amino acids
b. hexoses
c. minerals
d. fatty acids
e. water-soluble vitamins

199. *Diffusion capacity of the lung is best measured using:*

a. carbon monoxide
b. oxygen
c. nitrogen
d. carbon dioxide
e. helium

200. *The rate of diffusion of a gas in tissue is inversely related to the molecular weight of the gas, as described in the equation, Rate of Diffusion = :*

a. 2 x molecular weight
b. square root of molecular weight

c. molecular weight $\div$ 2
d. molecular weight^2
e. molecular weight $\div$ 10

201. *The second heart sound is produced by closure of which heart valves?*

a. aortic and mitral
b. mitral and pulmonary
c. mitral and tricuspid
d. pulmonary and aortic
e. pulmonary and tricuspid

202. *The first heart sound is produced by closure of which heart valves?*

a. aortic and mitral
b. mitral and pulmonary
c. mitral and tricuspid
d. pulmonary and aortic
e. pulmonary and tricuspid

203. *Which vessel normally carries blood with a high level of carbon dioxide?*

a. aorta
b. carotid artery
c. pulmonary vein
d. umbilical vein
e. vena cava

204. *The most numerous blood cell is the:*

a. basophil
b. eosinophil
c. erythrocyte
d. lymphocyte
e. monocyte

205. *A muscle that increases the angle between 2 bones is known as:*

a. an abductor
b. an adductor
c. a circumductor
d. an extensor
e. a flexor

Correct answers are on pages 237-241.

206. *Most of the filtering, humidifying and warming of inspired air occurs in the:*

a. larynx
b. nares
c. nasal passages
d. pharynx
e. trachea

207. *Which of the following is **not** a function of the respiratory system?*

a. acid-base regulation
b. olfaction
c. phonation
d. prehension
e. temperature regulation

208. *Oxygen and carbon dioxide are transferred between inspired air and blood in the lung by the process of:*

a. flow down the pressure gradient
b. diffusion
c. ion pumping
d. nitrogenation
e. osmosis

209. *Stimulation of the parasympathetic portion of the autonomic nervous system causes:*

a. dilation of airways in the lung
b. dilation of the pupil of the eye
c. increased gastrointestinal function
d. increased blood pressure
e. increased heart rate

210. *Stimulation of the sympathetic portion of the autonomic nervous system causes all of the following **except**:*

a. dilation of airways in the lung
b. dilation of the pupil of the eye
c. increased gastrointestinal function
d. increased heart rate
e. piloerection

211. *Which part of the central nervous system initiates conscious movements of the body?*

a. brachial plexus
b. brainstem
c. cerebellum
d. cerebrum
e. spinal cord

212. *Damage to which part of the nervous system is most likely to produce instant death in an animal?*

a. brachial plexus
b. brainstem
c. cerebellum
d. cerebrum
e. spinal cord

213. *Which hormone is produced by the anterior pituitary gland?*

a. antidiuretic hormone
b. calcitonin
c. luteinizing hormone
d. oxytocin
e. progesterone

214. *Which hormone is released by the posterior pituitary gland?*

a. adrenocorticotropic hormone
b. calcitonin
c. luteinizing hormone
d. oxytocin
e. prolactin

215. *Which endocrine gland releases the hormone that causes milk letdown from the mammary gland?*

a. adrenal cortex
b. anterior pituitary gland
c. ovary
d. posterior pituitary gland
e. thyroid gland

For Questions 216 through 219, select the correct answer from the 5 choices below.

a. chemical
b. electromagnetic
c. mechanical
d. thermal
e. vestibular

216. *The kinesthetic (movement, position) sense reacts to which general type of stimuli?*

217. *The visual (sight) sense reacts to which general type of stimuli?*

218. *The gustatory (taste) sense reacts to which general type of stimuli?*

219. *The auditory (hearing) sense reacts to which general type of stimuli?*

220. *Rotary motion of the head is detected by which sensory structure?*

a. cochlea
b. malleus
c. organ of Corti
d. semicircular canal
e. vestibule

221. *Accommodation for near and far vision is accomplished by contraction or relaxation of muscles in the:*

a. ciliary body
b. conjunctiva
c. iris
d. limbus
e. retina

222. *The kidney helps control water balance in the body under the influence of:*

a. adrenocorticotropic hormone
b. antidiuretic hormone
c. calcitonin
d. oxytocin
e. parathormone

223. *Spermatogenesis takes place in the:*

a. epididymis
b. prostate gland
c. seminal vesicles
d. seminiferous tubules
e. vas deferens

224. *What is the correct sequence of development of ovarian structures in a normal cycle?*

a. corpus albicans, corpus luteum, corpus hemorrhagicum
b. corpus hemorrhagicum, graafian follicle, corpus luteum
c. corpus luteum, graafian follicle, corpus hemorrhagicum
d. graafian follicle, corpus hemorrhagicum, corpus lutuem
e. graafian follicle, corpus luteum, corpus hemorrhagicum

225. *Which anterior pituitary hormone stimulates spermatogenesis in males?*

a. estrogen
b. follicle-stimulating hormone
c. growth hormone
d. luteinizing hormone
e. prolactin

Answers

1. c
2. b
3. a
4. d

5. d
6. d
7. c
8. a

9. **d**	50. **e**
10. **b**	51. **c**
11. **d**	52. **d**
12. **b**	53. **a**
13. **e**	54. **d**
14. **c**	55. **d**
15. **d**	56. **e**
16. **e**	57. **d**
17. **e**	58. **d**
18. **c**	59. **d**
19. **d**	60. **a**
20. **d**	61. **e**
21. **d**	62. **d**
22. **c**	63. **d**
23. **b**	64. **a**
24. **a**	65. **c**
25. **d**	66. **b**
26. **a**	67. **b**
27. **b**	68. **e**
28. **e**	69. **a**
29. **a**	70. **a**
30. **d**	71. **b**
31. **b**	72. **d**
32. **e**	73. **a**
33. **d**	74. **e**
34. **b**	75. **d**
35. **e**	76. **b**
36. **a**	77. **e**
37. **c**	78. **e**
38. **c**	79. **c**
39. **a**	80. **b**
40. **b**	81. **a**
41. **c**	82. **e**
42. **d**	83. **d**
43. **e**	84. **c**
44. **e**	85. **d**
45. **d**	86. **a**
46. **c**	87. **d**
47. **e**	88. **b**
48. **b**	89. **e**
49. **d**	90. **d**

91. **b**

92. **e**

93. **c**

94. **d**

95. **b**

96. **d**

97. **e**

98. **d**

99. **d** 100% saturation of 1 g of hemoglobin requires 1.39 ml of oxygen. 1.39 x 15 = 20.85.

100. **b**

101. **e**

102. **d**

103. **a**

104. **d**

105. **a**

106. **e**

107. **c**

108. **a**

109. **e**

110. **e**

111. **c**

112. **a**

113. **b**

114. **e**

115. **b**

116. **d**

117. **b**

118. **a**

119. **d**

120. **c**

121. **d**

122. **d**

123. **c**

124. **a**

125. **e**

126. **e**

127. **d**

128. **c**

129. **e**

130. **a**

131. **b**

132. **c**

133. **e**

134. **e**

135. **c**

136. **d**

137. **d**

138. **a**

139. **e**

140. **b**

141. **b**

142. **e**

143. **a**

144. **a**

145. **d**

146. **b**

147. **d**

148. **a**

149. **e**

150. **c**

151. **c**

152. **d**

153. **d**

154. **d**

155. **c**

156. **c**

157. **b**

158. **b**

159. **d**

160. **b**

161. **b**

162. **d**

163. **a**

164. **d**

165. **d**

166. **b**

167. **d**

168. **c**

169. **b**

170. **e**

171. **d**

172. **d**

173. **e**

174. **b**

175. **e**

176. **d**

177. **b**

178. **a**

179. **d**

180. **d**

181. **b**

182. **c**

183. **e**

184. **d**

185. **c**

186. **d**

187. **d**

188. **c**

189. **d**

190. **e**

191. **d**

192. **c**

193. **d**

194. **e**

195. **a**

196. **e**

197. **c**

198. **b**

199. **a**

200. **b**

201. **d** The second heart sound is produced by closure of the 2 ventricular outflow valves (pulmonary and aortic).

202. **c** The first heart sound is produced by closure of the 2 atrioventricular valves (mitral and tricuspid).

203. **e** All of the other vessels normally carry oxygen-rich blood.

204. **c** All of the other cells listed are white blood cells that are much less numerous.

205. **d** An extensor muscle increases the angle between 2 bones at a joint.

206. **c** The large surface area, extensive venous plexus, and active cilia of the nasal passages significantly condition inspired air.

207. **d** Prehension is the act of grasping.

208. **b** The gases diffuse from an area of high concentration to an area of low concentration through the thin alveolar and capillary walls.

209. **c** The parasympathetic nervous system is the "business as usual system" that helps support basic body functions, such as digestion.

210. **c** The sympathetic nervous system is the "fight or flight" system that prepares the body for intense short-term activity.

211. **d** The cerebrum is the only portion of the nervous system that can initiate conscious body movements. The others serve to transmit and/or modify nerve impulses that produce movements.

212. **b** The brainstem contains control centers for many basic body functions, such as respiration and cardiovascular function. Damage to those control centers results in rapid death.

213. **c** All of the other hormones listed are produced in other endocrine glands.

214. **d** Oxytocin is produced in the hypothalamus and transmitted along specialized nerve fibers to the posterior pituitary gland for storage and release.

215. **d** Oxytocin, the hormone that produces milk letdown, is produced in the hypothalamus and transported to the posterior pituitary gland along nerve fibers for storage and release.

216. **c** The kinesthetic (movement, position) sense receives information from mechanical receptors in muscles and joints.

217. **b** The visual sense (sight) converts light waves (electromagnetic radiation) into nerve impulses.

218. **a** The gustatory sense (taste) reacts to chemical substances in the mouth.

219. **c** The auditory sense (hearing) converts mechanical vibrations of air molecules (sound waves) into nerve impulses.

220. **d** The semicircular canals in each inner ear are arranged in different planes, so one or more is stimulated by rotary motion of the head in any direction.

221. **a** Muscles of the ciliary body cause stretching and relaxation of the lens of the eye.

222. **b** Antidiuretic hormone is secreted when the body becomes dehydrated. It increases water resorption from the kidney tubules.

223. **d** The seminiferous tubules are long U-shaped tubes in the testes where spermatozoa are produced before moving into the epididymis for storage. The other structures listed are part of the system that transports spermatozoa during ejaculation and produces the components of semen.

224. **d** Rupture of a graafian follicle (ovulation) results in formation of a corpus hemorrhagicum, which soon evolves into a corpus luteum.

225. **b** Though it is named for its effect in the female, follicle-stimulating hormone promotes spermatogenesis in the male.

Notes

Notes

Section 10

Terminology

P.W. Pratt

Recommended Reading

Blood DC and Studdert VP: *Bailliere's Comprehensive Veterinary Dictionary*. Saunders, Philadelphia, 1989.

Cochran PE: *Guide to Veterinary Medical Terminology*. American Veterinary Publications, Goleta, CA, 1991.

Prendergast A: *Medical Terminology: A Text/Workbook*. 2nd ed. Addison-Wesley Publishing, Menlo Park, CA, 1983.

Wroble EM: *Terminology for the Health Professions*. Lippincott, Philadelphia, 1982.

Practice answer sheet is on page 271.

Questions

For Questions 1 through 5, select the correct answer from the 5 choices below.

  a. dys –
  b. poly –
  c. micro –
  d. hydro –
  e. cryo –

1. *Prefix meaning very small.*

2. *Prefix relating to use of ultra-cold liquids.*

3. *Prefix relating to water.*

4. *Prefix meaning impaired or difficult.*

5. *Prefix meaning too much, in excess, many, or multiple.*

For Questions 6 through 10, select the correct answer from the 5 choices below.

  a. – phagia
  b. – emia
  c. – ectomy
  d. – uria
  e. – itis

6. *Suffix meaning inflammation of.*

7. *Suffix meaning excision or surgical removal of.*

8. *Suffix relating to ingestion or swallowing.*

Correct answers are on pages 248-249.

9. *Suffix relating to urine or urination.*

10. *Suffix relating to blood or blood cells.*

For Questions 11 through 15, select the correct answer from the 5 choices below.

    a. – tomy
    b. – stomy
    c. – rrhaphy
    d. – pexy
    e. – plasty

11. *Suffix meaning to surgically repair by joining in a seam or by suturing together.*

12. *Suffix meaning to shape or surgically form.*

13. *Suffix meaning to surgically create a new opening in a hollow organ, connecting it to the outside of the body or to another hollow organ.*

14. *Suffix meaning to incise or cut into.*

15. *Suffix relating to surgical fixation by suturing.*

For Questions 16 through 20, select the correct answer from the 5 choices below.

    a. – algia
    b. – cele
    c. – ectasia
    d. – iasis
    e. – pathy

16. *Suffix relating to pain.*

17. *Suffix relating to infestation or infection.*

18. *Suffix relating to dilation, expansion or distention.*

19. *Suffix relating to a disorder or disease condition.*

20. *Suffix relating to a swelling, especially one with a cavity or associated with a hernia.*

For Questions 21 through 25, select the correct answer from the 5 choices below.

    a. an –
    b. brady –
    c. contra –
    d. hypo –
    e. pyo –

21. *Prefix meaning against or opposed.*

22. *Prefix meaning insufficient or abnormally low.*

23. *Prefix meaning without or not having.*

24. *Prefix meaning abnormally slow.*

25. *Prefix relating to pus.*

For Questions 26 through 30, select the correct answer from the 5 choices below.

    a. salpingo –
    b. phlebo –
    c. orchi –
    d. hystero –
    e. episio –

26. *Combining form relating to the uterus.*

27. *Combining form relating to veins.*

28. *Combining form relating to the vulva.*

29. *Combining form relating to the oviducts.*

30. *Combining form relating to the testes.*

For Questions 31 through 35, select the correct answer from the 5 choices below.

   a. costo –
   b. adipo –
   c. myringo –
   d. gnatho –
   e. chordo –

31. *Combining form relating to fat.*

32. *Combining form relating to the jaw.*

33. *Combining form relating to the spinal cord.*

34. *Combining form relating to the ribs.*

35. *Combining form relating to the eardrum.*

For Questions 36 through 40, select the correct answer from the 5 choices below.

   a. histo –
   b. syndesmo –
   c. spondylo –
   d. pilo –
   e. onycho –

36. *Combining form relating to the claw or hoof.*

37. *Combining form relating to hair.*

38. *Combining form relating to ligaments or connective tissue.*

39. *Combining form relating to tissue.*

40. *Combining form relating to the vertebrae or spinal column.*

For Questions 41 through 45, select the correct answer from the 5 choices below.

   a. sclero –
   b. megalo –
   c. ankylo –
   d. crypto –
   e. litho –

41. *Prefix meaning bent, looped or fused.*

42. *Prefix relating to a stone or calculus.*

43. *Prefix relating to hardening.*

44. *Prefix meaning hidden, concealed or a depression on a surface.*

45. *Prefix meaning abnormally large.*

For Questions 46 through 50, select the correct answer from the 5 choices below.

   a. – paresis
   b. – lysis
   c. – plasia
   d. – plegia
   e. – rrhexis

46. *Suffix relating to paralysis.*

47. *Suffix relating to destruction of.*

48. *Suffix meaning rupture.*

49. *Suffix relating to weakness or partial paralysis.*

50. *Suffix relating to development or cell numbers.*

Correct answers are on pages 248-249.

For Questions 51 through 55, select the correct answer from the 5 choices below.

  a. mesial
  b. axial
  c. supine
  d. sagittal
  e. oblique

51. *In dorsal recumbency.*

52. *On a plane parallel to the median plane.*

53. *Contact surface of a tooth, closest to the midline of the dental arcade.*

54. *Pertaining to or situated near a longitudinal line about which a body or structure would rotate.*

55. *On a plane not parallel to 1 of the 3 major directional axes.*

For Questions 56 through 60, select the correct answer from the 5 choices below.

  a. amb –
  b. ecto –
  c. para –
  d. meta –
  e. infra –

56. *Prefix meaning outer or on the outside.*

57. *Prefix meaning beneath or below.*

58. *Prefix meaning both or on both sides.*

59. *Prefix meaning beside, beyond, accessory to, or apart from.*

60. *Prefix meaning change, exchange or transformation.*

For Questions 61 through 65, select the correct answer from the 5 choices below.

  a. *Streptobacillus*
  b. *Staphylococcus*
  c. *Bacillus*
  d. *Streptococcus*
  e. *Diplococcus*

61. *Spherical bacterium found in pairs.*

62. *Rod-shaped bacterium found singly or in chains that are not twisted.*

63. *Spherical bacterium found grouped in clusters or bunches.*

64. *Rod-shaped bacterium found grouped in twisted chains.*

65. *Spherical bacterium found grouped in chains.*

For Questions 66 through 70, select the correct answer from the 5 choices below.

  a. chloro –
  b. leuko –
  c. cyano –
  d. melano –
  e. xantho –

66. *Prefix relating to the color blue.*

67. *Prefix relating to the color yellow.*

68. *Prefix relating to the color green.*

69. *Prefix relating to the color white.*

70. *Prefix relating to the color black.*

For Questions 71 through 75, select the correct answer from the 5 choices below.

  a. picornavirus
  b. rotavirus
  c. papovavirus
  d. oncornavirus
  e. coronavirus

71. *Virus resembling a wheel.*

72. *RNA virus that causes neoplasia.*

73. *Small RNA virus.*

74. *Virus that causes papillomas, poliomas and vacuolization.*

75. *Virus resembling a crown.*

For Questions 76 through 80, select the correct answer from the 5 choices below.

  a. intra –
  b. syn –
  c. toco –
  d. amblyo –
  e. aniso –

76. *Prefix meaning together, union or in association with.*

77. *Prefix meaning within or inside.*

78. *Prefix meaning unequal or dissimilar.*

79. *Prefix meaning dull, dim or not clear.*

80. *Prefix relating to birth.*

For Questions 81 through 85, select the correct answer from the 5 choices below.

  a. prn
  b. qd
  c. qh
  d. od
  e. qid

81. *In prescriptions and medical records, the abbreviation meaning every day.*

82. *In prescriptions and medical records, the abbreviation meaning 4 times a day.*

83. *In prescriptions and medical records, the abbreviation meaning right eye.*

84. *In prescriptions and medical records, the abbreviation meaning every hour.*

85. *In prescriptions and medical records, the abbreviation meaning as needed.*

For Questions 86 through 90, select the correct answer from the 5 choices below.

  a. $\leq$
  b. μ
  c. $\propto$
  d. γ
  e. $>$

86. *Symbol meaning gamma.*

87. *Symbol meaning less than or equal to.*

88. *Symbol meaning micron.*

89. *Symbol meaning greater than.*

90. *Symbol meaning proportional to.*

Correct answers are on pages 248-249.

For Questions 91 through 95, select the correct answer from the 5 choices below.

   a. dacryo –

   b. kerato –

   c. oligo –

   d. dactylo –

   e. xero –

91. *Combining form meaning dry.*

92. *Combining form relating to the digits or toes.*

93. *Combining form relating to tears or the lacrimal gland.*

94. *Combining form meaning few or scanty.*

95. *Combining form relating to horny tissue or the cornea.*

For Questions 96 through 100, select the correct answer from the 5 choices below.

   a. lavage

   b. phytobezoar

   c. scoliosis

   d. petechia

   e. morbidity

96. *A concretion or solid mass of vegetable matter found in the stomach or intestine.*

97. *Lateral deviation of the spine.*

98. *A pinpoint, circular hemorrhage on the skin or on a serosal surface.*

99. *To irrigate or flush out an organ or cavity.*

100. *The proportion of sick animals to healthy animals in a population.*

Answers

1. **c**	17. **d**
2. **e**	18. **c**
3. **d**	19. **e**
4. **a**	20. **b**
5. **b**	21. **c**
6. **e**	22. **d**
7. **c**	23. **a**
8. **a**	24. **b**
9. **d**	25. **e**
10. **b**	26. **d**
11. **c**	27. **b**
12. **e**	28. **e**
13. **b**	29. **a**
14. **a**	30. **c**
15. **d**	31. **b**
16. **a**	32. **d**

---

33. **e**	67. **e**
34. **a**	68. **a**
35. **c**	69. **b**
36. **e**	70. **d**
37. **d**	71. **b**
38. **b**	72. **d**
39. **a**	73. **a**
40. **c**	74. **c**
41. **c**	75. **e**
42. **e**	76. **b**
43. **a**	77. **a**
44. **d**	78. **e**
45. **b**	79. **d**
46. **d**	80. **c**
47. **b**	81. **b**
48. **e**	82. **e**
49. **a**	83. **d**
50. **c**	84. **c**
51. **c**	85. **a**
52. **d**	86. **d**
53. **a**	87. **a**
54. **b**	88. **b**
55. **e**	89. **e**
56. **b**	90. **c**
57. **e**	91. **e**
58. **a**	92. **d**
59. **c**	93. **a**
60. **d**	94. **c**
61. **e**	95. **b**
62. **c**	96. **b**
63. **b**	97. **c**
64. **a**	98. **d**
65. **d**	99. **a**
66. **c**	100. **e**

Notes

Section 1
Biochemistry

Fill in a circled letter to indicate your answer choice.

1. ⓐ ⓑ ⓒ ⓓ ⓔ	47. ⓐ ⓑ ⓒ ⓓ ⓔ	93. ⓐ ⓑ ⓒ ⓓ ⓔ	139. ⓐ ⓑ ⓒ ⓓ ⓔ
2. ⓐ ⓑ ⓒ ⓓ ⓔ	48. ⓐ ⓑ ⓒ ⓓ ⓔ	94. ⓐ ⓑ ⓒ ⓓ ⓔ	140. ⓐ ⓑ ⓒ ⓓ ⓔ
3. ⓐ ⓑ ⓒ ⓓ ⓔ	49. ⓐ ⓑ ⓒ ⓓ ⓔ	95. ⓐ ⓑ ⓒ ⓓ ⓔ	141. ⓐ ⓑ ⓒ ⓓ ⓔ
4. ⓐ ⓑ ⓒ ⓓ ⓔ	50. ⓐ ⓑ ⓒ ⓓ ⓔ	96. ⓐ ⓑ ⓒ ⓓ ⓔ	142. ⓐ ⓑ ⓒ ⓓ ⓔ
5. ⓐ ⓑ ⓒ ⓓ ⓔ	51. ⓐ ⓑ ⓒ ⓓ ⓔ	97. ⓐ ⓑ ⓒ ⓓ ⓔ	143. ⓐ ⓑ ⓒ ⓓ ⓔ
6. ⓐ ⓑ ⓒ ⓓ ⓔ	52. ⓐ ⓑ ⓒ ⓓ ⓔ	98. ⓐ ⓑ ⓒ ⓓ ⓔ	144. ⓐ ⓑ ⓒ ⓓ ⓔ
7. ⓐ ⓑ ⓒ ⓓ ⓔ	53. ⓐ ⓑ ⓒ ⓓ ⓔ	99. ⓐ ⓑ ⓒ ⓓ ⓔ	145. ⓐ ⓑ ⓒ ⓓ ⓔ
8. ⓐ ⓑ ⓒ ⓓ ⓔ	54. ⓐ ⓑ ⓒ ⓓ ⓔ	100. ⓐ ⓑ ⓒ ⓓ ⓔ	146. ⓐ ⓑ ⓒ ⓓ ⓔ
9. ⓐ ⓑ ⓒ ⓓ ⓔ	55. ⓐ ⓑ ⓒ ⓓ ⓔ	101. ⓐ ⓑ ⓒ ⓓ ⓔ	147. ⓐ ⓑ ⓒ ⓓ ⓔ
10. ⓐ ⓑ ⓒ ⓓ ⓔ	56. ⓐ ⓑ ⓒ ⓓ ⓔ	102. ⓐ ⓑ ⓒ ⓓ ⓔ	148. ⓐ ⓑ ⓒ ⓓ ⓔ
11. ⓐ ⓑ ⓒ ⓓ ⓔ	57. ⓐ ⓑ ⓒ ⓓ ⓔ	103. ⓐ ⓑ ⓒ ⓓ ⓔ	149. ⓐ ⓑ ⓒ ⓓ ⓔ
12. ⓐ ⓑ ⓒ ⓓ ⓔ	58. ⓐ ⓑ ⓒ ⓓ ⓔ	104. ⓐ ⓑ ⓒ ⓓ ⓔ	150. ⓐ ⓑ ⓒ ⓓ ⓔ
13. ⓐ ⓑ ⓒ ⓓ ⓔ	59. ⓐ ⓑ ⓒ ⓓ ⓔ	105. ⓐ ⓑ ⓒ ⓓ ⓔ	151. ⓐ ⓑ ⓒ ⓓ ⓔ
14. ⓐ ⓑ ⓒ ⓓ ⓔ	60. ⓐ ⓑ ⓒ ⓓ ⓔ	106. ⓐ ⓑ ⓒ ⓓ ⓔ	152. ⓐ ⓑ ⓒ ⓓ ⓔ
15. ⓐ ⓑ ⓒ ⓓ ⓔ	61. ⓐ ⓑ ⓒ ⓓ ⓔ	107. ⓐ ⓑ ⓒ ⓓ ⓔ	153. ⓐ ⓑ ⓒ ⓓ ⓔ
16. ⓐ ⓑ ⓒ ⓓ ⓔ	62. ⓐ ⓑ ⓒ ⓓ ⓔ	108. ⓐ ⓑ ⓒ ⓓ ⓔ	154. ⓐ ⓑ ⓒ ⓓ ⓔ
17. ⓐ ⓑ ⓒ ⓓ ⓔ	63. ⓐ ⓑ ⓒ ⓓ ⓔ	109. ⓐ ⓑ ⓒ ⓓ ⓔ	155. ⓐ ⓑ ⓒ ⓓ ⓔ
18. ⓐ ⓑ ⓒ ⓓ ⓔ	64. ⓐ ⓑ ⓒ ⓓ ⓔ	110. ⓐ ⓑ ⓒ ⓓ ⓔ	156. ⓐ ⓑ ⓒ ⓓ ⓔ
19. ⓐ ⓑ ⓒ ⓓ ⓔ	65. ⓐ ⓑ ⓒ ⓓ ⓔ	111. ⓐ ⓑ ⓒ ⓓ ⓔ	157. ⓐ ⓑ ⓒ ⓓ ⓔ
20. ⓐ ⓑ ⓒ ⓓ ⓔ	66. ⓐ ⓑ ⓒ ⓓ ⓔ	112. ⓐ ⓑ ⓒ ⓓ ⓔ	158. ⓐ ⓑ ⓒ ⓓ ⓔ
21. ⓐ ⓑ ⓒ ⓓ ⓔ	67. ⓐ ⓑ ⓒ ⓓ ⓔ	113. ⓐ ⓑ ⓒ ⓓ ⓔ	159. ⓐ ⓑ ⓒ ⓓ ⓔ
22. ⓐ ⓑ ⓒ ⓓ ⓔ	68. ⓐ ⓑ ⓒ ⓓ ⓔ	114. ⓐ ⓑ ⓒ ⓓ ⓔ	160. ⓐ ⓑ ⓒ ⓓ ⓔ
23. ⓐ ⓑ ⓒ ⓓ ⓔ	69. ⓐ ⓑ ⓒ ⓓ ⓔ	115. ⓐ ⓑ ⓒ ⓓ ⓔ	161. ⓐ ⓑ ⓒ ⓓ ⓔ
24. ⓐ ⓑ ⓒ ⓓ ⓔ	70. ⓐ ⓑ ⓒ ⓓ ⓔ	116. ⓐ ⓑ ⓒ ⓓ ⓔ	162. ⓐ ⓑ ⓒ ⓓ ⓔ
25. ⓐ ⓑ ⓒ ⓓ ⓔ	71. ⓐ ⓑ ⓒ ⓓ ⓔ	117. ⓐ ⓑ ⓒ ⓓ ⓔ	163. ⓐ ⓑ ⓒ ⓓ ⓔ
26. ⓐ ⓑ ⓒ ⓓ ⓔ	72. ⓐ ⓑ ⓒ ⓓ ⓔ	118. ⓐ ⓑ ⓒ ⓓ ⓔ	164. ⓐ ⓑ ⓒ ⓓ ⓔ
27. ⓐ ⓑ ⓒ ⓓ ⓔ	73. ⓐ ⓑ ⓒ ⓓ ⓔ	119. ⓐ ⓑ ⓒ ⓓ ⓔ	165. ⓐ ⓑ ⓒ ⓓ ⓔ
28. ⓐ ⓑ ⓒ ⓓ ⓔ	74. ⓐ ⓑ ⓒ ⓓ ⓔ	120. ⓐ ⓑ ⓒ ⓓ ⓔ	166. ⓐ ⓑ ⓒ ⓓ ⓔ
29. ⓐ ⓑ ⓒ ⓓ ⓔ	75. ⓐ ⓑ ⓒ ⓓ ⓔ	121. ⓐ ⓑ ⓒ ⓓ ⓔ	167. ⓐ ⓑ ⓒ ⓓ ⓔ
30. ⓐ ⓑ ⓒ ⓓ ⓔ	76. ⓐ ⓑ ⓒ ⓓ ⓔ	122. ⓐ ⓑ ⓒ ⓓ ⓔ	168. ⓐ ⓑ ⓒ ⓓ ⓔ
31. ⓐ ⓑ ⓒ ⓓ ⓔ	77. ⓐ ⓑ ⓒ ⓓ ⓔ	123. ⓐ ⓑ ⓒ ⓓ ⓔ	169. ⓐ ⓑ ⓒ ⓓ ⓔ
32. ⓐ ⓑ ⓒ ⓓ ⓔ	78. ⓐ ⓑ ⓒ ⓓ ⓔ	124. ⓐ ⓑ ⓒ ⓓ ⓔ	170. ⓐ ⓑ ⓒ ⓓ ⓔ
33. ⓐ ⓑ ⓒ ⓓ ⓔ	79. ⓐ ⓑ ⓒ ⓓ ⓔ	125. ⓐ ⓑ ⓒ ⓓ ⓔ	171. ⓐ ⓑ ⓒ ⓓ ⓔ
34. ⓐ ⓑ ⓒ ⓓ ⓔ	80. ⓐ ⓑ ⓒ ⓓ ⓔ	126. ⓐ ⓑ ⓒ ⓓ ⓔ	172. ⓐ ⓑ ⓒ ⓓ ⓔ
35. ⓐ ⓑ ⓒ ⓓ ⓔ	81. ⓐ ⓑ ⓒ ⓓ ⓔ	127. ⓐ ⓑ ⓒ ⓓ ⓔ	173. ⓐ ⓑ ⓒ ⓓ ⓔ
36. ⓐ ⓑ ⓒ ⓓ ⓔ	82. ⓐ ⓑ ⓒ ⓓ ⓔ	128. ⓐ ⓑ ⓒ ⓓ ⓔ	174. ⓐ ⓑ ⓒ ⓓ ⓔ
37. ⓐ ⓑ ⓒ ⓓ ⓔ	83. ⓐ ⓑ ⓒ ⓓ ⓔ	129. ⓐ ⓑ ⓒ ⓓ ⓔ	175. ⓐ ⓑ ⓒ ⓓ ⓔ
38. ⓐ ⓑ ⓒ ⓓ ⓔ	84. ⓐ ⓑ ⓒ ⓓ ⓔ	130. ⓐ ⓑ ⓒ ⓓ ⓔ	176. ⓐ ⓑ ⓒ ⓓ ⓔ
39. ⓐ ⓑ ⓒ ⓓ ⓔ	85. ⓐ ⓑ ⓒ ⓓ ⓔ	131. ⓐ ⓑ ⓒ ⓓ ⓔ	177. ⓐ ⓑ ⓒ ⓓ ⓔ
40. ⓐ ⓑ ⓒ ⓓ ⓔ	86. ⓐ ⓑ ⓒ ⓓ ⓔ	132. ⓐ ⓑ ⓒ ⓓ ⓔ	178. ⓐ ⓑ ⓒ ⓓ ⓔ
41. ⓐ ⓑ ⓒ ⓓ ⓔ	87. ⓐ ⓑ ⓒ ⓓ ⓔ	133. ⓐ ⓑ ⓒ ⓓ ⓔ	179. ⓐ ⓑ ⓒ ⓓ ⓔ
42. ⓐ ⓑ ⓒ ⓓ ⓔ	88. ⓐ ⓑ ⓒ ⓓ ⓔ	134. ⓐ ⓑ ⓒ ⓓ ⓔ	180. ⓐ ⓑ ⓒ ⓓ ⓔ
43. ⓐ ⓑ ⓒ ⓓ ⓔ	89. ⓐ ⓑ ⓒ ⓓ ⓔ	135. ⓐ ⓑ ⓒ ⓓ ⓔ	181. ⓐ ⓑ ⓒ ⓓ ⓔ
44. ⓐ ⓑ ⓒ ⓓ ⓔ	90. ⓐ ⓑ ⓒ ⓓ ⓔ	136. ⓐ ⓑ ⓒ ⓓ ⓔ	182. ⓐ ⓑ ⓒ ⓓ ⓔ
45. ⓐ ⓑ ⓒ ⓓ ⓔ	91. ⓐ ⓑ ⓒ ⓓ ⓔ	137. ⓐ ⓑ ⓒ ⓓ ⓔ	183. ⓐ ⓑ ⓒ ⓓ ⓔ
46. ⓐ ⓑ ⓒ ⓓ ⓔ	92. ⓐ ⓑ ⓒ ⓓ ⓔ	138. ⓐ ⓑ ⓒ ⓓ ⓔ	184. ⓐ ⓑ ⓒ ⓓ ⓔ

Continued

185. ⓐ ⓑ ⓒ ⓓ ⓔ
186. ⓐ ⓑ ⓒ ⓓ ⓔ
187. ⓐ ⓑ ⓒ ⓓ ⓔ
188. ⓐ ⓑ ⓒ ⓓ ⓔ

189. ⓐ ⓑ ⓒ ⓓ ⓔ
190. ⓐ ⓑ ⓒ ⓓ ⓔ
191. ⓐ ⓑ ⓒ ⓓ ⓔ
192. ⓐ ⓑ ⓒ ⓓ ⓔ

193. ⓐ ⓑ ⓒ ⓓ ⓔ
194. ⓐ ⓑ ⓒ ⓓ ⓔ
195. ⓐ ⓑ ⓒ ⓓ ⓔ
196. ⓐ ⓑ ⓒ ⓓ ⓔ

197. ⓐ ⓑ ⓒ ⓓ ⓔ
198. ⓐ ⓑ ⓒ ⓓ ⓔ
199. ⓐ ⓑ ⓒ ⓓ ⓔ
200. ⓐ ⓑ ⓒ ⓓ ⓔ

Section 2

Embryology

Fill in a circled letter to indicate your answer choice.

1. ⓐ ⓑ ⓒ ⓓ ⓔ	9. ⓐ ⓑ ⓒ ⓓ ⓔ	17. ⓐ ⓑ ⓒ ⓓ ⓔ	25. ⓐ ⓑ ⓒ ⓓ ⓔ
2. ⓐ ⓑ ⓒ ⓓ ⓔ	10. ⓐ ⓑ ⓒ ⓓ ⓔ	18. ⓐ ⓑ ⓒ ⓓ ⓔ	
3. ⓐ ⓑ ⓒ ⓓ ⓔ	11. ⓐ ⓑ ⓒ ⓓ ⓔ	19. ⓐ ⓑ ⓒ ⓓ ⓔ	
4. ⓐ ⓑ ⓒ ⓓ ⓔ	12. ⓐ ⓑ ⓒ ⓓ ⓔ	20. ⓐ ⓑ ⓒ ⓓ ⓔ	
5. ⓐ ⓑ ⓒ ⓓ ⓔ	13. ⓐ ⓑ ⓒ ⓓ ⓔ	21. ⓐ ⓑ ⓒ ⓓ ⓔ	
6. ⓐ ⓑ ⓒ ⓓ ⓔ	14. ⓐ ⓑ ⓒ ⓓ ⓔ	22. ⓐ ⓑ ⓒ ⓓ ⓔ	
7. ⓐ ⓑ ⓒ ⓓ ⓔ	15. ⓐ ⓑ ⓒ ⓓ ⓔ	23. ⓐ ⓑ ⓒ ⓓ ⓔ	
8. ⓐ ⓑ ⓒ ⓓ ⓔ	16. ⓐ ⓑ ⓒ ⓓ ⓔ	24. ⓐ ⓑ ⓒ ⓓ ⓔ	

This page intentionally left blank.

Section 3

Gross Anatomy

Fill in a circled letter to indicate your answer choice.

1. ⓐ ⓑ ⓒ ⓓ ⓔ	47. ⓐ ⓑ ⓒ ⓓ ⓔ	93. ⓐ ⓑ ⓒ ⓓ ⓔ	139. ⓐ ⓑ ⓒ ⓓ ⓔ
2. ⓐ ⓑ ⓒ ⓓ ⓔ	48. ⓐ ⓑ ⓒ ⓓ ⓔ	94. ⓐ ⓑ ⓒ ⓓ ⓔ	140. ⓐ ⓑ ⓒ ⓓ ⓔ
3. ⓐ ⓑ ⓒ ⓓ ⓔ	49. ⓐ ⓑ ⓒ ⓓ ⓔ	95. ⓐ ⓑ ⓒ ⓓ ⓔ	141. ⓐ ⓑ ⓒ ⓓ ⓔ
4. ⓐ ⓑ ⓒ ⓓ ⓔ	50. ⓐ ⓑ ⓒ ⓓ ⓔ	96. ⓐ ⓑ ⓒ ⓓ ⓔ	142. ⓐ ⓑ ⓒ ⓓ ⓔ
5. ⓐ ⓑ ⓒ ⓓ ⓔ	51. ⓐ ⓑ ⓒ ⓓ ⓔ	97. ⓐ ⓑ ⓒ ⓓ ⓔ	143. ⓐ ⓑ ⓒ ⓓ ⓔ
6. ⓐ ⓑ ⓒ ⓓ ⓔ	52. ⓐ ⓑ ⓒ ⓓ ⓔ	98. ⓐ ⓑ ⓒ ⓓ ⓔ	144. ⓐ ⓑ ⓒ ⓓ ⓔ
7. ⓐ ⓑ ⓒ ⓓ ⓔ	53. ⓐ ⓑ ⓒ ⓓ ⓔ	99. ⓐ ⓑ ⓒ ⓓ ⓔ	145. ⓐ ⓑ ⓒ ⓓ ⓔ
8. ⓐ ⓑ ⓒ ⓓ ⓔ	54. ⓐ ⓑ ⓒ ⓓ ⓔ	100. ⓐ ⓑ ⓒ ⓓ ⓔ	146. ⓐ ⓑ ⓒ ⓓ ⓔ
9. ⓐ ⓑ ⓒ ⓓ ⓔ	55. ⓐ ⓑ ⓒ ⓓ ⓔ	101. ⓐ ⓑ ⓒ ⓓ ⓔ	147. ⓐ ⓑ ⓒ ⓓ ⓔ
10. ⓐ ⓑ ⓒ ⓓ ⓔ	56. ⓐ ⓑ ⓒ ⓓ ⓔ	102. ⓐ ⓑ ⓒ ⓓ ⓔ	148. ⓐ ⓑ ⓒ ⓓ ⓔ
11. ⓐ ⓑ ⓒ ⓓ ⓔ	57. ⓐ ⓑ ⓒ ⓓ ⓔ	103. ⓐ ⓑ ⓒ ⓓ ⓔ	149. ⓐ ⓑ ⓒ ⓓ ⓔ
12. ⓐ ⓑ ⓒ ⓓ ⓔ	58. ⓐ ⓑ ⓒ ⓓ ⓔ	104. ⓐ ⓑ ⓒ ⓓ ⓔ	150. ⓐ ⓑ ⓒ ⓓ ⓔ
13. ⓐ ⓑ ⓒ ⓓ ⓔ	59. ⓐ ⓑ ⓒ ⓓ ⓔ	105. ⓐ ⓑ ⓒ ⓓ ⓔ	151. ⓐ ⓑ ⓒ ⓓ ⓔ
14. ⓐ ⓑ ⓒ ⓓ ⓔ	60. ⓐ ⓑ ⓒ ⓓ ⓔ	106. ⓐ ⓑ ⓒ ⓓ ⓔ	152. ⓐ ⓑ ⓒ ⓓ ⓔ
15. ⓐ ⓑ ⓒ ⓓ ⓔ	61. ⓐ ⓑ ⓒ ⓓ ⓔ	107. ⓐ ⓑ ⓒ ⓓ ⓔ	153. ⓐ ⓑ ⓒ ⓓ ⓔ
16. ⓐ ⓑ ⓒ ⓓ ⓔ	62. ⓐ ⓑ ⓒ ⓓ ⓔ	108. ⓐ ⓑ ⓒ ⓓ ⓔ	154. ⓐ ⓑ ⓒ ⓓ ⓔ
17. ⓐ ⓑ ⓒ ⓓ ⓔ	63. ⓐ ⓑ ⓒ ⓓ ⓔ	109. ⓐ ⓑ ⓒ ⓓ ⓔ	155. ⓐ ⓑ ⓒ ⓓ ⓔ
18. ⓐ ⓑ ⓒ ⓓ ⓔ	64. ⓐ ⓑ ⓒ ⓓ ⓔ	110. ⓐ ⓑ ⓒ ⓓ ⓔ	156. ⓐ ⓑ ⓒ ⓓ ⓔ
19. ⓐ ⓑ ⓒ ⓓ ⓔ	65. ⓐ ⓑ ⓒ ⓓ ⓔ	111. ⓐ ⓑ ⓒ ⓓ ⓔ	157. ⓐ ⓑ ⓒ ⓓ ⓔ
20. ⓐ ⓑ ⓒ ⓓ ⓔ	66. ⓐ ⓑ ⓒ ⓓ ⓔ	112. ⓐ ⓑ ⓒ ⓓ ⓔ	158. ⓐ ⓑ ⓒ ⓓ ⓔ
21. ⓐ ⓑ ⓒ ⓓ ⓔ	67. ⓐ ⓑ ⓒ ⓓ ⓔ	113. ⓐ ⓑ ⓒ ⓓ ⓔ	159. ⓐ ⓑ ⓒ ⓓ ⓔ
22. ⓐ ⓑ ⓒ ⓓ ⓔ	68. ⓐ ⓑ ⓒ ⓓ ⓔ	114. ⓐ ⓑ ⓒ ⓓ ⓔ	160. ⓐ ⓑ ⓒ ⓓ ⓔ
23. ⓐ ⓑ ⓒ ⓓ ⓔ	69. ⓐ ⓑ ⓒ ⓓ ⓔ	115. ⓐ ⓑ ⓒ ⓓ ⓔ	161. ⓐ ⓑ ⓒ ⓓ ⓔ
24. ⓐ ⓑ ⓒ ⓓ ⓔ	70. ⓐ ⓑ ⓒ ⓓ ⓔ	116. ⓐ ⓑ ⓒ ⓓ ⓔ	162. ⓐ ⓑ ⓒ ⓓ ⓔ
25. ⓐ ⓑ ⓒ ⓓ ⓔ	71. ⓐ ⓑ ⓒ ⓓ ⓔ	117. ⓐ ⓑ ⓒ ⓓ ⓔ	163. ⓐ ⓑ ⓒ ⓓ ⓔ
26. ⓐ ⓑ ⓒ ⓓ ⓔ	72. ⓐ ⓑ ⓒ ⓓ ⓔ	118. ⓐ ⓑ ⓒ ⓓ ⓔ	164. ⓐ ⓑ ⓒ ⓓ ⓔ
27. ⓐ ⓑ ⓒ ⓓ ⓔ	73. ⓐ ⓑ ⓒ ⓓ ⓔ	119. ⓐ ⓑ ⓒ ⓓ ⓔ	165. ⓐ ⓑ ⓒ ⓓ ⓔ
28. ⓐ ⓑ ⓒ ⓓ ⓔ	74. ⓐ ⓑ ⓒ ⓓ ⓔ	120. ⓐ ⓑ ⓒ ⓓ ⓔ	166. ⓐ ⓑ ⓒ ⓓ ⓔ
29. ⓐ ⓑ ⓒ ⓓ ⓔ	75. ⓐ ⓑ ⓒ ⓓ ⓔ	121. ⓐ ⓑ ⓒ ⓓ ⓔ	167. ⓐ ⓑ ⓒ ⓓ ⓔ
30. ⓐ ⓑ ⓒ ⓓ ⓔ	76. ⓐ ⓑ ⓒ ⓓ ⓔ	122. ⓐ ⓑ ⓒ ⓓ ⓔ	168. ⓐ ⓑ ⓒ ⓓ ⓔ
31. ⓐ ⓑ ⓒ ⓓ ⓔ	77. ⓐ ⓑ ⓒ ⓓ ⓔ	123. ⓐ ⓑ ⓒ ⓓ ⓔ	169. ⓐ ⓑ ⓒ ⓓ ⓔ
32. ⓐ ⓑ ⓒ ⓓ ⓔ	78. ⓐ ⓑ ⓒ ⓓ ⓔ	124. ⓐ ⓑ ⓒ ⓓ ⓔ	170. ⓐ ⓑ ⓒ ⓓ ⓔ
33. ⓐ ⓑ ⓒ ⓓ ⓔ	79. ⓐ ⓑ ⓒ ⓓ ⓔ	125. ⓐ ⓑ ⓒ ⓓ ⓔ	171. ⓐ ⓑ ⓒ ⓓ ⓔ
34. ⓐ ⓑ ⓒ ⓓ ⓔ	80. ⓐ ⓑ ⓒ ⓓ ⓔ	126. ⓐ ⓑ ⓒ ⓓ ⓔ	172. ⓐ ⓑ ⓒ ⓓ ⓔ
35. ⓐ ⓑ ⓒ ⓓ ⓔ	81. ⓐ ⓑ ⓒ ⓓ ⓔ	127. ⓐ ⓑ ⓒ ⓓ ⓔ	173. ⓐ ⓑ ⓒ ⓓ ⓔ
36. ⓐ ⓑ ⓒ ⓓ ⓔ	82. ⓐ ⓑ ⓒ ⓓ ⓔ	128. ⓐ ⓑ ⓒ ⓓ ⓔ	174. ⓐ ⓑ ⓒ ⓓ ⓔ
37. ⓐ ⓑ ⓒ ⓓ ⓔ	83. ⓐ ⓑ ⓒ ⓓ ⓔ	129. ⓐ ⓑ ⓒ ⓓ ⓔ	175. ⓐ ⓑ ⓒ ⓓ ⓔ
38. ⓐ ⓑ ⓒ ⓓ ⓔ	84. ⓐ ⓑ ⓒ ⓓ ⓔ	130. ⓐ ⓑ ⓒ ⓓ ⓔ	176. ⓐ ⓑ ⓒ ⓓ ⓔ
39. ⓐ ⓑ ⓒ ⓓ ⓔ	85. ⓐ ⓑ ⓒ ⓓ ⓔ	131. ⓐ ⓑ ⓒ ⓓ ⓔ	177. ⓐ ⓑ ⓒ ⓓ ⓔ
40. ⓐ ⓑ ⓒ ⓓ ⓔ	86. ⓐ ⓑ ⓒ ⓓ ⓔ	132. ⓐ ⓑ ⓒ ⓓ ⓔ	178. ⓐ ⓑ ⓒ ⓓ ⓔ
41. ⓐ ⓑ ⓒ ⓓ ⓔ	87. ⓐ ⓑ ⓒ ⓓ ⓔ	133. ⓐ ⓑ ⓒ ⓓ ⓔ	179. ⓐ ⓑ ⓒ ⓓ ⓔ
42. ⓐ ⓑ ⓒ ⓓ ⓔ	88. ⓐ ⓑ ⓒ ⓓ ⓔ	134. ⓐ ⓑ ⓒ ⓓ ⓔ	180. ⓐ ⓑ ⓒ ⓓ ⓔ
43. ⓐ ⓑ ⓒ ⓓ ⓔ	89. ⓐ ⓑ ⓒ ⓓ ⓔ	135. ⓐ ⓑ ⓒ ⓓ ⓔ	181. ⓐ ⓑ ⓒ ⓓ ⓔ
44. ⓐ ⓑ ⓒ ⓓ ⓔ	90. ⓐ ⓑ ⓒ ⓓ ⓔ	136. ⓐ ⓑ ⓒ ⓓ ⓔ	182. ⓐ ⓑ ⓒ ⓓ ⓔ
45. ⓐ ⓑ ⓒ ⓓ ⓔ	91. ⓐ ⓑ ⓒ ⓓ ⓔ	137. ⓐ ⓑ ⓒ ⓓ ⓔ	183. ⓐ ⓑ ⓒ ⓓ ⓔ
46. ⓐ ⓑ ⓒ ⓓ ⓔ	92. ⓐ ⓑ ⓒ ⓓ ⓔ	138. ⓐ ⓑ ⓒ ⓓ ⓔ	184. ⓐ ⓑ ⓒ ⓓ ⓔ

Continued

185. (a) (b) (c) (d) (e)
186. (a) (b) (c) (d) (e)
187. (a) (b) (c) (d) (e)
188. (a) (b) (c) (d) (e)
189. (a) (b) (c) (d) (e)
190. (a) (b) (c) (d) (e)
191. (a) (b) (c) (d) (e)
192. (a) (b) (c) (d) (e)
193. (a) (b) (c) (d) (e)
194. (a) (b) (c) (d) (e)
195. (a) (b) (c) (d) (e)
196. (a) (b) (c) (d) (e)
197. (a) (b) (c) (d) (e)
198. (a) (b) (c) (d) (e)
199. (a) (b) (c) (d) (e)
200. (a) (b) (c) (d) (e)
201. (a) (b) (c) (d) (e)
202. (a) (b) (c) (d) (e)
203. (a) (b) (c) (d) (e)
204. (a) (b) (c) (d) (e)
205. (a) (b) (c) (d) (e)
206. (a) (b) (c) (d) (e)
207. (a) (b) (c) (d) (e)
208. (a) (b) (c) (d) (e)
209. (a) (b) (c) (d) (e)
210. (a) (b) (c) (d) (e)
211. (a) (b) (c) (d) (e)
212. (a) (b) (c) (d) (e)
213. (a) (b) (c) (d) (e)
214. (a) (b) (c) (d) (e)
215. (a) (b) (c) (d) (e)
216. (a) (b) (c) (d) (e)
217. (a) (b) (c) (d) (e)
218. (a) (b) (c) (d) (e)
219. (a) (b) (c) (d) (e)
220. (a) (b) (c) (d) (e)
221. (a) (b) (c) (d) (e)
222. (a) (b) (c) (d) (e)
223. (a) (b) (c) (d) (e)
224. (a) (b) (c) (d) (e)
225. (a) (b) (c) (d) (e)
226. (a) (b) (c) (d) (e)
227. (a) (b) (c) (d) (e)
228. (a) (b) (c) (d) (e)
229. (a) (b) (c) (d) (e)
230. (a) (b) (c) (d) (e)

231. (a) (b) (c) (d) (e)
232. (a) (b) (c) (d) (e)
233. (a) (b) (c) (d) (e)
234. (a) (b) (c) (d) (e)
235. (a) (b) (c) (d) (e)
236. (a) (b) (c) (d) (e)
237. (a) (b) (c) (d) (e)
238. (a) (b) (c) (d) (e)
239. (a) (b) (c) (d) (e)
240. (a) (b) (c) (d) (e)
241. (a) (b) (c) (d) (e)
242. (a) (b) (c) (d) (e)
243. (a) (b) (c) (d) (e)
244. (a) (b) (c) (d) (e)
245. (a) (b) (c) (d) (e)
246. (a) (b) (c) (d) (e)
247. (a) (b) (c) (d) (e)
248. (a) (b) (c) (d) (e)
249. (a) (b) (c) (d) (e)
250. (a) (b) (c) (d) (e)
251. (a) (b) (c) (d) (e)
252. (a) (b) (c) (d) (e)
253. (a) (b) (c) (d) (e)
254. (a) (b) (c) (d) (e)
255. (a) (b) (c) (d) (e)
256. (a) (b) (c) (d) (e)
257. (a) (b) (c) (d) (e)
258. (a) (b) (c) (d) (e)
259. (a) (b) (c) (d) (e)
260. (a) (b) (c) (d) (e)
261. (a) (b) (c) (d) (e)
262. (a) (b) (c) (d) (e)
263. (a) (b) (c) (d) (e)
264. (a) (b) (c) (d) (e)
265. (a) (b) (c) (d) (e)
266. (a) (b) (c) (d) (e)
267. (a) (b) (c) (d) (e)
268. (a) (b) (c) (d) (e)
269. (a) (b) (c) (d) (e)
270. (a) (b) (c) (d) (e)
271. (a) (b) (c) (d) (e)
272. (a) (b) (c) (d) (e)
273. (a) (b) (c) (d) (e)
274. (a) (b) (c) (d) (e)
275. (a) (b) (c) (d) (e)
276. (a) (b) (c) (d) (e)

277. (a) (b) (c) (d) (e)
278. (a) (b) (c) (d) (e)
279. (a) (b) (c) (d) (e)
280. (a) (b) (c) (d) (e)
281. (a) (b) (c) (d) (e)
282. (a) (b) (c) (d) (e)
283. (a) (b) (c) (d) (e)
284. (a) (b) (c) (d) (e)
285. (a) (b) (c) (d) (e)
286. (a) (b) (c) (d) (e)
287. (a) (b) (c) (d) (e)
288. (a) (b) (c) (d) (e)
289. (a) (b) (c) (d) (e)
290. (a) (b) (c) (d) (e)
291. (a) (b) (c) (d) (e)
292. (a) (b) (c) (d) (e)
293. (a) (b) (c) (d) (e)
294. (a) (b) (c) (d) (e)
295. (a) (b) (c) (d) (e)
296. (a) (b) (c) (d) (e)
297. (a) (b) (c) (d) (e)
298. (a) (b) (c) (d) (e)
299. (a) (b) (c) (d) (e)
300. (a) (b) (c) (d) (e)
301. (a) (b) (c) (d) (e)
302. (a) (b) (c) (d) (e)
303. (a) (b) (c) (d) (e)
304. (a) (b) (c) (d) (e)
305. (a) (b) (c) (d) (e)
306. (a) (b) (c) (d) (e)
307. (a) (b) (c) (d) (e)
308. (a) (b) (c) (d) (e)
309. (a) (b) (c) (d) (e)
310. (a) (b) (c) (d) (e)
311. (a) (b) (c) (d) (e)
312. (a) (b) (c) (d) (e)
313. (a) (b) (c) (d) (e)
314. (a) (b) (c) (d) (e)
315. (a) (b) (c) (d) (e)
316. (a) (b) (c) (d) (e)
317. (a) (b) (c) (d) (e)
318. (a) (b) (c) (d) (e)
319. (a) (b) (c) (d) (e)
320. (a) (b) (c) (d) (e)
321. (a) (b) (c) (d) (e)
322. (a) (b) (c) (d) (e)

323. (a) (b) (c) (d) (e)
324. (a) (b) (c) (d) (e)
325. (a) (b) (c) (d) (e)
326. (a) (b) (c) (d) (e)
327. (a) (b) (c) (d) (e)
328. (a) (b) (c) (d) (e)
329. (a) (b) (c) (d) (e)
330. (a) (b) (c) (d) (e)
331. (a) (b) (c) (d) (e)
332. (a) (b) (c) (d) (e)
333. (a) (b) (c) (d) (e)
334. (a) (b) (c) (d) (e)
335. (a) (b) (c) (d) (e)
336. (a) (b) (c) (d) (e)
337. (a) (b) (c) (d) (e)
338. (a) (b) (c) (d) (e)
339. (a) (b) (c) (d) (e)
340. (a) (b) (c) (d) (e)
341. (a) (b) (c) (d) (e)
342. (a) (b) (c) (d) (e)
343. (a) (b) (c) (d) (e)
344. (a) (b) (c) (d) (e)
345. (a) (b) (c) (d) (e)
346. (a) (b) (c) (d) (e)
347. (a) (b) (c) (d) (e)
348. (a) (b) (c) (d) (e)
349. (a) (b) (c) (d) (e)
350. (a) (b) (c) (d) (e)
351. (a) (b) (c) (d) (e)
352. (a) (b) (c) (d) (e)
353. (a) (b) (c) (d) (e)
354. (a) (b) (c) (d) (e)
355. (a) (b) (c) (d) (e)
356. (a) (b) (c) (d) (e)
357. (a) (b) (c) (d) (e)
358. (a) (b) (c) (d) (e)
359. (a) (b) (c) (d) (e)
360. (a) (b) (c) (d) (e)
361. (a) (b) (c) (d) (e)
362. (a) (b) (c) (d) (e)
363. (a) (b) (c) (d) (e)
364. (a) (b) (c) (d) (e)
365. (a) (b) (c) (d) (e)
366. (a) (b) (c) (d) (e)
367. (a) (b) (c) (d) (e)
368. (a) (b) (c) (d) (e)

Continued

369. ⓐ ⓑ ⓒ ⓓ ⓔ	393. ⓐ ⓑ ⓒ ⓓ ⓔ	417. ⓐ ⓑ ⓒ ⓓ ⓔ	441. ⓐ ⓑ ⓒ ⓓ ⓔ
370. ⓐ ⓑ ⓒ ⓓ ⓔ	394. ⓐ ⓑ ⓒ ⓓ ⓔ	418. ⓐ ⓑ ⓒ ⓓ ⓔ	442. ⓐ ⓑ ⓒ ⓓ ⓔ
371. ⓐ ⓑ ⓒ ⓓ ⓔ	395. ⓐ ⓑ ⓒ ⓓ ⓔ	419. ⓐ ⓑ ⓒ ⓓ ⓔ	443. ⓐ ⓑ ⓒ ⓓ ⓔ
372. ⓐ ⓑ ⓒ ⓓ ⓔ	396. ⓐ ⓑ ⓒ ⓓ ⓔ	420. ⓐ ⓑ ⓒ ⓓ ⓔ	444. ⓐ ⓑ ⓒ ⓓ ⓔ
373. ⓐ ⓑ ⓒ ⓓ ⓔ	397. ⓐ ⓑ ⓒ ⓓ ⓔ	421. ⓐ ⓑ ⓒ ⓓ ⓔ	445. ⓐ ⓑ ⓒ ⓓ ⓔ
374. ⓐ ⓑ ⓒ ⓓ ⓔ	398. ⓐ ⓑ ⓒ ⓓ ⓔ	422. ⓐ ⓑ ⓒ ⓓ ⓔ	446. ⓐ ⓑ ⓒ ⓓ ⓔ
375. ⓐ ⓑ ⓒ ⓓ ⓔ	399. ⓐ ⓑ ⓒ ⓓ ⓔ	423. ⓐ ⓑ ⓒ ⓓ ⓔ	447. ⓐ ⓑ ⓒ ⓓ ⓔ
376. ⓐ ⓑ ⓒ ⓓ ⓔ	400. ⓐ ⓑ ⓒ ⓓ ⓔ	424. ⓐ ⓑ ⓒ ⓓ ⓔ	448. ⓐ ⓑ ⓒ ⓓ ⓔ
377. ⓐ ⓑ ⓒ ⓓ ⓔ	401. ⓐ ⓑ ⓒ ⓓ ⓔ	425. ⓐ ⓑ ⓒ ⓓ ⓔ	449. ⓐ ⓑ ⓒ ⓓ ⓔ
378. ⓐ ⓑ ⓒ ⓓ ⓔ	402. ⓐ ⓑ ⓒ ⓓ ⓔ	426. ⓐ ⓑ ⓒ ⓓ ⓔ	450. ⓐ ⓑ ⓒ ⓓ ⓔ
379. ⓐ ⓑ ⓒ ⓓ ⓔ	403. ⓐ ⓑ ⓒ ⓓ ⓔ	427. ⓐ ⓑ ⓒ ⓓ ⓔ	451. ⓐ ⓑ ⓒ ⓓ ⓔ
380. ⓐ ⓑ ⓒ ⓓ ⓔ	404. ⓐ ⓑ ⓒ ⓓ ⓔ	428. ⓐ ⓑ ⓒ ⓓ ⓔ	452. ⓐ ⓑ ⓒ ⓓ ⓔ
381. ⓐ ⓑ ⓒ ⓓ ⓔ	405. ⓐ ⓑ ⓒ ⓓ ⓔ	429. ⓐ ⓑ ⓒ ⓓ ⓔ	453. ⓐ ⓑ ⓒ ⓓ ⓔ
382. ⓐ ⓑ ⓒ ⓓ ⓔ	406. ⓐ ⓑ ⓒ ⓓ ⓔ	430. ⓐ ⓑ ⓒ ⓓ ⓔ	454. ⓐ ⓑ ⓒ ⓓ ⓔ
383. ⓐ ⓑ ⓒ ⓓ ⓔ	407. ⓐ ⓑ ⓒ ⓓ ⓔ	431. ⓐ ⓑ ⓒ ⓓ ⓔ	455. ⓐ ⓑ ⓒ ⓓ ⓔ
384. ⓐ ⓑ ⓒ ⓓ ⓔ	408. ⓐ ⓑ ⓒ ⓓ ⓔ	432. ⓐ ⓑ ⓒ ⓓ ⓔ	456. ⓐ ⓑ ⓒ ⓓ ⓔ
385. ⓐ ⓑ ⓒ ⓓ ⓔ	409. ⓐ ⓑ ⓒ ⓓ ⓔ	433. ⓐ ⓑ ⓒ ⓓ ⓔ	457. ⓐ ⓑ ⓒ ⓓ ⓔ
386. ⓐ ⓑ ⓒ ⓓ ⓔ	410. ⓐ ⓑ ⓒ ⓓ ⓔ	434. ⓐ ⓑ ⓒ ⓓ ⓔ	458. ⓐ ⓑ ⓒ ⓓ ⓔ
387. ⓐ ⓑ ⓒ ⓓ ⓔ	411. ⓐ ⓑ ⓒ ⓓ ⓔ	435. ⓐ ⓑ ⓒ ⓓ ⓔ	
388. ⓐ ⓑ ⓒ ⓓ ⓔ	412. ⓐ ⓑ ⓒ ⓓ ⓔ	436. ⓐ ⓑ ⓒ ⓓ ⓔ	
389. ⓐ ⓑ ⓒ ⓓ ⓔ	413. ⓐ ⓑ ⓒ ⓓ ⓔ	437. ⓐ ⓑ ⓒ ⓓ ⓔ	
390. ⓐ ⓑ ⓒ ⓓ ⓔ	414. ⓐ ⓑ ⓒ ⓓ ⓔ	438. ⓐ ⓑ ⓒ ⓓ ⓔ	
391. ⓐ ⓑ ⓒ ⓓ ⓔ	415. ⓐ ⓑ ⓒ ⓓ ⓔ	439. ⓐ ⓑ ⓒ ⓓ ⓔ	
392. ⓐ ⓑ ⓒ ⓓ ⓔ	416. ⓐ ⓑ ⓒ ⓓ ⓔ	440. ⓐ ⓑ ⓒ ⓓ ⓔ	

This page intentionally left blank.

Section 4
Microbiology

Fill in a circled letter to indicate your answer choice.

1. ⓐ ⓑ ⓒ ⓓ ⓔ	47. ⓐ ⓑ ⓒ ⓓ ⓔ	93. ⓐ ⓑ ⓒ ⓓ ⓔ	139. ⓐ ⓑ ⓒ ⓓ ⓔ
2. ⓐ ⓑ ⓒ ⓓ ⓔ	48. ⓐ ⓑ ⓒ ⓓ ⓔ	94. ⓐ ⓑ ⓒ ⓓ ⓔ	140. ⓐ ⓑ ⓒ ⓓ ⓔ
3. ⓐ ⓑ ⓒ ⓓ ⓔ	49. ⓐ ⓑ ⓒ ⓓ ⓔ	95. ⓐ ⓑ ⓒ ⓓ ⓔ	141. ⓐ ⓑ ⓒ ⓓ ⓔ
4. ⓐ ⓑ ⓒ ⓓ ⓔ	50. ⓐ ⓑ ⓒ ⓓ ⓔ	96. ⓐ ⓑ ⓒ ⓓ ⓔ	142. ⓐ ⓑ ⓒ ⓓ ⓔ
5. ⓐ ⓑ ⓒ ⓓ ⓔ	51. ⓐ ⓑ ⓒ ⓓ ⓔ	97. ⓐ ⓑ ⓒ ⓓ ⓔ	143. ⓐ ⓑ ⓒ ⓓ ⓔ
6. ⓐ ⓑ ⓒ ⓓ ⓔ	52. ⓐ ⓑ ⓒ ⓓ ⓔ	98. ⓐ ⓑ ⓒ ⓓ ⓔ	144. ⓐ ⓑ ⓒ ⓓ ⓔ
7. ⓐ ⓑ ⓒ ⓓ ⓔ	53. ⓐ ⓑ ⓒ ⓓ ⓔ	99. ⓐ ⓑ ⓒ ⓓ ⓔ	145. ⓐ ⓑ ⓒ ⓓ ⓔ
8. ⓐ ⓑ ⓒ ⓓ ⓔ	54. ⓐ ⓑ ⓒ ⓓ ⓔ	100. ⓐ ⓑ ⓒ ⓓ ⓔ	146. ⓐ ⓑ ⓒ ⓓ ⓔ
9. ⓐ ⓑ ⓒ ⓓ ⓔ	55. ⓐ ⓑ ⓒ ⓓ ⓔ	101. ⓐ ⓑ ⓒ ⓓ ⓔ	147. ⓐ ⓑ ⓒ ⓓ ⓔ
10. ⓐ ⓑ ⓒ ⓓ ⓔ	56. ⓐ ⓑ ⓒ ⓓ ⓔ	102. ⓐ ⓑ ⓒ ⓓ ⓔ	148. ⓐ ⓑ ⓒ ⓓ ⓔ
11. ⓐ ⓑ ⓒ ⓓ ⓔ	57. ⓐ ⓑ ⓒ ⓓ ⓔ	103. ⓐ ⓑ ⓒ ⓓ ⓔ	149. ⓐ ⓑ ⓒ ⓓ ⓔ
12. ⓐ ⓑ ⓒ ⓓ ⓔ	58. ⓐ ⓑ ⓒ ⓓ ⓔ	104. ⓐ ⓑ ⓒ ⓓ ⓔ	150. ⓐ ⓑ ⓒ ⓓ ⓔ
13. ⓐ ⓑ ⓒ ⓓ ⓔ	59. ⓐ ⓑ ⓒ ⓓ ⓔ	105. ⓐ ⓑ ⓒ ⓓ ⓔ	151. ⓐ ⓑ ⓒ ⓓ ⓔ
14. ⓐ ⓑ ⓒ ⓓ ⓔ	60. ⓐ ⓑ ⓒ ⓓ ⓔ	106. ⓐ ⓑ ⓒ ⓓ ⓔ	152. ⓐ ⓑ ⓒ ⓓ ⓔ
15. ⓐ ⓑ ⓒ ⓓ ⓔ	61. ⓐ ⓑ ⓒ ⓓ ⓔ	107. ⓐ ⓑ ⓒ ⓓ ⓔ	153. ⓐ ⓑ ⓒ ⓓ ⓔ
16. ⓐ ⓑ ⓒ ⓓ ⓔ	62. ⓐ ⓑ ⓒ ⓓ ⓔ	108. ⓐ ⓑ ⓒ ⓓ ⓔ	154. ⓐ ⓑ ⓒ ⓓ ⓔ
17. ⓐ ⓑ ⓒ ⓓ ⓔ	63. ⓐ ⓑ ⓒ ⓓ ⓔ	109. ⓐ ⓑ ⓒ ⓓ ⓔ	155. ⓐ ⓑ ⓒ ⓓ ⓔ
18. ⓐ ⓑ ⓒ ⓓ ⓔ	64. ⓐ ⓑ ⓒ ⓓ ⓔ	110. ⓐ ⓑ ⓒ ⓓ ⓔ	156. ⓐ ⓑ ⓒ ⓓ ⓔ
19. ⓐ ⓑ ⓒ ⓓ ⓔ	65. ⓐ ⓑ ⓒ ⓓ ⓔ	111. ⓐ ⓑ ⓒ ⓓ ⓔ	157. ⓐ ⓑ ⓒ ⓓ ⓔ
20. ⓐ ⓑ ⓒ ⓓ ⓔ	66. ⓐ ⓑ ⓒ ⓓ ⓔ	112. ⓐ ⓑ ⓒ ⓓ ⓔ	158. ⓐ ⓑ ⓒ ⓓ ⓔ
21. ⓐ ⓑ ⓒ ⓓ ⓔ	67. ⓐ ⓑ ⓒ ⓓ ⓔ	113. ⓐ ⓑ ⓒ ⓓ ⓔ	159. ⓐ ⓑ ⓒ ⓓ ⓔ
22. ⓐ ⓑ ⓒ ⓓ ⓔ	68. ⓐ ⓑ ⓒ ⓓ ⓔ	114. ⓐ ⓑ ⓒ ⓓ ⓔ	160. ⓐ ⓑ ⓒ ⓓ ⓔ
23. ⓐ ⓑ ⓒ ⓓ ⓔ	69. ⓐ ⓑ ⓒ ⓓ ⓔ	115. ⓐ ⓑ ⓒ ⓓ ⓔ	161. ⓐ ⓑ ⓒ ⓓ ⓔ
24. ⓐ ⓑ ⓒ ⓓ ⓔ	70. ⓐ ⓑ ⓒ ⓓ ⓔ	116. ⓐ ⓑ ⓒ ⓓ ⓔ	162. ⓐ ⓑ ⓒ ⓓ ⓔ
25. ⓐ ⓑ ⓒ ⓓ ⓔ	71. ⓐ ⓑ ⓒ ⓓ ⓔ	117. ⓐ ⓑ ⓒ ⓓ ⓔ	163. ⓐ ⓑ ⓒ ⓓ ⓔ
26. ⓐ ⓑ ⓒ ⓓ ⓔ	72. ⓐ ⓑ ⓒ ⓓ ⓔ	118. ⓐ ⓑ ⓒ ⓓ ⓔ	164. ⓐ ⓑ ⓒ ⓓ ⓔ
27. ⓐ ⓑ ⓒ ⓓ ⓔ	73. ⓐ ⓑ ⓒ ⓓ ⓔ	119. ⓐ ⓑ ⓒ ⓓ ⓔ	165. ⓐ ⓑ ⓒ ⓓ ⓔ
28. ⓐ ⓑ ⓒ ⓓ ⓔ	74. ⓐ ⓑ ⓒ ⓓ ⓔ	120. ⓐ ⓑ ⓒ ⓓ ⓔ	166. ⓐ ⓑ ⓒ ⓓ ⓔ
29. ⓐ ⓑ ⓒ ⓓ ⓔ	75. ⓐ ⓑ ⓒ ⓓ ⓔ	121. ⓐ ⓑ ⓒ ⓓ ⓔ	167. ⓐ ⓑ ⓒ ⓓ ⓔ
30. ⓐ ⓑ ⓒ ⓓ ⓔ	76. ⓐ ⓑ ⓒ ⓓ ⓔ	122. ⓐ ⓑ ⓒ ⓓ ⓔ	168. ⓐ ⓑ ⓒ ⓓ ⓔ
31. ⓐ ⓑ ⓒ ⓓ ⓔ	77. ⓐ ⓑ ⓒ ⓓ ⓔ	123. ⓐ ⓑ ⓒ ⓓ ⓔ	169. ⓐ ⓑ ⓒ ⓓ ⓔ
32. ⓐ ⓑ ⓒ ⓓ ⓔ	78. ⓐ ⓑ ⓒ ⓓ ⓔ	124. ⓐ ⓑ ⓒ ⓓ ⓔ	170. ⓐ ⓑ ⓒ ⓓ ⓔ
33. ⓐ ⓑ ⓒ ⓓ ⓔ	79. ⓐ ⓑ ⓒ ⓓ ⓔ	125. ⓐ ⓑ ⓒ ⓓ ⓔ	171. ⓐ ⓑ ⓒ ⓓ ⓔ
34. ⓐ ⓑ ⓒ ⓓ ⓔ	80. ⓐ ⓑ ⓒ ⓓ ⓔ	126. ⓐ ⓑ ⓒ ⓓ ⓔ	172. ⓐ ⓑ ⓒ ⓓ ⓔ
35. ⓐ ⓑ ⓒ ⓓ ⓔ	81. ⓐ ⓑ ⓒ ⓓ ⓔ	127. ⓐ ⓑ ⓒ ⓓ ⓔ	173. ⓐ ⓑ ⓒ ⓓ ⓔ
36. ⓐ ⓑ ⓒ ⓓ ⓔ	82. ⓐ ⓑ ⓒ ⓓ ⓔ	128. ⓐ ⓑ ⓒ ⓓ ⓔ	174. ⓐ ⓑ ⓒ ⓓ ⓔ
37. ⓐ ⓑ ⓒ ⓓ ⓔ	83. ⓐ ⓑ ⓒ ⓓ ⓔ	129. ⓐ ⓑ ⓒ ⓓ ⓔ	175. ⓐ ⓑ ⓒ ⓓ ⓔ
38. ⓐ ⓑ ⓒ ⓓ ⓔ	84. ⓐ ⓑ ⓒ ⓓ ⓔ	130. ⓐ ⓑ ⓒ ⓓ ⓔ	176. ⓐ ⓑ ⓒ ⓓ ⓔ
39. ⓐ ⓑ ⓒ ⓓ ⓔ	85. ⓐ ⓑ ⓒ ⓓ ⓔ	131. ⓐ ⓑ ⓒ ⓓ ⓔ	177. ⓐ ⓑ ⓒ ⓓ ⓔ
40. ⓐ ⓑ ⓒ ⓓ ⓔ	86. ⓐ ⓑ ⓒ ⓓ ⓔ	132. ⓐ ⓑ ⓒ ⓓ ⓔ	178. ⓐ ⓑ ⓒ ⓓ ⓔ
41. ⓐ ⓑ ⓒ ⓓ ⓔ	87. ⓐ ⓑ ⓒ ⓓ ⓔ	133. ⓐ ⓑ ⓒ ⓓ ⓔ	179. ⓐ ⓑ ⓒ ⓓ ⓔ
42. ⓐ ⓑ ⓒ ⓓ ⓔ	88. ⓐ ⓑ ⓒ ⓓ ⓔ	134. ⓐ ⓑ ⓒ ⓓ ⓔ	180. ⓐ ⓑ ⓒ ⓓ ⓔ
43. ⓐ ⓑ ⓒ ⓓ ⓔ	89. ⓐ ⓑ ⓒ ⓓ ⓔ	135. ⓐ ⓑ ⓒ ⓓ ⓔ	181. ⓐ ⓑ ⓒ ⓓ ⓔ
44. ⓐ ⓑ ⓒ ⓓ ⓔ	90. ⓐ ⓑ ⓒ ⓓ ⓔ	136. ⓐ ⓑ ⓒ ⓓ ⓔ	182. ⓐ ⓑ ⓒ ⓓ ⓔ
45. ⓐ ⓑ ⓒ ⓓ ⓔ	91. ⓐ ⓑ ⓒ ⓓ ⓔ	137. ⓐ ⓑ ⓒ ⓓ ⓔ	183. ⓐ ⓑ ⓒ ⓓ ⓔ
46. ⓐ ⓑ ⓒ ⓓ ⓔ	92. ⓐ ⓑ ⓒ ⓓ ⓔ	138. ⓐ ⓑ ⓒ ⓓ ⓔ	184. ⓐ ⓑ ⓒ ⓓ ⓔ

Continued

185. ⓐ ⓑ ⓒ ⓓ
186. ⓐ ⓑ ⓒ ⓓ
187. ⓐ ⓑ ⓒ ⓓ
188. ⓐ ⓑ ⓒ ⓓ
189. ⓐ ⓑ ⓒ ⓓ ⓔ
190. ⓐ ⓑ ⓒ ⓓ ⓔ
191. ⓐ ⓑ ⓒ ⓓ ⓔ
192. ⓐ ⓑ ⓒ ⓓ ⓔ
193. ⓐ ⓑ ⓒ ⓓ ⓔ
194. ⓐ ⓑ ⓒ ⓓ ⓔ
195. ⓐ ⓑ ⓒ ⓓ ⓔ
196. ⓐ ⓑ ⓒ ⓓ ⓔ
197. ⓐ ⓑ ⓒ ⓓ ⓔ
198. ⓐ ⓑ ⓒ ⓓ ⓔ
199. ⓐ ⓑ ⓒ ⓓ ⓔ
200. ⓐ ⓑ ⓒ ⓓ ⓔ
201. ⓐ ⓑ ⓒ ⓓ ⓔ
202. ⓐ ⓑ ⓒ ⓓ ⓔ

203. ⓐ ⓑ ⓒ ⓓ ⓔ
204. ⓐ ⓑ ⓒ ⓓ ⓔ
205. ⓐ ⓑ ⓒ ⓓ ⓔ
206. ⓐ ⓑ ⓒ ⓓ ⓔ
207. ⓐ ⓑ ⓒ ⓓ ⓔ
208. ⓐ ⓑ ⓒ ⓓ ⓔ
209. ⓐ ⓑ ⓒ ⓓ ⓔ
210. ⓐ ⓑ ⓒ ⓓ
211. ⓐ ⓑ ⓒ ⓓ
212. ⓐ ⓑ ⓒ ⓓ
213. ⓐ ⓑ ⓒ ⓓ
214. ⓐ ⓑ ⓒ ⓓ ⓔ
215. ⓐ ⓑ ⓒ ⓓ ⓔ
216. ⓐ ⓑ ⓒ ⓓ ⓔ
217. ⓐ ⓑ ⓒ ⓓ ⓔ
218. ⓐ ⓑ ⓒ ⓓ
219. ⓐ ⓑ ⓒ ⓓ
220. ⓐ ⓑ ⓒ ⓓ

221. ⓐ ⓑ ⓒ ⓓ
222. ⓐ ⓑ ⓒ ⓓ
223. ⓐ ⓑ ⓒ ⓓ
224. ⓐ ⓑ ⓒ ⓓ
225. ⓐ ⓑ ⓒ ⓓ
226. ⓐ ⓑ ⓒ ⓓ ⓔ
227. ⓐ ⓑ ⓒ ⓓ ⓔ
228. ⓐ ⓑ ⓒ ⓓ ⓔ
229. ⓐ ⓑ ⓒ ⓓ ⓔ
230. ⓐ ⓑ ⓒ ⓓ ⓔ
231. ⓐ ⓑ ⓒ ⓓ ⓔ
232. ⓐ ⓑ ⓒ ⓓ ⓔ
233. ⓐ ⓑ ⓒ ⓓ ⓔ
234. ⓐ ⓑ ⓒ ⓓ ⓔ
235. ⓐ ⓑ ⓒ ⓓ ⓔ
236. ⓐ ⓑ ⓒ ⓓ ⓔ
237. ⓐ ⓑ ⓒ ⓓ ⓔ
238. ⓐ ⓑ ⓒ ⓓ ⓔ

239. ⓐ ⓑ ⓒ ⓓ ⓔ
240. ⓐ ⓑ ⓒ ⓓ ⓔ
241. ⓐ ⓑ ⓒ ⓓ ⓔ
242. ⓐ ⓑ ⓒ ⓓ ⓔ
243. ⓐ ⓑ ⓒ ⓓ ⓔ
244. ⓐ ⓑ ⓒ ⓓ ⓔ
245. ⓐ ⓑ ⓒ ⓓ ⓔ
246. ⓐ ⓑ ⓒ ⓓ ⓔ
247. ⓐ ⓑ ⓒ ⓓ ⓔ
248. ⓐ ⓑ ⓒ ⓓ ⓔ
249. ⓐ ⓑ ⓒ ⓓ ⓔ
250. ⓐ ⓑ ⓒ ⓓ ⓔ
251. ⓐ ⓑ ⓒ ⓓ ⓔ
252. ⓐ ⓑ ⓒ ⓓ ⓔ

Section 5
Microscopic Anatomy

Fill in a circled letter to indicate your answer choice.

1. ⓐ ⓑ ⓒ ⓓ ⓔ	29. ⓐ ⓑ ⓒ ⓓ ⓔ	57. ⓐ ⓑ ⓒ ⓓ ⓔ	85. ⓐ ⓑ ⓒ ⓓ ⓔ
2. ⓐ ⓑ ⓒ ⓓ ⓔ	30. ⓐ ⓑ ⓒ ⓓ ⓔ	58. ⓐ ⓑ ⓒ ⓓ ⓔ	86. ⓐ ⓑ ⓒ ⓓ ⓔ
3. ⓐ ⓑ ⓒ ⓓ ⓔ	31. ⓐ ⓑ ⓒ ⓓ ⓔ	59. ⓐ ⓑ ⓒ ⓓ ⓔ	87. ⓐ ⓑ ⓒ ⓓ ⓔ
4. ⓐ ⓑ ⓒ ⓓ ⓔ	32. ⓐ ⓑ ⓒ ⓓ ⓔ	60. ⓐ ⓑ ⓒ ⓓ ⓔ	88. ⓐ ⓑ ⓒ ⓓ ⓔ
5. ⓐ ⓑ ⓒ ⓓ ⓔ	33. ⓐ ⓑ ⓒ ⓓ ⓔ	61. ⓐ ⓑ ⓒ ⓓ ⓔ	89. ⓐ ⓑ ⓒ ⓓ ⓔ
6. ⓐ ⓑ ⓒ ⓓ ⓔ	34. ⓐ ⓑ ⓒ ⓓ ⓔ	62. ⓐ ⓑ ⓒ ⓓ ⓔ	90. ⓐ ⓑ ⓒ ⓓ ⓔ
7. ⓐ ⓑ ⓒ ⓓ ⓔ	35. ⓐ ⓑ ⓒ ⓓ ⓔ	63. ⓐ ⓑ ⓒ ⓓ ⓔ	91. ⓐ ⓑ ⓒ ⓓ ⓔ
8. ⓐ ⓑ ⓒ ⓓ ⓔ	36. ⓐ ⓑ ⓒ ⓓ ⓔ	64. ⓐ ⓑ ⓒ ⓓ ⓔ	92. ⓐ ⓑ ⓒ ⓓ ⓔ
9. ⓐ ⓑ ⓒ ⓓ ⓔ	37. ⓐ ⓑ ⓒ ⓓ ⓔ	65. ⓐ ⓑ ⓒ ⓓ ⓔ	93. ⓐ ⓑ ⓒ ⓓ ⓔ
10. ⓐ ⓑ ⓒ ⓓ ⓔ	38. ⓐ ⓑ ⓒ ⓓ ⓔ	66. ⓐ ⓑ ⓒ ⓓ ⓔ	94. ⓐ ⓑ ⓒ ⓓ ⓔ
11. ⓐ ⓑ ⓒ ⓓ ⓔ	39. ⓐ ⓑ ⓒ ⓓ ⓔ	67. ⓐ ⓑ ⓒ ⓓ ⓔ	95. ⓐ ⓑ ⓒ ⓓ ⓔ
12. ⓐ ⓑ ⓒ ⓓ ⓔ	40. ⓐ ⓑ ⓒ ⓓ ⓔ	68. ⓐ ⓑ ⓒ ⓓ ⓔ	96. ⓐ ⓑ ⓒ ⓓ ⓔ
13. ⓐ ⓑ ⓒ ⓓ ⓔ	41. ⓐ ⓑ ⓒ ⓓ ⓔ	69. ⓐ ⓑ ⓒ ⓓ ⓔ	97. ⓐ ⓑ ⓒ ⓓ ⓔ
14. ⓐ ⓑ ⓒ ⓓ ⓔ	42. ⓐ ⓑ ⓒ ⓓ ⓔ	70. ⓐ ⓑ ⓒ ⓓ ⓔ	98. ⓐ ⓑ ⓒ ⓓ ⓔ
15. ⓐ ⓑ ⓒ ⓓ ⓔ	43. ⓐ ⓑ ⓒ ⓓ ⓔ	71. ⓐ ⓑ ⓒ ⓓ ⓔ	99. ⓐ ⓑ ⓒ ⓓ ⓔ
16. ⓐ ⓑ ⓒ ⓓ ⓔ	44. ⓐ ⓑ ⓒ ⓓ ⓔ	72. ⓐ ⓑ ⓒ ⓓ ⓔ	100. ⓐ ⓑ ⓒ ⓓ ⓔ
17. ⓐ ⓑ ⓒ ⓓ ⓔ	45. ⓐ ⓑ ⓒ ⓓ ⓔ	73. ⓐ ⓑ ⓒ ⓓ ⓔ	101. ⓐ ⓑ ⓒ ⓓ ⓔ
18. ⓐ ⓑ ⓒ ⓓ ⓔ	46. ⓐ ⓑ ⓒ ⓓ ⓔ	74. ⓐ ⓑ ⓒ ⓓ ⓔ	102. ⓐ ⓑ ⓒ ⓓ ⓔ
19. ⓐ ⓑ ⓒ ⓓ ⓔ	47. ⓐ ⓑ ⓒ ⓓ ⓔ	75. ⓐ ⓑ ⓒ ⓓ ⓔ	103. ⓐ ⓑ ⓒ ⓓ ⓔ
20. ⓐ ⓑ ⓒ ⓓ ⓔ	48. ⓐ ⓑ ⓒ ⓓ ⓔ	76. ⓐ ⓑ ⓒ ⓓ ⓔ	104. ⓐ ⓑ ⓒ ⓓ ⓔ
21. ⓐ ⓑ ⓒ ⓓ ⓔ	49. ⓐ ⓑ ⓒ ⓓ ⓔ	77. ⓐ ⓑ ⓒ ⓓ ⓔ	105. ⓐ ⓑ ⓒ ⓓ ⓔ
22. ⓐ ⓑ ⓒ ⓓ ⓔ	50. ⓐ ⓑ ⓒ ⓓ ⓔ	78. ⓐ ⓑ ⓒ ⓓ ⓔ	106. ⓐ ⓑ ⓒ ⓓ ⓔ
23. ⓐ ⓑ ⓒ ⓓ ⓔ	51. ⓐ ⓑ ⓒ ⓓ ⓔ	79. ⓐ ⓑ ⓒ ⓓ ⓔ	107. ⓐ ⓑ ⓒ ⓓ ⓔ
24. ⓐ ⓑ ⓒ ⓓ ⓔ	52. ⓐ ⓑ ⓒ ⓓ ⓔ	80. ⓐ ⓑ ⓒ ⓓ ⓔ	108. ⓐ ⓑ ⓒ ⓓ ⓔ
25. ⓐ ⓑ ⓒ ⓓ ⓔ	53. ⓐ ⓑ ⓒ ⓓ ⓔ	81. ⓐ ⓑ ⓒ ⓓ ⓔ	109. ⓐ ⓑ ⓒ ⓓ ⓔ
26. ⓐ ⓑ ⓒ ⓓ ⓔ	54. ⓐ ⓑ ⓒ ⓓ ⓔ	82. ⓐ ⓑ ⓒ ⓓ ⓔ	110. ⓐ ⓑ ⓒ ⓓ ⓔ
27. ⓐ ⓑ ⓒ ⓓ ⓔ	55. ⓐ ⓑ ⓒ ⓓ ⓔ	83. ⓐ ⓑ ⓒ ⓓ ⓔ	
28. ⓐ ⓑ ⓒ ⓓ ⓔ	56. ⓐ ⓑ ⓒ ⓓ ⓔ	84. ⓐ ⓑ ⓒ ⓓ ⓔ	

This page intentionally left blank.

Section 6

Neuroanatomy

Fill in a circled letter to indicate your answer choice.

1. ⓐ ⓑ ⓒ ⓓ ⓔ	15. ⓐ ⓑ ⓒ ⓓ ⓔ	29. ⓐ ⓑ ⓒ ⓓ ⓔ	43. ⓐ ⓑ ⓒ ⓓ ⓔ
2. ⓐ ⓑ ⓒ ⓓ ⓔ	16. ⓐ ⓑ ⓒ ⓓ ⓔ	30. ⓐ ⓑ ⓒ ⓓ ⓔ	44. ⓐ ⓑ ⓒ ⓓ ⓔ
3. ⓐ ⓑ ⓒ ⓓ ⓔ	17. ⓐ ⓑ ⓒ ⓓ ⓔ	31. ⓐ ⓑ ⓒ ⓓ ⓔ	45. ⓐ ⓑ ⓒ ⓓ ⓔ
4. ⓐ ⓑ ⓒ ⓓ ⓔ	18. ⓐ ⓑ ⓒ ⓓ ⓔ	32. ⓐ ⓑ ⓒ ⓓ ⓔ	46. ⓐ ⓑ ⓒ ⓓ ⓔ
5. ⓐ ⓑ ⓒ ⓓ ⓔ	19. ⓐ ⓑ ⓒ ⓓ ⓔ	33. ⓐ ⓑ ⓒ ⓓ ⓔ	47. ⓐ ⓑ ⓒ ⓓ ⓔ
6. ⓐ ⓑ ⓒ ⓓ ⓔ	20. ⓐ ⓑ ⓒ ⓓ ⓔ	34. ⓐ ⓑ ⓒ ⓓ ⓔ	48. ⓐ ⓑ ⓒ ⓓ ⓔ
7. ⓐ ⓑ ⓒ ⓓ ⓔ	21. ⓐ ⓑ ⓒ ⓓ ⓔ	35. ⓐ ⓑ ⓒ ⓓ ⓔ	49. ⓐ ⓑ ⓒ ⓓ ⓔ
8. ⓐ ⓑ ⓒ ⓓ ⓔ	22. ⓐ ⓑ ⓒ ⓓ ⓔ	36. ⓐ ⓑ ⓒ ⓓ ⓔ	50. ⓐ ⓑ ⓒ ⓓ ⓔ
9. ⓐ ⓑ ⓒ ⓓ ⓔ	23. ⓐ ⓑ ⓒ ⓓ ⓔ	37. ⓐ ⓑ ⓒ ⓓ ⓔ	
10. ⓐ ⓑ ⓒ ⓓ ⓔ	24. ⓐ ⓑ ⓒ ⓓ ⓔ	38. ⓐ ⓑ ⓒ ⓓ ⓔ	
11. ⓐ ⓑ ⓒ ⓓ ⓔ	25. ⓐ ⓑ ⓒ ⓓ ⓔ	39. ⓐ ⓑ ⓒ ⓓ ⓔ	
12. ⓐ ⓑ ⓒ ⓓ ⓔ	26. ⓐ ⓑ ⓒ ⓓ ⓔ	40. ⓐ ⓑ ⓒ ⓓ ⓔ	
13. ⓐ ⓑ ⓒ ⓓ ⓔ	27. ⓐ ⓑ ⓒ ⓓ ⓔ	41. ⓐ ⓑ ⓒ ⓓ ⓔ	
14. ⓐ ⓑ ⓒ ⓓ ⓔ	28. ⓐ ⓑ ⓒ ⓓ ⓔ	42. ⓐ ⓑ ⓒ ⓓ ⓔ	

This page intentionally left blank.

Section 7
Parasitology

Fill in a circled letter to indicate your answer choice.

1. ⓐ ⓑ ⓒ ⓓ ⓔ	47. ⓐ ⓑ ⓒ ⓓ ⓔ	93. ⓐ ⓑ ⓒ ⓓ ⓔ	139. ⓐ ⓑ ⓒ ⓓ ⓔ
2. ⓐ ⓑ ⓒ ⓓ ⓔ	48. ⓐ ⓑ ⓒ ⓓ ⓔ	94. ⓐ ⓑ ⓒ ⓓ ⓔ	140. ⓐ ⓑ ⓒ ⓓ ⓔ
3. ⓐ ⓑ ⓒ ⓓ ⓔ	49. ⓐ ⓑ ⓒ ⓓ ⓔ	95. ⓐ ⓑ ⓒ ⓓ ⓔ	141. ⓐ ⓑ ⓒ ⓓ ⓔ
4. ⓐ ⓑ ⓒ ⓓ ⓔ	50. ⓐ ⓑ ⓒ ⓓ ⓔ	96. ⓐ ⓑ ⓒ ⓓ ⓔ	142. ⓐ ⓑ ⓒ ⓓ ⓔ
5. ⓐ ⓑ ⓒ ⓓ ⓔ	51. ⓐ ⓑ ⓒ ⓓ ⓔ	97. ⓐ ⓑ ⓒ ⓓ ⓔ	143. ⓐ ⓑ ⓒ ⓓ ⓔ
6. ⓐ ⓑ ⓒ ⓓ ⓔ	52. ⓐ ⓑ ⓒ ⓓ ⓔ	98. ⓐ ⓑ ⓒ ⓓ ⓔ	144. ⓐ ⓑ ⓒ ⓓ ⓔ
7. ⓐ ⓑ ⓒ ⓓ ⓔ	53. ⓐ ⓑ ⓒ ⓓ ⓔ	99. ⓐ ⓑ ⓒ ⓓ ⓔ	145. ⓐ ⓑ ⓒ ⓓ ⓔ
8. ⓐ ⓑ ⓒ ⓓ ⓔ	54. ⓐ ⓑ ⓒ ⓓ ⓔ	100. ⓐ ⓑ ⓒ ⓓ ⓔ	146. ⓐ ⓑ ⓒ ⓓ ⓔ
9. ⓐ ⓑ ⓒ ⓓ ⓔ	55. ⓐ ⓑ ⓒ ⓓ ⓔ	101. ⓐ ⓑ ⓒ ⓓ ⓔ	147. ⓐ ⓑ ⓒ ⓓ ⓔ
10. ⓐ ⓑ ⓒ ⓓ ⓔ	56. ⓐ ⓑ ⓒ ⓓ ⓔ	102. ⓐ ⓑ ⓒ ⓓ ⓔ	148. ⓐ ⓑ ⓒ ⓓ ⓔ
11. ⓐ ⓑ ⓒ ⓓ ⓔ	57. ⓐ ⓑ ⓒ ⓓ ⓔ	103. ⓐ ⓑ ⓒ ⓓ ⓔ	149. ⓐ ⓑ ⓒ ⓓ ⓔ
12. ⓐ ⓑ ⓒ ⓓ ⓔ	58. ⓐ ⓑ ⓒ ⓓ ⓔ	104. ⓐ ⓑ ⓒ ⓓ ⓔ	150. ⓐ ⓑ ⓒ ⓓ ⓔ
13. ⓐ ⓑ ⓒ ⓓ ⓔ	59. ⓐ ⓑ ⓒ ⓓ ⓔ	105. ⓐ ⓑ ⓒ ⓓ ⓔ	151. ⓐ ⓑ ⓒ ⓓ ⓔ
14. ⓐ ⓑ ⓒ ⓓ ⓔ	60. ⓐ ⓑ ⓒ ⓓ ⓔ	106. ⓐ ⓑ ⓒ ⓓ ⓔ	152. ⓐ ⓑ ⓒ ⓓ ⓔ
15. ⓐ ⓑ ⓒ ⓓ ⓔ	61. ⓐ ⓑ ⓒ ⓓ ⓔ	107. ⓐ ⓑ ⓒ ⓓ ⓔ	153. ⓐ ⓑ ⓒ ⓓ ⓔ
16. ⓐ ⓑ ⓒ ⓓ ⓔ	62. ⓐ ⓑ ⓒ ⓓ ⓔ	108. ⓐ ⓑ ⓒ ⓓ ⓔ	154. ⓐ ⓑ ⓒ ⓓ ⓔ
17. ⓐ ⓑ ⓒ ⓓ ⓔ	63. ⓐ ⓑ ⓒ ⓓ ⓔ	109. ⓐ ⓑ ⓒ ⓓ ⓔ	155. ⓐ ⓑ ⓒ ⓓ ⓔ
18. ⓐ ⓑ ⓒ ⓓ ⓔ	64. ⓐ ⓑ ⓒ ⓓ ⓔ	110. ⓐ ⓑ ⓒ ⓓ ⓔ	156. ⓐ ⓑ ⓒ ⓓ ⓔ
19. ⓐ ⓑ ⓒ ⓓ ⓔ	65. ⓐ ⓑ ⓒ ⓓ ⓔ	111. ⓐ ⓑ ⓒ ⓓ ⓔ	157. ⓐ ⓑ ⓒ ⓓ ⓔ
20. ⓐ ⓑ ⓒ ⓓ ⓔ	66. ⓐ ⓑ ⓒ ⓓ ⓔ	112. ⓐ ⓑ ⓒ ⓓ ⓔ	158. ⓐ ⓑ ⓒ ⓓ ⓔ
21. ⓐ ⓑ ⓒ ⓓ ⓔ	67. ⓐ ⓑ ⓒ ⓓ ⓔ	113. ⓐ ⓑ ⓒ ⓓ ⓔ	159. ⓐ ⓑ ⓒ ⓓ ⓔ
22. ⓐ ⓑ ⓒ ⓓ ⓔ	68. ⓐ ⓑ ⓒ ⓓ ⓔ	114. ⓐ ⓑ ⓒ ⓓ ⓔ	160. ⓐ ⓑ ⓒ ⓓ ⓔ
23. ⓐ ⓑ ⓒ ⓓ ⓔ	69. ⓐ ⓑ ⓒ ⓓ ⓔ	115. ⓐ ⓑ ⓒ ⓓ ⓔ	161. ⓐ ⓑ ⓒ ⓓ ⓔ
24. ⓐ ⓑ ⓒ ⓓ ⓔ	70. ⓐ ⓑ ⓒ ⓓ ⓔ	116. ⓐ ⓑ ⓒ ⓓ ⓔ	162. ⓐ ⓑ ⓒ ⓓ ⓔ
25. ⓐ ⓑ ⓒ ⓓ ⓔ	71. ⓐ ⓑ ⓒ ⓓ ⓔ	117. ⓐ ⓑ ⓒ ⓓ ⓔ	163. ⓐ ⓑ ⓒ ⓓ ⓔ
26. ⓐ ⓑ ⓒ ⓓ ⓔ	72. ⓐ ⓑ ⓒ ⓓ ⓔ	118. ⓐ ⓑ ⓒ ⓓ ⓔ	164. ⓐ ⓑ ⓒ ⓓ ⓔ
27. ⓐ ⓑ ⓒ ⓓ ⓔ	73. ⓐ ⓑ ⓒ ⓓ ⓔ	119. ⓐ ⓑ ⓒ ⓓ ⓔ	165. ⓐ ⓑ ⓒ ⓓ ⓔ
28. ⓐ ⓑ ⓒ ⓓ ⓔ	74. ⓐ ⓑ ⓒ ⓓ ⓔ	120. ⓐ ⓑ ⓒ ⓓ ⓔ	166. ⓐ ⓑ ⓒ ⓓ ⓔ
29. ⓐ ⓑ ⓒ ⓓ ⓔ	75. ⓐ ⓑ ⓒ ⓓ ⓔ	121. ⓐ ⓑ ⓒ ⓓ ⓔ	167. ⓐ ⓑ ⓒ ⓓ ⓔ
30. ⓐ ⓑ ⓒ ⓓ ⓔ	76. ⓐ ⓑ ⓒ ⓓ ⓔ	122. ⓐ ⓑ ⓒ ⓓ ⓔ	168. ⓐ ⓑ ⓒ ⓓ ⓔ
31. ⓐ ⓑ ⓒ ⓓ ⓔ	77. ⓐ ⓑ ⓒ ⓓ ⓔ	123. ⓐ ⓑ ⓒ ⓓ ⓔ	169. ⓐ ⓑ ⓒ ⓓ ⓔ
32. ⓐ ⓑ ⓒ ⓓ ⓔ	78. ⓐ ⓑ ⓒ ⓓ ⓔ	124. ⓐ ⓑ ⓒ ⓓ ⓔ	170. ⓐ ⓑ ⓒ ⓓ ⓔ
33. ⓐ ⓑ ⓒ ⓓ ⓔ	79. ⓐ ⓑ ⓒ ⓓ ⓔ	125. ⓐ ⓑ ⓒ ⓓ ⓔ	171. ⓐ ⓑ ⓒ ⓓ ⓔ
34. ⓐ ⓑ ⓒ ⓓ ⓔ	80. ⓐ ⓑ ⓒ ⓓ ⓔ	126. ⓐ ⓑ ⓒ ⓓ ⓔ	172. ⓐ ⓑ ⓒ ⓓ ⓔ
35. ⓐ ⓑ ⓒ ⓓ ⓔ	81. ⓐ ⓑ ⓒ ⓓ ⓔ	127. ⓐ ⓑ ⓒ ⓓ ⓔ	173. ⓐ ⓑ ⓒ ⓓ ⓔ
36. ⓐ ⓑ ⓒ ⓓ ⓔ	82. ⓐ ⓑ ⓒ ⓓ ⓔ	128. ⓐ ⓑ ⓒ ⓓ ⓔ	174. ⓐ ⓑ ⓒ ⓓ ⓔ
37. ⓐ ⓑ ⓒ ⓓ ⓔ	83. ⓐ ⓑ ⓒ ⓓ ⓔ	129. ⓐ ⓑ ⓒ ⓓ ⓔ	175. ⓐ ⓑ ⓒ ⓓ ⓔ
38. ⓐ ⓑ ⓒ ⓓ ⓔ	84. ⓐ ⓑ ⓒ ⓓ ⓔ	130. ⓐ ⓑ ⓒ ⓓ ⓔ	176. ⓐ ⓑ ⓒ ⓓ ⓔ
39. ⓐ ⓑ ⓒ ⓓ ⓔ	85. ⓐ ⓑ ⓒ ⓓ ⓔ	131. ⓐ ⓑ ⓒ ⓓ ⓔ	177. ⓐ ⓑ ⓒ ⓓ ⓔ
40. ⓐ ⓑ ⓒ ⓓ ⓔ	86. ⓐ ⓑ ⓒ ⓓ ⓔ	132. ⓐ ⓑ ⓒ ⓓ ⓔ	178. ⓐ ⓑ ⓒ ⓓ ⓔ
41. ⓐ ⓑ ⓒ ⓓ ⓔ	87. ⓐ ⓑ ⓒ ⓓ ⓔ	133. ⓐ ⓑ ⓒ ⓓ ⓔ	179. ⓐ ⓑ ⓒ ⓓ ⓔ
42. ⓐ ⓑ ⓒ ⓓ ⓔ	88. ⓐ ⓑ ⓒ ⓓ ⓔ	134. ⓐ ⓑ ⓒ ⓓ ⓔ	180. ⓐ ⓑ ⓒ ⓓ ⓔ
43. ⓐ ⓑ ⓒ ⓓ ⓔ	89. ⓐ ⓑ ⓒ ⓓ ⓔ	135. ⓐ ⓑ ⓒ ⓓ ⓔ	181. ⓐ ⓑ ⓒ ⓓ ⓔ
44. ⓐ ⓑ ⓒ ⓓ ⓔ	90. ⓐ ⓑ ⓒ ⓓ ⓔ	136. ⓐ ⓑ ⓒ ⓓ ⓔ	182. ⓐ ⓑ ⓒ ⓓ ⓔ
45. ⓐ ⓑ ⓒ ⓓ ⓔ	91. ⓐ ⓑ ⓒ ⓓ ⓔ	137. ⓐ ⓑ ⓒ ⓓ ⓔ	183. ⓐ ⓑ ⓒ ⓓ ⓔ
46. ⓐ ⓑ ⓒ ⓓ ⓔ	92. ⓐ ⓑ ⓒ ⓓ ⓔ	138. ⓐ ⓑ ⓒ ⓓ ⓔ	184. ⓐ ⓑ ⓒ ⓓ ⓔ

Continued

185. ⓐ ⓑ ⓒ ⓓ ⓔ   189. ⓐ ⓑ ⓒ ⓓ ⓔ   193. ⓐ ⓑ ⓒ ⓓ ⓔ   197. ⓐ ⓑ ⓒ ⓓ ⓔ
186. ⓐ ⓑ ⓒ ⓓ ⓔ   190. ⓐ ⓑ ⓒ ⓓ ⓔ   194. ⓐ ⓑ ⓒ ⓓ ⓔ   198. ⓐ ⓑ ⓒ ⓓ ⓔ
187. ⓐ ⓑ ⓒ ⓓ ⓔ   191. ⓐ ⓑ ⓒ ⓓ ⓔ   195. ⓐ ⓑ ⓒ ⓓ ⓔ   199. ⓐ ⓑ ⓒ ⓓ ⓔ
188. ⓐ ⓑ ⓒ ⓓ ⓔ   192. ⓐ ⓑ ⓒ ⓓ ⓔ   196. ⓐ ⓑ ⓒ ⓓ ⓔ   200. ⓐ ⓑ ⓒ ⓓ ⓔ

Section 8
Pathology

Fill in a circled letter to indicate your answer choice.

1. (a) (b) (c) (d) (e)	47. (a) (b) (c) (d) (e)	93. (a) (b) (c) (d) (e)	139. (a) (b) (c) (d) (e)
2. (a) (b) (c) (d) (e)	48. (a) (b) (c) (d) (e)	94. (a) (b) (c) (d) (e)	140. (a) (b) (c) (d) (e)
3. (a) (b) (c) (d) (e)	49. (a) (b) (c) (d) (e)	95. (a) (b) (c) (d) (e)	141. (a) (b) (c) (d) (e)
4. (a) (b) (c) (d) (e)	50. (a) (b) (c) (d) (e)	96. (a) (b) (c) (d) (e)	142. (a) (b) (c) (d) (e)
5. (a) (b) (c) (d) (e)	51. (a) (b) (c) (d) (e)	97. (a) (b) (c) (d) (e)	143. (a) (b) (c) (d) (e)
6. (a) (b) (c) (d) (e)	52. (a) (b) (c) (d) (e)	98. (a) (b) (c) (d) (e)	144. (a) (b) (c) (d) (e)
7. (a) (b) (c) (d) (e)	53. (a) (b) (c) (d) (e)	99. (a) (b) (c) (d) (e)	145. (a) (b) (c) (d) (e)
8. (a) (b) (c) (d) (e)	54. (a) (b) (c) (d) (e)	100. (a) (b) (c) (d) (e)	146. (a) (b) (c) (d) (e)
9. (a) (b) (c) (d) (e)	55. (a) (b) (c) (d) (e)	101. (a) (b) (c) (d) (e)	147. (a) (b) (c) (d) (e)
10. (a) (b) (c) (d) (e)	56. (a) (b) (c) (d) (e)	102. (a) (b) (c) (d) (e)	148. (a) (b) (c) (d) (e)
11. (a) (b) (c) (d) (e)	57. (a) (b) (c) (d) (e)	103. (a) (b) (c) (d) (e)	149. (a) (b) (c) (d) (e)
12. (a) (b) (c) (d) (e)	58. (a) (b) (c) (d) (e)	104. (a) (b) (c) (d) (e)	150. (a) (b) (c) (d) (e)
13. (a) (b) (c) (d) (e)	59. (a) (b) (c) (d) (e)	105. (a) (b) (c) (d) (e)	151. (a) (b) (c) (d) (e)
14. (a) (b) (c) (d) (e)	60. (a) (b) (c) (d) (e)	106. (a) (b) (c) (d) (e)	152. (a) (b) (c) (d) (e)
15. (a) (b) (c) (d) (e)	61. (a) (b) (c) (d) (e)	107. (a) (b) (c) (d) (e)	153. (a) (b) (c) (d) (e)
16. (a) (b) (c) (d) (e)	62. (a) (b) (c) (d) (e)	108. (a) (b) (c) (d) (e)	154. (a) (b) (c) (d) (e)
17. (a) (b) (c) (d) (e)	63. (a) (b) (c) (d) (e)	109. (a) (b) (c) (d) (e)	155. (a) (b) (c) (d) (e)
18. (a) (b) (c) (d) (e)	64. (a) (b) (c) (d) (e)	110. (a) (b) (c) (d) (e)	156. (a) (b) (c) (d) (e)
19. (a) (b) (c) (d) (e)	65. (a) (b) (c) (d) (e)	111. (a) (b) (c) (d) (e)	157. (a) (b) (c) (d) (e)
20. (a) (b) (c) (d) (e)	66. (a) (b) (c) (d) (e)	112. (a) (b) (c) (d) (e)	158. (a) (b) (c) (d) (e)
21. (a) (b) (c) (d) (e)	67. (a) (b) (c) (d) (e)	113. (a) (b) (c) (d) (e)	159. (a) (b) (c) (d) (e)
22. (a) (b) (c) (d) (e)	68. (a) (b) (c) (d) (e)	114. (a) (b) (c) (d) (e)	160. (a) (b) (c) (d) (e)
23. (a) (b) (c) (d) (e)	69. (a) (b) (c) (d) (e)	115. (a) (b) (c) (d) (e)	161. (a) (b) (c) (d) (e)
24. (a) (b) (c) (d) (e)	70. (a) (b) (c) (d) (e)	116. (a) (b) (c) (d) (e)	162. (a) (b) (c) (d) (e)
25. (a) (b) (c) (d) (e)	71. (a) (b) (c) (d) (e)	117. (a) (b) (c) (d) (e)	163. (a) (b) (c) (d) (e)
26. (a) (b) (c) (d) (e)	72. (a) (b) (c) (d) (e)	118. (a) (b) (c) (d) (e)	164. (a) (b) (c) (d) (e)
27. (a) (b) (c) (d) (e)	73. (a) (b) (c) (d) (e)	119. (a) (b) (c) (d) (e)	165. (a) (b) (c) (d) (e)
28. (a) (b) (c) (d) (e)	74. (a) (b) (c) (d) (e)	120. (a) (b) (c) (d) (e)	166. (a) (b) (c) (d) (e)
29. (a) (b) (c) (d) (e)	75. (a) (b) (c) (d) (e)	121. (a) (b) (c) (d) (e)	167. (a) (b) (c) (d) (e)
30. (a) (b) (c) (d) (e)	76. (a) (b) (c) (d) (e)	122. (a) (b) (c) (d) (e)	168. (a) (b) (c) (d) (e)
31. (a) (b) (c) (d) (e)	77. (a) (b) (c) (d) (e)	123. (a) (b) (c) (d) (e)	169. (a) (b) (c) (d) (e)
32. (a) (b) (c) (d) (e)	78. (a) (b) (c) (d) (e)	124. (a) (b) (c) (d) (e)	170. (a) (b) (c) (d) (e)
33. (a) (b) (c) (d) (e)	79. (a) (b) (c) (d) (e)	125. (a) (b) (c) (d) (e)	171. (a) (b) (c) (d) (e)
34. (a) (b) (c) (d) (e)	80. (a) (b) (c) (d) (e)	126. (a) (b) (c) (d) (e)	172. (a) (b) (c) (d) (e)
35. (a) (b) (c) (d) (e)	81. (a) (b) (c) (d) (e)	127. (a) (b) (c) (d) (e)	173. (a) (b) (c) (d) (e)
36. (a) (b) (c) (d) (e)	82. (a) (b) (c) (d) (e)	128. (a) (b) (c) (d) (e)	174. (a) (b) (c) (d) (e)
37. (a) (b) (c) (d) (e)	83. (a) (b) (c) (d) (e)	129. (a) (b) (c) (d) (e)	175. (a) (b) (c) (d) (e)
38. (a) (b) (c) (d) (e)	84. (a) (b) (c) (d) (e)	130. (a) (b) (c) (d) (e)	176. (a) (b) (c) (d) (e)
39. (a) (b) (c) (d) (e)	85. (a) (b) (c) (d) (e)	131. (a) (b) (c) (d) (e)	177. (a) (b) (c) (d) (e)
40. (a) (b) (c) (d) (e)	86. (a) (b) (c) (d) (e)	132. (a) (b) (c) (d) (e)	178. (a) (b) (c) (d) (e)
41. (a) (b) (c) (d) (e)	87. (a) (b) (c) (d) (e)	133. (a) (b) (c) (d) (e)	179. (a) (b) (c) (d) (e)
42. (a) (b) (c) (d) (e)	88. (a) (b) (c) (d) (e)	134. (a) (b) (c) (d) (e)	180. (a) (b) (c) (d) (e)
43. (a) (b) (c) (d) (e)	89. (a) (b) (c) (d) (e)	135. (a) (b) (c) (d) (e)	181. (a) (b) (c) (d) (e)
44. (a) (b) (c) (d) (e)	90. (a) (b) (c) (d) (e)	136. (a) (b) (c) (d) (e)	182. (a) (b) (c) (d) (e)
45. (a) (b) (c) (d) (e)	91. (a) (b) (c) (d) (e)	137. (a) (b) (c) (d) (e)	183. (a) (b) (c) (d) (e)
46. (a) (b) (c) (d) (e)	92. (a) (b) (c) (d) (e)	138. (a) (b) (c) (d) (e)	184. (a) (b) (c) (d) (e)

Continued

185. ⓐ ⓑ ⓒ ⓓ ⓔ
186. ⓐ ⓑ ⓒ ⓓ ⓔ
187. ⓐ ⓑ ⓒ ⓓ ⓔ
188. ⓐ ⓑ ⓒ ⓓ ⓔ
189. ⓐ ⓑ ⓒ ⓓ ⓔ
190. ⓐ ⓑ ⓒ ⓓ ⓔ

191. ⓐ ⓑ ⓒ ⓓ ⓔ
192. ⓐ ⓑ ⓒ ⓓ ⓔ
193. ⓐ ⓑ ⓒ ⓓ ⓔ
194. ⓐ ⓑ ⓒ ⓓ ⓔ
195. ⓐ ⓑ ⓒ ⓓ ⓔ
196. ⓐ ⓑ ⓒ ⓓ ⓔ

197. ⓐ ⓑ ⓒ ⓓ ⓔ
198. ⓐ ⓑ ⓒ ⓓ ⓔ
199. ⓐ ⓑ ⓒ ⓓ ⓔ
200. ⓐ ⓑ ⓒ ⓓ ⓔ
201. ⓐ ⓑ ⓒ ⓓ ⓔ
202. ⓐ ⓑ ⓒ ⓓ ⓔ

203. ⓐ ⓑ ⓒ ⓓ ⓔ
204. ⓐ ⓑ ⓒ ⓓ ⓔ
205. ⓐ ⓑ ⓒ ⓓ ⓔ
206. ⓐ ⓑ ⓒ ⓓ ⓔ
207. ⓐ ⓑ ⓒ ⓓ ⓔ
208. ⓐ ⓑ ⓒ ⓓ ⓔ

Section 9

Physiology

Fill in a circled letter to indicate your answer choice.

#	Answer	#	Answer	#	Answer	#	Answer
1.	ⓐ ⓑ ⓒ ⓓ ⓔ	47.	ⓐ ⓑ ⓒ ⓓ ⓔ	93.	ⓐ ⓑ ⓒ ⓓ ⓔ	139.	ⓐ ⓑ ⓒ ⓓ ⓔ
2.	ⓐ ⓑ ⓒ ⓓ ⓔ	48.	ⓐ ⓑ ⓒ ⓓ ⓔ	94.	ⓐ ⓑ ⓒ ⓓ ⓔ	140.	ⓐ ⓑ ⓒ ⓓ ⓔ
3.	ⓐ ⓑ ⓒ ⓓ ⓔ	49.	ⓐ ⓑ ⓒ ⓓ ⓔ	95.	ⓐ ⓑ ⓒ ⓓ ⓔ	141.	ⓐ ⓑ ⓒ ⓓ ⓔ
4.	ⓐ ⓑ ⓒ ⓓ ⓔ	50.	ⓐ ⓑ ⓒ ⓓ ⓔ	96.	ⓐ ⓑ ⓒ ⓓ ⓔ	142.	ⓐ ⓑ ⓒ ⓓ ⓔ
5.	ⓐ ⓑ ⓒ ⓓ ⓔ	51.	ⓐ ⓑ ⓒ ⓓ ⓔ	97.	ⓐ ⓑ ⓒ ⓓ ⓔ	143.	ⓐ ⓑ ⓒ ⓓ ⓔ
6.	ⓐ ⓑ ⓒ ⓓ ⓔ	52.	ⓐ ⓑ ⓒ ⓓ ⓔ	98.	ⓐ ⓑ ⓒ ⓓ ⓔ	144.	ⓐ ⓑ ⓒ ⓓ ⓔ
7.	ⓐ ⓑ ⓒ ⓓ ⓔ	53.	ⓐ ⓑ ⓒ ⓓ ⓔ	99.	ⓐ ⓑ ⓒ ⓓ ⓔ	145.	ⓐ ⓑ ⓒ ⓓ ⓔ
8.	ⓐ ⓑ ⓒ ⓓ ⓔ	54.	ⓐ ⓑ ⓒ ⓓ ⓔ	100.	ⓐ ⓑ ⓒ ⓓ ⓔ	146.	ⓐ ⓑ ⓒ ⓓ ⓔ
9.	ⓐ ⓑ ⓒ ⓓ ⓔ	55.	ⓐ ⓑ ⓒ ⓓ ⓔ	101.	ⓐ ⓑ ⓒ ⓓ ⓔ	147.	ⓐ ⓑ ⓒ ⓓ ⓔ
10.	ⓐ ⓑ ⓒ ⓓ ⓔ	56.	ⓐ ⓑ ⓒ ⓓ ⓔ	102.	ⓐ ⓑ ⓒ ⓓ ⓔ	148.	ⓐ ⓑ ⓒ ⓓ ⓔ
11.	ⓐ ⓑ ⓒ ⓓ ⓔ	57.	ⓐ ⓑ ⓒ ⓓ ⓔ	103.	ⓐ ⓑ ⓒ ⓓ ⓔ	149.	ⓐ ⓑ ⓒ ⓓ ⓔ
12.	ⓐ ⓑ ⓒ ⓓ ⓔ	58.	ⓐ ⓑ ⓒ ⓓ ⓔ	104.	ⓐ ⓑ ⓒ ⓓ ⓔ	150.	ⓐ ⓑ ⓒ ⓓ ⓔ
13.	ⓐ ⓑ ⓒ ⓓ ⓔ	59.	ⓐ ⓑ ⓒ ⓓ ⓔ	105.	ⓐ ⓑ ⓒ ⓓ ⓔ	151.	ⓐ ⓑ ⓒ ⓓ ⓔ
14.	ⓐ ⓑ ⓒ ⓓ ⓔ	60.	ⓐ ⓑ ⓒ ⓓ ⓔ	106.	ⓐ ⓑ ⓒ ⓓ ⓔ	152.	ⓐ ⓑ ⓒ ⓓ ⓔ
15.	ⓐ ⓑ ⓒ ⓓ ⓔ	61.	ⓐ ⓑ ⓒ ⓓ ⓔ	107.	ⓐ ⓑ ⓒ ⓓ ⓔ	153.	ⓐ ⓑ ⓒ ⓓ ⓔ
16.	ⓐ ⓑ ⓒ ⓓ ⓔ	62.	ⓐ ⓑ ⓒ ⓓ ⓔ	108.	ⓐ ⓑ ⓒ ⓓ ⓔ	154.	ⓐ ⓑ ⓒ ⓓ ⓔ
17.	ⓐ ⓑ ⓒ ⓓ ⓔ	63.	ⓐ ⓑ ⓒ ⓓ ⓔ	109.	ⓐ ⓑ ⓒ ⓓ ⓔ	155.	ⓐ ⓑ ⓒ ⓓ ⓔ
18.	ⓐ ⓑ ⓒ ⓓ ⓔ	64.	ⓐ ⓑ ⓒ ⓓ ⓔ	110.	ⓐ ⓑ ⓒ ⓓ ⓔ	156.	ⓐ ⓑ ⓒ ⓓ ⓔ
19.	ⓐ ⓑ ⓒ ⓓ ⓔ	65.	ⓐ ⓑ ⓒ ⓓ ⓔ	111.	ⓐ ⓑ ⓒ ⓓ ⓔ	157.	ⓐ ⓑ ⓒ ⓓ ⓔ
20.	ⓐ ⓑ ⓒ ⓓ ⓔ	66.	ⓐ ⓑ ⓒ ⓓ ⓔ	112.	ⓐ ⓑ ⓒ ⓓ ⓔ	158.	ⓐ ⓑ ⓒ ⓓ ⓔ
21.	ⓐ ⓑ ⓒ ⓓ ⓔ	67.	ⓐ ⓑ ⓒ ⓓ ⓔ	113.	ⓐ ⓑ ⓒ ⓓ ⓔ	159.	ⓐ ⓑ ⓒ ⓓ ⓔ
22.	ⓐ ⓑ ⓒ ⓓ ⓔ	68.	ⓐ ⓑ ⓒ ⓓ ⓔ	114.	ⓐ ⓑ ⓒ ⓓ ⓔ	160.	ⓐ ⓑ ⓒ ⓓ ⓔ
23.	ⓐ ⓑ ⓒ ⓓ ⓔ	69.	ⓐ ⓑ ⓒ ⓓ ⓔ	115.	ⓐ ⓑ ⓒ ⓓ ⓔ	161.	ⓐ ⓑ ⓒ ⓓ ⓔ
24.	ⓐ ⓑ ⓒ ⓓ ⓔ	70.	ⓐ ⓑ ⓒ ⓓ ⓔ	116.	ⓐ ⓑ ⓒ ⓓ ⓔ	162.	ⓐ ⓑ ⓒ ⓓ ⓔ
25.	ⓐ ⓑ ⓒ ⓓ ⓔ	71.	ⓐ ⓑ ⓒ ⓓ ⓔ	117.	ⓐ ⓑ ⓒ ⓓ ⓔ	163.	ⓐ ⓑ ⓒ ⓓ ⓔ
26.	ⓐ ⓑ ⓒ ⓓ ⓔ	72.	ⓐ ⓑ ⓒ ⓓ ⓔ	118.	ⓐ ⓑ ⓒ ⓓ ⓔ	164.	ⓐ ⓑ ⓒ ⓓ ⓔ
27.	ⓐ ⓑ ⓒ ⓓ ⓔ	73.	ⓐ ⓑ ⓒ ⓓ ⓔ	119.	ⓐ ⓑ ⓒ ⓓ ⓔ	165.	ⓐ ⓑ ⓒ ⓓ ⓔ
28.	ⓐ ⓑ ⓒ ⓓ ⓔ	74.	ⓐ ⓑ ⓒ ⓓ ⓔ	120.	ⓐ ⓑ ⓒ ⓓ ⓔ	166.	ⓐ ⓑ ⓒ ⓓ ⓔ
29.	ⓐ ⓑ ⓒ ⓓ ⓔ	75.	ⓐ ⓑ ⓒ ⓓ ⓔ	121.	ⓐ ⓑ ⓒ ⓓ ⓔ	167.	ⓐ ⓑ ⓒ ⓓ ⓔ
30.	ⓐ ⓑ ⓒ ⓓ ⓔ	76.	ⓐ ⓑ ⓒ ⓓ ⓔ	122.	ⓐ ⓑ ⓒ ⓓ ⓔ	168.	ⓐ ⓑ ⓒ ⓓ ⓔ
31.	ⓐ ⓑ ⓒ ⓓ ⓔ	77.	ⓐ ⓑ ⓒ ⓓ ⓔ	123.	ⓐ ⓑ ⓒ ⓓ ⓔ	169.	ⓐ ⓑ ⓒ ⓓ ⓔ
32.	ⓐ ⓑ ⓒ ⓓ ⓔ	78.	ⓐ ⓑ ⓒ ⓓ ⓔ	124.	ⓐ ⓑ ⓒ ⓓ ⓔ	170.	ⓐ ⓑ ⓒ ⓓ ⓔ
33.	ⓐ ⓑ ⓒ ⓓ ⓔ	79.	ⓐ ⓑ ⓒ ⓓ ⓔ	125.	ⓐ ⓑ ⓒ ⓓ ⓔ	171.	ⓐ ⓑ ⓒ ⓓ ⓔ
34.	ⓐ ⓑ ⓒ ⓓ ⓔ	80.	ⓐ ⓑ ⓒ ⓓ ⓔ	126.	ⓐ ⓑ ⓒ ⓓ ⓔ	172.	ⓐ ⓑ ⓒ ⓓ ⓔ
35.	ⓐ ⓑ ⓒ ⓓ ⓔ	81.	ⓐ ⓑ ⓒ ⓓ ⓔ	127.	ⓐ ⓑ ⓒ ⓓ ⓔ	173.	ⓐ ⓑ ⓒ ⓓ ⓔ
36.	ⓐ ⓑ ⓒ ⓓ ⓔ	82.	ⓐ ⓑ ⓒ ⓓ ⓔ	128.	ⓐ ⓑ ⓒ ⓓ ⓔ	174.	ⓐ ⓑ ⓒ ⓓ ⓔ
37.	ⓐ ⓑ ⓒ ⓓ ⓔ	83.	ⓐ ⓑ ⓒ ⓓ ⓔ	129.	ⓐ ⓑ ⓒ ⓓ ⓔ	175.	ⓐ ⓑ ⓒ ⓓ ⓔ
38.	ⓐ ⓑ ⓒ ⓓ ⓔ	84.	ⓐ ⓑ ⓒ ⓓ ⓔ	130.	ⓐ ⓑ ⓒ ⓓ ⓔ	176.	ⓐ ⓑ ⓒ ⓓ ⓔ
39.	ⓐ ⓑ ⓒ ⓓ ⓔ	85.	ⓐ ⓑ ⓒ ⓓ ⓔ	131.	ⓐ ⓑ ⓒ ⓓ ⓔ	177.	ⓐ ⓑ ⓒ ⓓ ⓔ
40.	ⓐ ⓑ ⓒ ⓓ ⓔ	86.	ⓐ ⓑ ⓒ ⓓ ⓔ	132.	ⓐ ⓑ ⓒ ⓓ ⓔ	178.	ⓐ ⓑ ⓒ ⓓ ⓔ
41.	ⓐ ⓑ ⓒ ⓓ ⓔ	87.	ⓐ ⓑ ⓒ ⓓ ⓔ	133.	ⓐ ⓑ ⓒ ⓓ ⓔ	179.	ⓐ ⓑ ⓒ ⓓ ⓔ
42.	ⓐ ⓑ ⓒ ⓓ ⓔ	88.	ⓐ ⓑ ⓒ ⓓ ⓔ	134.	ⓐ ⓑ ⓒ ⓓ ⓔ	180.	ⓐ ⓑ ⓒ ⓓ ⓔ
43.	ⓐ ⓑ ⓒ ⓓ ⓔ	89.	ⓐ ⓑ ⓒ ⓓ ⓔ	135.	ⓐ ⓑ ⓒ ⓓ ⓔ	181.	ⓐ ⓑ ⓒ ⓓ ⓔ
44.	ⓐ ⓑ ⓒ ⓓ ⓔ	90.	ⓐ ⓑ ⓒ ⓓ ⓔ	136.	ⓐ ⓑ ⓒ ⓓ ⓔ	182.	ⓐ ⓑ ⓒ ⓓ ⓔ
45.	ⓐ ⓑ ⓒ ⓓ ⓔ	91.	ⓐ ⓑ ⓒ ⓓ ⓔ	137.	ⓐ ⓑ ⓒ ⓓ ⓔ	183.	ⓐ ⓑ ⓒ ⓓ ⓔ
46.	ⓐ ⓑ ⓒ ⓓ ⓔ	92.	ⓐ ⓑ ⓒ ⓓ ⓔ	138.	ⓐ ⓑ ⓒ ⓓ ⓔ	184.	ⓐ ⓑ ⓒ ⓓ ⓔ

Continued

185. ⓐ ⓑ ⓒ ⓓ ⓔ	197. ⓐ ⓑ ⓒ ⓓ ⓔ	209. ⓐ ⓑ ⓒ ⓓ ⓔ	221. ⓐ ⓑ ⓒ ⓓ ⓔ
186. ⓐ ⓑ ⓒ ⓓ ⓔ	198. ⓐ ⓑ ⓒ ⓓ ⓔ	210. ⓐ ⓑ ⓒ ⓓ ⓔ	222. ⓐ ⓑ ⓒ ⓓ ⓔ
187. ⓐ ⓑ ⓒ ⓓ ⓔ	199. ⓐ ⓑ ⓒ ⓓ ⓔ	211. ⓐ ⓑ ⓒ ⓓ ⓔ	223. ⓐ ⓑ ⓒ ⓓ ⓔ
188. ⓐ ⓑ ⓒ ⓓ ⓔ	200. ⓐ ⓑ ⓒ ⓓ ⓔ	212. ⓐ ⓑ ⓒ ⓓ ⓔ	224. ⓐ ⓑ ⓒ ⓓ ⓔ
189. ⓐ ⓑ ⓒ ⓓ ⓔ	201. ⓐ ⓑ ⓒ ⓓ ⓔ	213. ⓐ ⓑ ⓒ ⓓ ⓔ	225. ⓐ ⓑ ⓒ ⓓ ⓔ
190. ⓐ ⓑ ⓒ ⓓ ⓔ	202. ⓐ ⓑ ⓒ ⓓ ⓔ	214. ⓐ ⓑ ⓒ ⓓ ⓔ	
191. ⓐ ⓑ ⓒ ⓓ ⓔ	203. ⓐ ⓑ ⓒ ⓓ ⓔ	215. ⓐ ⓑ ⓒ ⓓ ⓔ	
192. ⓐ ⓑ ⓒ ⓓ ⓔ	204. ⓐ ⓑ ⓒ ⓓ ⓔ	216. ⓐ ⓑ ⓒ ⓓ ⓔ	
193. ⓐ ⓑ ⓒ ⓓ ⓔ	205. ⓐ ⓑ ⓒ ⓓ ⓔ	217. ⓐ ⓑ ⓒ ⓓ ⓔ	
194. ⓐ ⓑ ⓒ ⓓ ⓔ	206. ⓐ ⓑ ⓒ ⓓ ⓔ	218. ⓐ ⓑ ⓒ ⓓ ⓔ	
195. ⓐ ⓑ ⓒ ⓓ ⓔ	207. ⓐ ⓑ ⓒ ⓓ ⓔ	219. ⓐ ⓑ ⓒ ⓓ ⓔ	
196. ⓐ ⓑ ⓒ ⓓ ⓔ	208. ⓐ ⓑ ⓒ ⓓ ⓔ	220. ⓐ ⓑ ⓒ ⓓ ⓔ	

Section 10

Terminology

Fill in a circled letter to indicate your answer choice.

1. ⓐ ⓑ ⓒ ⓓ ⓔ	27. ⓐ ⓑ ⓒ ⓓ ⓔ	53. ⓐ ⓑ ⓒ ⓓ ⓔ	79. ⓐ ⓑ ⓒ ⓓ ⓔ
2. ⓐ ⓑ ⓒ ⓓ ⓔ	28. ⓐ ⓑ ⓒ ⓓ ⓔ	54. ⓐ ⓑ ⓒ ⓓ ⓔ	80. ⓐ ⓑ ⓒ ⓓ ⓔ
3. ⓐ ⓑ ⓒ ⓓ ⓔ	29. ⓐ ⓑ ⓒ ⓓ ⓔ	55. ⓐ ⓑ ⓒ ⓓ ⓔ	81. ⓐ ⓑ ⓒ ⓓ ⓔ
4. ⓐ ⓑ ⓒ ⓓ ⓔ	30. ⓐ ⓑ ⓒ ⓓ ⓔ	56. ⓐ ⓑ ⓒ ⓓ ⓔ	82. ⓐ ⓑ ⓒ ⓓ ⓔ
5. ⓐ ⓑ ⓒ ⓓ ⓔ	31. ⓐ ⓑ ⓒ ⓓ ⓔ	57. ⓐ ⓑ ⓒ ⓓ ⓔ	83. ⓐ ⓑ ⓒ ⓓ ⓔ
6. ⓐ ⓑ ⓒ ⓓ ⓔ	32. ⓐ ⓑ ⓒ ⓓ ⓔ	58. ⓐ ⓑ ⓒ ⓓ ⓔ	84. ⓐ ⓑ ⓒ ⓓ ⓔ
7. ⓐ ⓑ ⓒ ⓓ ⓔ	33. ⓐ ⓑ ⓒ ⓓ ⓔ	59. ⓐ ⓑ ⓒ ⓓ ⓔ	85. ⓐ ⓑ ⓒ ⓓ ⓔ
8. ⓐ ⓑ ⓒ ⓓ ⓔ	34. ⓐ ⓑ ⓒ ⓓ ⓔ	60. ⓐ ⓑ ⓒ ⓓ ⓔ	86. ⓐ ⓑ ⓒ ⓓ ⓔ
9. ⓐ ⓑ ⓒ ⓓ ⓔ	35. ⓐ ⓑ ⓒ ⓓ ⓔ	61. ⓐ ⓑ ⓒ ⓓ ⓔ	87. ⓐ ⓑ ⓒ ⓓ ⓔ
10. ⓐ ⓑ ⓒ ⓓ ⓔ	36. ⓐ ⓑ ⓒ ⓓ ⓔ	62. ⓐ ⓑ ⓒ ⓓ ⓔ	88. ⓐ ⓑ ⓒ ⓓ ⓔ
11. ⓐ ⓑ ⓒ ⓓ ⓔ	37. ⓐ ⓑ ⓒ ⓓ ⓔ	63. ⓐ ⓑ ⓒ ⓓ ⓔ	89. ⓐ ⓑ ⓒ ⓓ ⓔ
12. ⓐ ⓑ ⓒ ⓓ ⓔ	38. ⓐ ⓑ ⓒ ⓓ ⓔ	64. ⓐ ⓑ ⓒ ⓓ ⓔ	90. ⓐ ⓑ ⓒ ⓓ ⓔ
13. ⓐ ⓑ ⓒ ⓓ ⓔ	39. ⓐ ⓑ ⓒ ⓓ ⓔ	65. ⓐ ⓑ ⓒ ⓓ ⓔ	91. ⓐ ⓑ ⓒ ⓓ ⓔ
14. ⓐ ⓑ ⓒ ⓓ ⓔ	40. ⓐ ⓑ ⓒ ⓓ ⓔ	66. ⓐ ⓑ ⓒ ⓓ ⓔ	92. ⓐ ⓑ ⓒ ⓓ ⓔ
15. ⓐ ⓑ ⓒ ⓓ ⓔ	41. ⓐ ⓑ ⓒ ⓓ ⓔ	67. ⓐ ⓑ ⓒ ⓓ ⓔ	93. ⓐ ⓑ ⓒ ⓓ ⓔ
16. ⓐ ⓑ ⓒ ⓓ ⓔ	42. ⓐ ⓑ ⓒ ⓓ ⓔ	68. ⓐ ⓑ ⓒ ⓓ ⓔ	94. ⓐ ⓑ ⓒ ⓓ ⓔ
17. ⓐ ⓑ ⓒ ⓓ ⓔ	43. ⓐ ⓑ ⓒ ⓓ ⓔ	69. ⓐ ⓑ ⓒ ⓓ ⓔ	95. ⓐ ⓑ ⓒ ⓓ ⓔ
18. ⓐ ⓑ ⓒ ⓓ ⓔ	44. ⓐ ⓑ ⓒ ⓓ ⓔ	70. ⓐ ⓑ ⓒ ⓓ ⓔ	96. ⓐ ⓑ ⓒ ⓓ ⓔ
19. ⓐ ⓑ ⓒ ⓓ ⓔ	45. ⓐ ⓑ ⓒ ⓓ ⓔ	71. ⓐ ⓑ ⓒ ⓓ ⓔ	97. ⓐ ⓑ ⓒ ⓓ ⓔ
20. ⓐ ⓑ ⓒ ⓓ ⓔ	46. ⓐ ⓑ ⓒ ⓓ ⓔ	72. ⓐ ⓑ ⓒ ⓓ ⓔ	98. ⓐ ⓑ ⓒ ⓓ ⓔ
21. ⓐ ⓑ ⓒ ⓓ ⓔ	47. ⓐ ⓑ ⓒ ⓓ ⓔ	73. ⓐ ⓑ ⓒ ⓓ ⓔ	99. ⓐ ⓑ ⓒ ⓓ ⓔ
22. ⓐ ⓑ ⓒ ⓓ ⓔ	48. ⓐ ⓑ ⓒ ⓓ ⓔ	74. ⓐ ⓑ ⓒ ⓓ ⓔ	100. ⓐ ⓑ ⓒ ⓓ ⓔ
23. ⓐ ⓑ ⓒ ⓓ ⓔ	49. ⓐ ⓑ ⓒ ⓓ ⓔ	75. ⓐ ⓑ ⓒ ⓓ ⓔ	
24. ⓐ ⓑ ⓒ ⓓ ⓔ	50. ⓐ ⓑ ⓒ ⓓ ⓔ	76. ⓐ ⓑ ⓒ ⓓ ⓔ	
25. ⓐ ⓑ ⓒ ⓓ ⓔ	51. ⓐ ⓑ ⓒ ⓓ ⓔ	77. ⓐ ⓑ ⓒ ⓓ ⓔ	
26. ⓐ ⓑ ⓒ ⓓ ⓔ	52. ⓐ ⓑ ⓒ ⓓ ⓔ	78. ⓐ ⓑ ⓒ ⓓ ⓔ	

We Welcome Your Comments

We value your opinion and encourage you to send us your comments, flattering or critical. Please let us know if you detect any errors or ambiguous statements, or if there is any way in which we can make *Review Questions & Answers For Veterinary Boards* more useful to you.

Paul W. Pratt, VMD
Editor and Publisher

Return to:
American Veterinary Publications
5782 Thornwood Drive
Goleta, CA 93117

Detach, fold and seal with tape.
No postage needed in the United States.

FOLD HERE

BUSINESS REPLY MAIL
FIRST CLASS MAIL PERMIT NO. 770 SANTA BARBARA, CA

POSTAGE WILL BE PAID BY ADDRESSEE

American Veterinary Publications
5782 Thornwood Drive
Goleta, CA 93117-9942

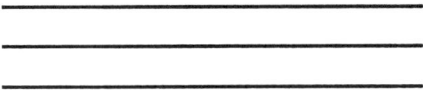

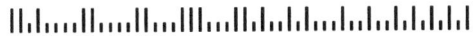

FOLD HERE

You may use this as a return
envelope. Detach at right and fold
as indicated. If a check is enclosed,
please tape the sides.

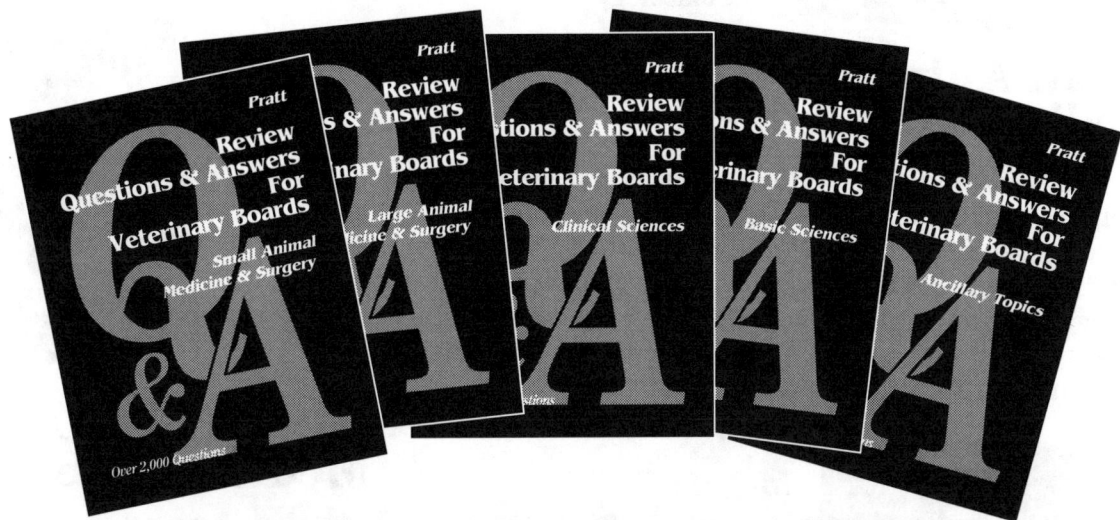

√ *Over 9,400 multiple-choice questions, with accompanying answers.*

√ *Written by 112 veterinary educators, content-area specialists and experienced clinicians.*

√ *5 volumes cover nearly every aspect of veterinary medicine.*

Basic Sciences

Over 1,800 questions on Biochemistry, Embryology, Gross Anatomy, Microbiology, Microscopic Anatomy, Neuroanatomy, Parasitology, Pathology, Physiology, Terminology.

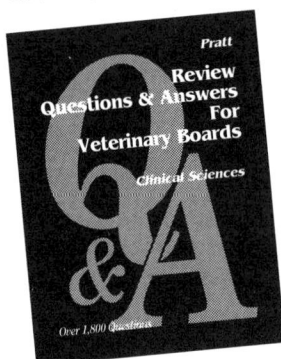

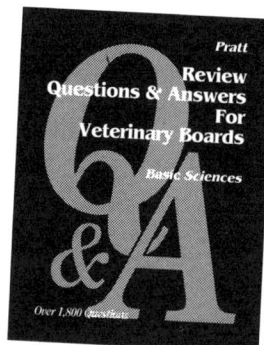

Clinical Sciences

Over 1,800 questions on Anesthesiology, Clinical Pathology, Cytology, Diagnostic Imaging, Hematology, Immunology, Nutrition, Pharmacology, Principles of Surgery, Theriogenology, Toxicology.

Small Animal Medicine & Surgery

Over 2,000 questions on medical and surgical diseases of dogs and cats. Disciplines include Anesthesiology, Cardiology, Clinical Pathology, Cytology, Dentistry, Dermatology, Hematology, Neurology, Oncology, Ophthalmology, Pharmacology, Preventive Medicine, Theriogenology, Urology/Nephrology. Questions on history taking, physical examination, diagnostic techniques, medical care, preoperative preparations, operative techniques, postoperative care, emergency care.

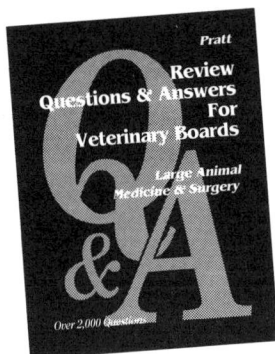

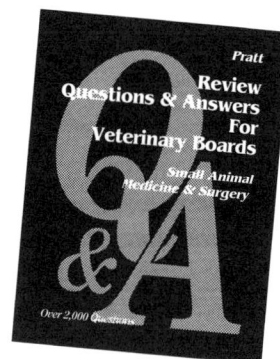

Large Animal Medicine & Surgery

Over 2,000 questions on medical and surgical diseases of horses, cattle, pigs, sheep and goats. Questions on history taking, physical examination, diagnostic techniques, medical care, preoperative preparations, operative techniques, postoperative care, emergency care.

Ancillary Topics

Over 1,800 questions on Behavior, Cage/Aviary Bird Medicine, Epidemiology, Ethics, Jurisprudence and Animal Welfare, Laboratory Animal Medicine, Necropsy, Physical Restraint, Poultry Medicine, Practice Management, Public Health and Regulatory Medicine, Zoo and Exotic Animal Medicine, Marine Mammal Medicine, Aquarium Fish.

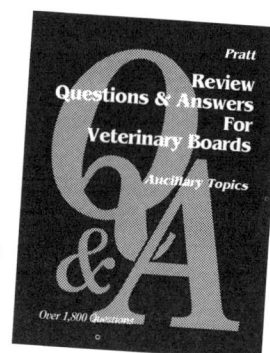

Order Form

Please send the following volumes of *Review Questions & Answers For Veterinary Boards:*

☐ *Basic Sciences*
☐ *Clinical Sciences*
☐ *Small Animal Medicine & Surgery*
☐ *Large Animal Medicine & Surgery*
☐ *Ancillary Topics*

Any 1 volume: $38 ($33 plus $5 shipping)
Any 2 volumes: $69 ($64 plus $5 shipping)
Any 3 volumes: $99 ($93 plus $6 shipping)
Any 4 volumes: $127 ($120 plus $7 shipping)
All 5 volumes: $152 ($145 plus $7 shipping)

(Non-U.S. orders, add $2 per volume.)

Payment or credit card information must be enclosed.
Sorry, we cannot bill you.

☐ Please charge my _____ VISA _____ MasterCard

Card # _____Expiration _____

Signature _____

☐ Payment enclosed *(U.S. funds only) (California residents please add 7.25% sales tax)*

Name _____

Street _____

           ☐ Business   ☐ Residence

City/State/Zip _____

Telephone (_____)_____

For fastest service, call
(805) 967-5988
8 AM – 4 PM
M-F, Pacific Time

Return to:
American Veterinary Publications
5782 Thornwood Dr.
Goleta, CA 93117

Detach order form, enclose payment, fold and seal with tape.
No postage needed if mailed in the United States.

FOLD HERE

BUSINESS REPLY MAIL
FIRST CLASS MAIL PERMIT NO. 770 SANTA BARBARA, CA

POSTAGE WILL BE PAID BY ADDRESSEE

American Veterinary Publications
5782 Thornwood Drive
Goleta, CA 93117-9942

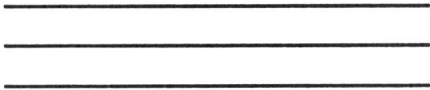

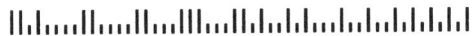

NO POSTAGE
NECESSARY
IF MAILED
IN THE
UNITED STATES

FOLD HERE

You may use this as a return
envelope. Detach at right and fold
as indicated. If a check is enclosed,
please tape the sides.